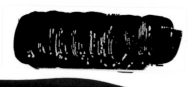

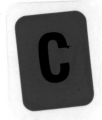

**Clothing and difference : embodied
identities in colonial and post-colonial
Africa**

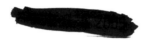

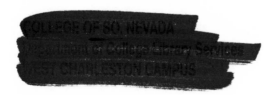

BODY, COMMODITY, TEXT

Studies of Objectifying Practice

A series edited by

Arjun Appadurai,

Jean Comaroff, and

Judith Farquhar

CLOTHING

AND DIFFERENCE

Embodied Identities in Colonial and

Post-Colonial Africa

Edited by HILDI HENDRICKSON

Duke University Press

Durham and London

1996

© 1996 Duke University Press
All rights reserved
Printed in the United States of America on acid-free paper ∞
Typeset in Minion by Keystone Typesetting, Inc.
Library of Congress Cataloging-in-Publication Data
appear on the last printed page of this book.

CONTENTS

FIGURES

ACKNOWLEDGMENTS

I extend my thanks to Fred Myers, Ed Wilmsen, Ivan Karp, and Ken Wissoker, whose support has been vital to the development of this volume. Conversations with Karin Barber, David William Cohen, and the Fellows at The Institute for Advanced Study and Research in the African Humanities at Northwestern in 1992 and 1994 were invaluable in helping me to develop my ideas. I thank the governments of Namibia and Botswana for permitting me to carry out my research in southern Africa.

I also acknowledge the Long Island University faculty seminar, "Classic Texts of Non-Western Cultures," funded by the National Endowment for the Humanities for providing a forum for wide-ranging discussions about culture and pedagogy and putting me in touch with my academic colleagues in other fields. The Long Island University Faculty Federation made release time available to me to complete this work.

Jean Comaroff, Leah Dilworth, Hannah Green, Arnold Krupat, Laurie Van Rooten, my fellow contributors, and the anonymous reviewers for Duke University Press provided welcome, insightful comments on the introductory essay. Gerald Meyer has been an especially generous critic. I appreciate the continuing support of Michael Hittman, Jean Howson, and Heidi Knecht for my work. Most of all, I thank my husband, Dean Jacobson, for being there through every phase of this project.

CLOTHING AND DIFFERENCE

INTRODUCTION

Hildi Hendrickson

Fashion has dualities in its formation, a reputation for snobbery and sin. . . . It is obsessive about outward appearances, yet speaks the unconscious and our deepest desires.—J. Ash and E. Wilson (1992, xi)

To be able to blend—that's what realness is. The idea of realness is to look as much as possible like your straight counterpart. . . . It's not a take-off or a satire—no, it's actually being able to *be* this. It's really a case of going back into the closet.—Dorian Corey on transvestism in the film *Paris is Burning,* dir. Jennie Livingston

If you wear the clothes of your enemy, the spirit of the enemy is weakened. You are then wearing the spirit of his brothers and then they are weakened.—Herero cultural commentator in southern Africa (cited in Hendrickson, this volume)

In this volume, we investigate popular, political, economic, and spiritual meanings assigned to treatments of the body surface in a variety of African colonial and post-colonial contexts. We explore the bodily and material engendering of women, spirits, youths, ancestors, and entrepreneurs; we consider fashion, spirit possession, commodity exchange, hygiene, and mourning, among other divergent spheres of action and meaning.

In studying treatments of the body surface in nineteenth- and twentieth-century African history, we sharpen our consciousness of both the constructed-ness and the interconnectedness of cultural systems. Our essays demonstrate that Africa and the West are mutually engaged in a semiotic web whose implications are not completely controlled by any of us. We illuminate performative processes critical to the creation of "tradition" and "modernity" through which national and international identities are negotiated. We challenge conceptions that divide too cleanly "first" and "third" worlds, colonizer and colonized, producer and consumer, indigene and tourist, or body and spirit.

By taking the body surface as our focus, we investigate one of the frontiers upon which individual and social identities are simultaneously created, and we join a variety of scholars studying bodily representation in other regions of the world. In particular, we address human processes for constituting the social self, social organization, and shared notions of authority and value. The body surface has been called "the symbolic stage upon which the drama of socialization is enacted" (Turner 1980, 12); it is a field for representation, which, being concrete, has lasting semiotic value. Being personal, it is susceptible to individual manipulation. Being public, it has social import.

By taking kin-based polities as our focus, we are reminded that self, family, class, community, political party, and state are interconnected entities. These African cases remind us that individual action is always shaped by family, gender, and residential groups, that political, spiritual, and economic activity are intertwined, and that it is social *groups* that affect cultural configurations.

Ultimately, our essays provide alternative views of the structures underpinning Western systems of commodification, postmodernism, and cultural differentiation. African social histories teach us that factors considered integral to Western social development—such as heterogeneity, migration, democratization, transnational exchange, and media representation—have existed elsewhere in different configurations and with different outcomes. In Africa, such transformative social processes can be considered afresh. Cultural and linguistic diversity, for example, can be studied as an age-old condition of everyday living in many parts of Africa. Meanwhile, nation-building, entrepreneurship, and mass consumerism can be explored as they continue to emerge in African societies.

In investigating African case material, the fact that "men make their own history, but they do not make it just as they please" (Marx [1852] in Tucker 1978, 595) can be seen from a new angle. Moreover, since Africans have been subject to Western imperialism and later made poor partners in Western industrial economies, the investigation of African history and experience helps to reveal the underside of Western politico-economic systems.

Most specifically, our essays provide new evidence for the ways that cross-cultural relations structure and evoke concepts of value. When we see Africans using *our* products to create *their* identities—and vice versa—we learn that the meaning of body or commodity is not inherent but is in fact symbolically created and contested by both producers and consumers. Clearly, the power of industrial systems to define those meanings—and of materialist analyses to account for them—is more limited than it may appear.

Treatments of the body surface are not just commodities circulating between and among social groups, nor are they simply markers of social status or identity. In the societies considered here, we find that bodies and dress also help to express and shape ideas about the most potent kinds of political and spiritual power thought to be available to human beings. These too are social facts that must be taken into account, even in the West. We learn from these African cases that, at this late-twentieth-century moment, acts of devotion to notions of identity belie postmodern cynicism about the tyrannies of the past, the emptiness of the present, and the disconnections of the future.

In this introduction, I first consider research and writing on dress in Western contexts to sharpen an understanding of how our African cases complement, extend, and challenge these analyses. Second, I identify methodological and conceptual differences in our social scientific investigation of this subject. Next, I present the individual papers and go on to place our contributions within the context of recent Africanist research. Finally, I consider the implications of our work for a semiotics of the body.

Western Dress and the Politics of Postmodernism

The essays collected here contribute to a widening body of research on the body surface as a principal site of social and political action in industrial society. While the analysis of dress has been undertaken by art historians, social psychologists, and social historians (e.g., Veblen [1899] 1957; Flugel 1930; Roach and Eicher 1965; Bell 1968; Hollander 1975), some of the most challenging recent work has emerged out of American and British feminist and cultural studies (e.g., Hebdige 1979; Gaines and Herzog 1990; Ash and Wilson 1992; Benstock and Ferriss 1994). Current works consider dress as both sign and commodity enmeshed in multiple webs of meaning and value. Subjects as diverse as high-fashion houses (Taylor 1992), paramilitary clothing in Northern Ireland (Herr 1994), female bodybuilding (Schultze 1990), and Hollywood costumers (Nielsen 1990) have been fruitfully analyzed.

Many of these new analyses focus on marginalized social groups—such as women, gays and lesbians, and ethnic minorities—in late-twentieth-century capitalist contexts. Such studies may explore the "repressive power" of fashion as a commodity (Benstock and Ferriss 1994, 8) or the ways that "the camera . . . support[s] (and sometimes subvert[s]) . . . notions of the feminine and of the female body (clothed or unclothed) as something-to-be-looked-at" (11). The theory asserts that the eye of the camera should be equated with the gaze of masculine power-holders, whose vantage point is unattainable for most of those viewed.

Jane Gaines (1990) traces this idea to the work of Laura Mulvey (1975) and John Berger (1972), the latter asserting, for example, that "men look at women and this is the visual organizing principle in oil painting, magazine advertising, and motion pictures" (Gaines 1990, 3). Gaines notes that earlier feminists "explained the danger of fashion culture in terms of patriarchy in league with capitalism. Femininity, in this analysis, was false consciousness" (4).

Gaines asserts that feminist thinking has taken a leap forward from a preoccupation with patriarchy (1990, 6) and from the cynicism of the position that "the image has swallowed reality whole" (5). She contends that since the 1980s, feminist theorists of dress have begun to analyze the pursuit of fantasy and pleasure in fashion. They have fruitfully applied to women theories of resistance and subculture taken from British cultural studies and investigated the place of women in consumer culture. Utopian dreams, deep ambivalence, and subtle forms of resistance have been uncovered in analyses of the empowered position of female consumers in thrift shops (Young 1994) or the ways that women may create a kind of bricolage of fashion, modifying the products and messages received from international designers (Partington 1992).

Elizabeth Wilson (1985, 1990, 1992) has written extensively on the ways that such populist phenomena, emerging particularly since the 1960s, are a part of what the Marxist cultural critic Fredric Jameson (1991) and others have called postmodernism. The language and imagery used to describe the postmodern social world are striking in their severity:

> The post-modern social landscape has a kind of ghastly kitsch excitement about it. Its "hallucinatory euphoria," and the glittering, depthless polish of the postmodern urban scene reflect a world denuded of feeling. . . . Postmodernism expresses at one level a horror at the destructive excess of Western consumerist society, yet in aestheticising this horror, we somehow convert it into a pleasurable object of consumption. (Wilson 1992, 4)

Wilson, like sociologist Fred Davis (1992), however, recognizes that in this context, dress serves both to dominate and to subvert—that "fashion, like postmodernism itself, remains ambivalent" (Wilson 1992, 14–15). In Wilson's analysis, however, people are not paralyzed by their postmodern condition. Rather, they are seen to express and pursue multiple, contradictory desires in the semiosis of dress.

Evidence for a wider, more popular interest in the linkages between postmodernism, dress, and the self can be found outside academic publications. For instance, in a New York Times interview with fashion designer Thierry Mugler, feminist art historian Linda Nochlin commented recently:

I would also tie [fashion] in to certain postmodern ideas about the self—that there is no self even. That the self is a condition of disguise and that we can move back and forth in terms of sexualities, in terms of social being, in terms of all kinds of sense of who we are. And I think fashion helps us wonderfully in this. That's why, in a sense, I would say that fashion is *the* postmodern art, because it helps to destabilize the self in such a wonderful way. (*Times Sunday Magazine*, 17 July 1994, 46, 49)

Marjorie Garber goes to the core of postmodern ambivalence about representation, the self, and society in her *Vested Interests: Cross-Dressing and Cultural Anxiety* (1992). Garber identifies numerous culturally unsettling instances of cross-dressing in literature, film, opera, and the popular arts, which she takes as central not only to postmodern society but to society itself. She turns the analytical spotlight on a fantastic array of female Peter Pans, male Salomes, discovered cross-dressed murderers, Shakespearean actors, transvestite female saints, and the "transvestite continuum" of Liberace, Rudolf Valentino, and Elvis, who inhabit the "ghastly kitsch world."

Garber suggests that if we refuse to elide the physical existence of these cross-dressers, we will notice that these figures perform a "necessary critique of binary thinking, whether particularized as male and female, black and white, yes and no, Republican and Democrat, self and other" (1992, 10–11). Garber draws upon Lacan's psychoanalytic theory about the tripartite functioning of the psyche to posit that the transvestite acts as a disruptive "third"—that is, an

> interruption . . . of things that "exist" in a theatrically conceived space and time but were not present onstage as agents before, [which] reconfigures the relationships between the original pair, and puts in question identities previously conceived as stable, unchallengeable, grounded, and "known."
> (1992, 12–13)

The transvestite is an essential, anxiety-producing index of a crisis of gender, class, racial, or other categories somewhere offstage, Garber contends. Ultimately, she argues that "transvestism creates culture [and] culture creates transvestites" (1992, 16). Her analysis explores how one cannot exist without the other, how both categorizing and category-confounding implicate and create one another.

What motivates actual people to occupy the pivotal cultural role of the cross-dresser is perhaps best understood by listening to transvestites' own words, as heard, for example, in the film *Paris Is Burning*. The lived world of the transvestite is animated by irony, desire, and belief. Gay, African American men, the participants in the New York transvestite balls that are the film's subject, struggle with prejudice against their race, gender, and sexual orientation. In response, they create temporary utopias—they pursue fantasy to the limits of its possibilities. They show that through active, bodily devotion to an alternate vision of the world—ultimately through belief—people alter and recreate that shared system of ideas we call culture. Though they are in profound ways bound by the symbolic and social systems within which they act (see Butler 1993), the "legendary mothers" and "children" of the drag world show that the dressing of the body can be empowering and creative, even if it does not become more deeply subversive.

The Analysis of Dress by Social Scientists

Work like that of Gaines, Garber, and Wilson illuminates the relation between some social groups and representation in Western industrial society. It is limited, however, by its singular cultural vantage point. It cannot provide a more general understanding of the human uses of dress and the body in social, economic, and political life. We need to know how widely concepts like "patriarchy," "the masculine gaze," "cultural anxiety," and "a world denuded of feeling" can be applied. They do not adequately describe the spectrum of non-Western social realities, and this raises questions about their comprehensiveness when applied to Western case material.

What is needed for a full understanding of these symbolic processes is the cross-cultural investigation of the desires, fantasies, representations, resistances, and capitalisms that are, have been, and may be possible for human societies and groups therein. By exploring a variety of African social histories and taking treatments of the body surface as a point of departure, the essays in this volume illuminate some of the ways in which dress is deeply connected to structure and agency in cultures, plural. Like Roach and Eicher (1965), Cordwell and Schwartz (1979), Appadurai (1986), Weiner and Schneider (1989), Barnes and Eicher (1992), and others before us, we bring to the discussion of cloth/clothing, commodities, and cultural change cross-cultural insights from the increasingly intertwined fields of anthropology and history.

As is true for other social scientists, our strongest contribution to the wider literature on dress and the body comes through our ethnographic methodology. Each chapter presented here consists of original observations and analysis resulting from recent and extended residence among and consultation with members of varying societies in their own languages whenever possible. Like earlier generations of anthropologists, we strive to translate terms in the symbolic experience of others who share this late-twentieth-century moment with us but who inhabit it with a different set of values, wishes, and representations.

The fact that an ethnographic methodology offers a way out of potentially circular auto-theorizing has recently been recognized by analysts accustomed to producing more subjective interpretations of cultural activity as text (e.g., Wright 1992). Ethnography has been embraced by the burgeoning, politically conscious field of cultural studies (Grossberg, Nelson, and Treichler 1992). The recent public appreciation for Anna Deavere Smith's powerful interview pastiche stems at least in part from the recognition that some of the critical stuff of life is in the spoken words of others—that testimony is where culture and self are mutually created and perpetuated, where both social action and motivation can be examined.

Moreover, this collection is, like the projects of cultural studies, "interdisciplinary, transdisciplinary, and sometimes counter-disciplinary" (Grossberg, Nelson, and Treichler 1992, 4). Our ethnographic techniques are combined with a range of other methodological approaches. We combine oral histories and archival data with the insights of a wide range of living speakers—men and women, young and old, insiders and outsiders, conservatives and mavericks—to illuminate both the present and the past. We use historical photographs, advertisements, and cartoons as data pertinent to the exploration of cultural systems. We participate in and analyze contexts for action as varied as tourist traps and funerals.

Like others in our fields, we borrow from literary criticism and cultural studies to further our study of the political nature of identity claims, the relation between symbolic form and meaning, and the analysis of media representations. We also attempt to span the theoretical distance between materialist and idealist social analyses, drawing on the insights not just of Marx and Michel Foucault but also the work of Max Weber, Emile Durkheim, and Claude Lévi-Strauss. Thus, we attend to the constructedness of authority and value, the power of collective action and ritual, the motivating role of spirituality and religion, and the systemic nature of representational thought as well as processes of commodification and consumption.

Our work also builds upon that of earlier anthropologists who have long grappled with issues of identity and difference—whose explicit mission in fact has been to identify cultural universals and to account for cross-cultural variation. Dress and the construction of self have long received attention within this literature, as the early work of Georg Simmel (1904) and Marcel Mauss ([1950] 1979) attests.

While Barthes ([1967] 1983), Kroeber (1963), Sahlins (1976), Hebdige (1979), and Bourdieu (1984) have turned their attention to clothing and fashion within complex societies, Terence Turner (1980) stands out among anthropologists investigating clothing and body adornment in pre-industrial societies. In his definitive analysis of Kayapo bodily ornamentation in South America, Turner explores the body surface as inscribed over historical time by many actors who thereby work to build up a social person. He underscores the importance of body treatments in creating the individual experience of the limitations and possibilities of social life: "through the symbolic medium of bodily adornment, the body of every Kayapo becomes a microcosm of the Kayapo body politic" (1980, 121).

The research considered here has also been shaped by the cross-cultural analyses by Weiner (1980, 1985, 1992) and Weiner and Schneider (1986, 1989) of cloth as a class of object with particular concrete characteristics and symbolic potentials. Cloth is now understood to have considerable semiotic value in the expression of both the fragility and the potency of social statuses and sociopolitical relations. Of particular importance for our studies here is the idea that cloth is critical in the representation and reproduction of society—that it is often a critical link between social groups across space and through time.

Dress and the Body in Eight African Societies

Authenticating social identities
The essays collected here explore the significance of the body surface in three processes central to social reproduction and representation: the authentication of social categories, the legitimation of authority, and the creation of value. The essays by Renne, James, and Masquelier focus on body coverings as essential in the constitution of the social identities of married women, traditionalist dancers, and supernatural spirits, respectively. Tracing change in Ekiti Yoruba ideas about a marriageable woman's bodily state and the cloth that is the sign of her moral virtue, Renne shows how ideas about the existence of hymenal bodily tissue and blood and the physiological state of virginity have long been conflated in Yoruba thought. The white cloth used to test a bride's virtue against this standard has been symbolically linked with these ideas. White cloth has become a sign of what was, especially in the past, the proper bodily state of a marrying woman.

Renne delineates the role of the body in the long-term exchange of cultural knowledge and the changing historical circumstances, which have affected the Yoruba conceptualization of women, virginity, and bodily practice. She explores the weakening of paternal control of young women's bodies, fertility, and movement within domestic space after British colonial policy legalized divorce. Virginity and marriage have come to be less strictly equated, and ideas about the virginity cloth, women, and women's bodies have taken a new turn. "Modern" women's bodies have come to be associated with sexual knowledge and fertility, virginity is now a sign of a backward or diseased body, and the cloth with which it is associated no longer receives great social attention.

James investigates the ways in which clothing serves to articulate differences in gender, age, and religion within a southern African community. She explores the complex content and use of notions of *sesotho* (*sotho* ways) in opposition to *sekgowa* (white ways) for Sotho speakers in the northern Transvaal of South Africa. She draws upon the life histories of women belonging to a group that since 1976 has performed dances and songs considered *sesotho* in style. The female performers wear dress that has come to reflect aspects of *sekgowa* style.

James argues that these performances at least temporarily empower women. They create a collective female identity that obscures the economic and other status differences between women, unifying the participants into an effective representation of Sotho historical identity. Ultimately, she asserts, these symbolic forms can "enunciate [women's] autonomy from male control." James analyzes the categories *sesotho* and *sekgowa* as historically emergent, contextually sensitive, and individually manipulated—as "conceptual tools . . . used as grids or templates to order experience in a variety of different settings." Indigenous notions of a Sotho ethnic identity have developed in opposition to and in tandem with the idea of *sekgowa,* and Sotho women have been particularly closely associated with the definition and perpetuation of *sesotho* identity.

Masquelier's essay focuses on clothing as a principal medium of communication between people and the spirits among the Hausaphone Mawri in Niger. Dress creates spiritual beings; specific spirits require particular types of attire, which must be provided by those faithful to them. Clothes express the commitment of the living to the spirits and the harmony between them. Clothes give substance to these incorporeal beings—they "extend the spirits' personae in space and time." The garments themselves come to have potency. A spirit's clothes can be used as a channel through which communication with the spirit can be effected in private, domestic contexts. By borrowing specific clothes, one may unknowingly inherit a spirit that is associated with them.

Masquelier notes that clothing aptly expresses the ephemeral nature of the link between living people and the spirits; both the garments and the relationship should be periodically renewed. She also links specific ritual uses of body coverings with the symbolism and use of everyday clothing. While the tying of clothing is metaphorically linked with marriage and reproduction and with the initiation of relationships and social statuses, untying speaks of relationships severed and death, when the deceased's clothes are given away. Dress is also found to express Muslim modesty and social deviance in a wider Mawri world.

Ideologies of authority
Bastian and Weiss trace the creation and perpetuation of systems of authority as well as challenges to them. Like Renne, Bastian investigates one strand within the complex web of cultures and histories upon which the nation-state of Nigeria has been founded. She explores the ways in which Igbo women and men test the limits of senior male authority by wearing types of body adornment associated with it and with Muslim Hausa elites to the north. Bastian argues that this constitutes a politically inspired "clothing practice" with implications for a late-twentieth-century imagination of gender and authority.

Using a cartoon from the Nigerian popular press among other data, Bastian outlines the possibilities that clothing provides women, as a relatively disempowered social group, in making satirical and potentially subversive statements about their identities in relation to power-holders. These possibilities turn on culturally shared conceptions of body shape and structure and ideas about a gendered treatment of the body, which cross-dressing women, for instance, confound.

Bastian goes on to show that another subordinated political group, young men, has also used clothing practice to challenge existing articulations of identity. Their enthusiasm for new styles of dress, especially in colors associated with both mourning practice and the suits of Europeans, is troublesome to their male elders. It signifies the engagement of junior men in social arenas that are potentially disruptive to traditional authority. Bastian concludes, however, that while such signifying practice challenges older regimes of value, it does not deeply threaten them—women will not soon be the power-holders they impersonate and junior men will someday themselves be elders on the other side of the power equation.

Weiss's essay introduces the idea that body treatments can act as mnemonic devices that help to construct and represent lasting relationships between generations and between the living and the dead. He discusses the importance of body treatments, including clothing and bark-cloth funerary shrouds, in the remembering and forgetting that are critical in intergenerational relationships, especially at death among the Haya in Tanzania. In his analysis, as in Masquelier's, clothes are seen to have the possibility of a history of their own.

Like Masquelier, Weiss also focuses on the links between dress and the dead, between notions of corporeality and spiritual potency. Among Haya mortuary observances, for instance, bark cloth is wrapped around both the corpse and his living clansmen, serving as a reminder of the long-term nurturance provided by these people and their relatives. Blankets and sheets given as bride-wealth years before are conceptually linked to these mortuary cloths. The Haya say that the cloths given at marriage replace those used by a mother to wrap her infant and are a form of recognition for the years of care a mother has provided to her marrying child. Weiss calls all these cloths "material recollections" which "invoke memories that are features of intergenerational relations."

Weiss goes on to delineate the broader meaning of body coverings for the Haya, contextualizing the meaning of these material symbols within a system of ideas about the closure and exposure of the body. At funerals, mourners are dissolute, unraveled. They wear special headcloths in an effort to regain their bodily integrity. The one large piece of bark cloth that is used to enclose both the mourners and the corpse contributes to this reintegration, expressing an "aesthetic of seamlessness" which also prompts the Haya to oil their skin. In these and other ways, bodily coverings help the Haya think about and personalize the past and the future, to remember that death comes at the end of long years of nurturance, that grief can be overcome, and that the next generation will sustain life.

The creation of value

The essays by Burke, Schoss, and myself delineate the processes whereby value is created in body treatments that derive from foreign sources. Schoss analyzes dress that marks two styles of culture brokering in the Swahili tourist trade in Malindi, Kenya. She identifies two styles of dress and comportment, one associated with the professionalized "tour guides," who have ties to tour operators, the other with the "beachboys," who offer their services to tourists on a free-lance basis.

Not only dress but bodily comportment and social behavior differ widely between these two groups. The tour guides present themselves in fastidious, European-style clothing that is either produced in Europe or custom-made locally. They comport themselves with restraint at all times in public, thereby emphasizing their control over the tourist economy and themselves. In contrast, the beachboys value the unconventional—their dress incorporates bright color; innovative, locally made designs; and Euro-American items such as jeans and fanny packs, which they acquire through trade with their clients. During their off-hours, they behave with abandon and excess, frequenting the discos, ostensibly run to attract the tourists themselves.

Schoss finds that both groups understand and move within a "cosmopolitan," multicultural world, between local mores and those of the wider world economic system. This competence is made apparent in their control of bodily practice. Further, she argues that despite the considerable knowledge of global culture that is acquired by these Kenyan businessmen, they remain a part of local social worlds as well—they are not marginalized at home by their competence with foreign commodities and lifestyles.

Focusing not on clothing per se but on skin treatments, Burke also considers the strategies employed by African people encountering the agents and products of a wider world economic system. Burke analyzes nineteenth- and twentieth-century commodity exchange in colonial Zimbabwe, tracing the development of ideas about the body, hygiene, and race that structured colonial relations there. He investigates how colonial bureaucrats, missionaries, travelers, and mercantilists linked order and rationality with cleanliness, defining African bodies—and African people in the process—as unclean, disorderly, depraved, and polluting.

Burke argues that these conceptions played an important part in the development of colonial policy. Hygiene was taken as a discipline through which the bodies and minds of African workers, mission converts, and pupils could be improved. Women's bodies in particular were scrutinized, and women's domestic practice became a subject of bureaucratic and mercantilist concern. But even as they were coerced and convinced to adopt European practices of hygiene and manners and so transform themselves into more properly socialized persons, Zimbabwean consumers used and symbolically constructed skin products in their own culturally idiosyncratic ways, which were never fully understood or controlled by capitalist producers.

Burke argues that "the" body should be seen as a particular construct of a nineteenth-century, European colonial world, which was preoccupied with control of the body. He cautions that the African bodies that were the collective object of colonial fascination and abhorrence must be seen as belonging to members of heterogeneous Shona, Ndebele, and Tonga groups and subgroups, each of which had their own aesthetics of body adornment and hygiene.

My own essay focuses on changing and differentiated conceptions of value, on developing representations of collective and gendered identity in nineteenth- and twentieth-century Namibian history. In oral histories, particular male Herero leaders are said to have reimagined morality and society in a nineteenth-century era of economic and political change. The commitment of individuals to newly defined ideas about moral social relations and male leadership, in particular, has been expressed and read in the practice of wearing tokens of colored cloth, first on hatbands and later on other parts of the body.

In spite of explicit attempts by Europeans to inculcate the use of banners as symbols of the unified polity, the Herero use of banners as individual bodily symbols has expressed a characteristically individual-centered relation of people to the wider collectivity. Herero notions of identity hinge upon the expressed commitment of individuals to the authority of male leaders and the moral values they live by. This is expressed in their use of individual bodies as flags.

The idiosyncratic Herero use of cloth banners and the issues of gendered authority that underlie them continue to be elaborated in the twentieth century. Annual Herero "troop" ceremonies celebrate the heroism of nineteenth-century paragons of masculinity and virtue. Further, they constitute an effort to unify Ovaherero behind a common history. Though these ceremonies are only one type of symbolic construction in a changing history of Herero representations of gender and identity, they have come to be seen as "traditional" by Ovaherero and varying groups of interested onlookers.

Dress and the Body Surface in
Africanist Scholarship

In these eight essays, we show that clothing and other treatments of the body surface are primary symbols in the performances through which modernity—and therefore history—have been conceived, constructed, and challenged in Africa. We have discovered a distinctive African modernity expressed and shaped through redefined body commodities, funerary ritual and dance, and spiritual practice. We find that both the "modern" and the "traditional" are powerfully and principally constituted in body treatments. We explore the fact that "the body . . . cannot escape being a vehicle of history, a metaphor and metonym of being-in-time" (Comaroff and Comaroff 1992, 79).

The performative nature of these processes is especially clear in the essays by Masquelier, James, and Weiss, which explicitly examine ritual uses of dress. Furthermore, the whole collection focuses on potent, public performances, which have contributed significantly to African social production and reproduction in the last two centuries. In taking ritual as a critical starting point in the analysis of African modernity, our work exemplifies a recent focus in historical and anthropological Africanist research (Hobsbawm and Ranger 1983; J. Comaroff 1985; Comaroff and Comaroff 1993).

In this effort, we also build upon the considerable insights of earlier analysts of African culture, for whom both quotidian and ritual dress have long been fruitful points of analysis. The symbolic interplay of bodily and social experience has been investigated within African societies by such authors as T. O. Beidelman (1968, 1986), Mary Douglas (1967, 1970), Michael Jackson (1983, 1989), and Hilda Kuper (1973a, 1973b).

Among the most recent analyses (e.g., Heath 1992), Karen Tranberg Hansen (1994) has shown how used clothing from abroad is redefined and recom-modified by Zambians empowered by the new consumer choices, economic opportunities, and ties to a wider cosmopolitan world that this clothing offers. As has been recognized in much of the other literature discussed here, however, the enjoyment of such freedoms is "tinged with ambivalence" (Hansen 1994, 522) for Africans wearied by the instability of their local economies and cog-nizant of their peripheralized position in a wider politico-economic world.

Like other recent researchers (Jackson and Karp 1990), we also follow Fortes (1973) and Riesman (1977, 1986) in exploring the relations between lived experi-ence and culturally constructed ideas about moral persons in Africa. It is the fertile ground between official and unofficial ideologies of personhood and identity (Jacobson-Widding 1990, 34) that we examine here. By investigating the symbolic use of the body surface, we are able to accomplish a fine-grained analysis of the ways in which both individual agency and sociocultural con-straint are operative in social life. We consider ways in which individual-centered notions of "fantasy" and "fashion," familiar in Western settings, are operative in African contexts as well.

Bodily Signs and Spiritual Representations

As discussed earlier, Garber has raised the provocative question of whether dressing across social boundaries is in fact essential to, or even constitutive of, culture. Our studies are not new in suggesting that opposing social categories always implicate each other; however, we do contribute evidence that cross-dressing, broadly defined, has indeed been a powerful symbolic tool in African contexts as well as Western ones. Whether it has involved women dressed as men, male commoners dressed as elites, colonized men dressing as colonizers, young men dressed as cosmopolitan tourists, spirits dressed as living people, or grandchildren dressed as grandparents, "cross-dressing" is here found to be cross-cultural. In Africa as in the West, dress has been an index of difference between social groups.

An index is a sign in which form and referent are linked physically as if by cause and effect (see C. S. Peirce in Buchler 1940). Our analyses suggest that cross-culturally, the body surface is an especially compelling indexical sign. Bodily signifiers present an ever-present semiotic possibility for expressing identity and intention, for asserting the legitimacy of the status quo or subverting it. In the African cases we discuss here, treatments of the body surface allude to linkages between oneself and people, power and knowledge beyond the immediate, local context. Such allusions are powerful because they can challenge the taken-for-granted categories into which the social world is divided.

Whether or not bodily signs are intended to be read as indicators of specific motivations and identities, they may be taken as such by onlookers. Bodily signs may be conservative because their symbolic forms are material and potentially lasting. Simultaneously, concrete bodily signs are potentially subversive, since they are literally manipulable by individuals or groups with differing motivations and access to power.

Moreover, our African case studies allow us to state that the body surface has been a powerful arena in which colonial relations have been enacted and contested. While colonial projects may entail the rigorous separation of social and economic interaction between colonizer and colonized, colonial domination ultimately is grounded in the face-to-face relations between local coresidents. The circumstances of physical contiguity that are central to the creation of ideologies and industries of "the other" are necessarily contexts in which the visually accessed languages of the body and body coverings are central.

Under these conditions, the body is a signifier that is shared cross-culturally yet assigned contrasting, simultaneous meanings. Especially in the absence of shared spoken language, colonial encounters can be seen as a particular kind of semiotic event in which a visual language of bodily forms is especially critical. The recognition of formal, material or physical commonalities between members of unlike groups or cultures may constitute an avenue of implicit resistance to developing ideologies of the other. Material symbolic forms, especially the body, draw cross-cultural notions of personal, moral, and social identity into metaphorical relation. Possibilities for resistance lie in the fact that this semiotic process can never be fully controlled, even by a dominating colonial power.

In the concrete processes of construction and decay to which they continuously allude, bodily signs also refer to the passage of time and processes of change that occur at rates different from that of the everyday. Object "events"— in the sense of the purposeful manipulation of material signs in an effort to alter social representations and therefore relations of power—happen at a slower pace than speech events. Paradoxically, this makes them persuasive agents for change. The body is perhaps the quintessential subversive object sign, since it refers almost inevitably to individual as well as to group intentions and identities, which are always at issue—and at risk—in a changing, plural, social and cultural world.

These essays also remind us that there are multiple ways of thinking about the relations between people, objects, and spiritual/social power. Cross-culturally, corporeality can itself be seen as containment of power. As is true among many of the people we discuss in this volume, the body may be one among many types of objects in which power is thought to reside. In these societies, restrictions on contact with spiritually powerful objects may follow from age, sex, marital status, lineage, or caste, but many categories of people and not just religious specialists have personal contact with the most potent containers of power. People in such societies thus enjoy considerable access to the sacred in their daily lives.

If, alternatively, power is thought to reside only in nonmaterial entities—as is common in the Protestant iconoclastic thought associated with Western industrial societies, for example—then people may have no personal contact with or control over the most potent forms of power at all. It is ironic that it is capitalist consumers who fetishize commodities, even while they are constrained from worshiping icons: they are encouraged to "believe" in the products they buy, but they are taught to separate the power of products from the power of gods.

It is to these cosmological matters that the analysis of the symbolic uses of the body surface ultimately reaches. The essays in this collection demonstrate anew that economic and spiritual matters mutually inform one another, and that cynicism is not the only tenor of these postmodern times. The world of spiritual belief, of what humanists might call desire and its fulfillment, may not be the social dead-end that Western cultural critics since Marx have suggested. In fact, it may be belief that rescues us from alienation. The feminist turn toward exploring the fantasy element in consumer behavior seems attuned to this idea. We must look outside our own societies to be reminded that even postmodern capitalist consumers act within an imagined world of potency and possibility which can affect concrete realities. To overlook this symbolic production is to obscure the creative processes through which ordinary people understand and shape their daily lives. Women and men make their own history and they do not make it just as they please, but they make it, we have learned, in powerful semiotic forms.

To fully understand Western economic, political, and spiritual life, we would do well to heed the African examples and give attention to issues of imagination and belief as they are associated with objects and manifested on the body. These cases remind us that what Garber calls cultural anxiety—awareness of the unresolved contradictions in a system of symbolic thought that guides daily life—is the common cultural conundrum with which all human societies must contend. Many who coexist with us in a postmodern world greet these conditions not with cynicism but with creativity and conviction.

I CREATING SOCIAL IDENTITIES

1 VIRGINITY CLOTHS AND VAGINAL COVERINGS IN EKITI, NIGERIA

Elisha P. Renne

The body is the innermost part of the material self in each of us; and certain parts of the body seem more intimately ours than the rest. The clothes come next.—W. James, *Principles of Psychology*

Introduction

Until relatively recently, it was taken for granted in American society that a concrete physiological marker—a thin, membranous tissue known as the hymen—constituted a woman's virginity, the state of never having had sexual intercourse with a man. Further evidence of virginity was the rupture of the hymen upon first intercourse, which resulted in a sign of blood. The unequivocal presence of this bodily marker (the hymen) in all virgins has since been questioned (Kahn and Holt 1990, 152), and its absence is no longer considered legally sufficient evidence of a nonvirgin state (Townsend 1974, 3). This reassessment of what signifies virginity underscores the political nature of such readings of the body, which, grounded in a particular social and historical context, "must be regarded as a narrative of culture in anatomical disguise" (Laqueur 1990, 236). Expanding on this insight in the Nigerian context, I analyze here the particularities of one such narrative, based on interviews with 95 Ekiti Yoruba women,[1] whose experience of the importance of a hymen-like tissue, the *ibale*—"a sort of biological undergarment protecting the female genitals" (Sissa 1990, 1)—has changed dramatically in the last seventy-five years. What is striking about their remarks is that they illustrate how the meaning attributed to a so-called anatomical given may shift in time. For these Ekiti Yoruba women, the shift in the perception of the *ibale*-hymen—from something whose presence was preserved and celebrated at marriage to something old-fashioned and traditional that should be quickly dispensed with—relates to changing ideas about what constitutes "enlightened" behavior and knowledge, which are in turn part of a shift in relations of power in Ekiti society in colonial and post-colonial Nigeria.

Ekiti views of virginity also illustrate the ways in which bodily states may be conflated with material objects—in this case, cloth and clothing—underscoring Durkheim's insights about the dialectical relation between ideas held by people which are embodied in things. Like the "leprosy of a mildewed garment" of the Old Testament, which was ritually cleansed as if it were a leper (Leviticus 14:1–9, 47–59), the white cloths used to test the presence of hymeneal blood were synonymous with the virgin herself. However, before discussing the related careers of the *ibale*-hymen and virginity cloths in Ekiti Yoruba social life, I would like to consider what these women meant by the term virginity, whose meaning—couched in terms of local knowledge of the body as well as influenced by social and political concerns—cannot be assumed.

Virginity in Ekiti

In the Ekiti Yoruba context, virginity is referred to generally by the term *ibale*,[2] which also refers more specifically to a part of the body. One traditional healer (*babalawo*) described its bodily manifestation as looking like a red "plastic-film wrapping" covering the vagina (*obo* or *oju ara*),[3] something like an "internal security system." This vaginal covering was also described by an older woman as being

> something like blood, very thick and as soon as the man is able to penetrate, the thing will just break, and that shows the girl has lost her virginity. It is called *ibale* and at the same time *ayere*. It is the thing that stained the white cloth and shows that one has lost her virginity.

Another younger woman compared it to the breaking of a palm kernel:

> It is usually difficult to be able to penetrate the first time. For about three hours the man will still be trying, because it will be very hard. And it is painful that day. It will just be as if someone were trying to crack a palm kernel. If the woman is still a virgin, as soon as the man is able to penetrate, blood will just stain the white cloth that has been spread on the bed. That shows that she has not known a man before.

Several other women mentioned this hardness of the *ibale*: "The place was hard and thick and when the man was able to penetrate, the place will soften, then blood will come out."

These descriptions are, to the best of my understanding, what physiologically constitutes the "hymen" for Yoruba women. The Western perception of virginity as a particular bodily state defined by the presence of a particular bit of anatomy, the membranous hymen which when pierced results in bleeding, while similar in some ways to the Yoruba perception of virginity, is not the same. For example, no woman mentioned the use of manual examinations to ascertain whether the *ibale*-membrane was intact. Rather, for them, the membrane—the reddish, plastic-like covering that is hard and then softens after penetration—and the resulting blood were conflated. If the *ibale*-membrane is present, there must be blood, as explained by one older woman:

Do you know of any example when a girl insisted that she was a virgin but she didn't bleed?
There was nothing like that because it was compulsory in the past that when you lost your virginity you must see blood. If blood was not seen, it meant that one had lost one's virginity before.

As if to emphasize this point, there is no linguistic distinction made in Yoruba between the hymen, hymeneal blood, and virginity. The word *ibale* refers to all three—to the membranous thing (*ibale*) that is pierced or penetrated (*ja*); to the blood-like thing (*ibale* or *ayere*), thick and dark, that stains the white cloth, which confirms a woman's virginity; to the state of virginity (ibale) itself.

This triple conflation of membrane, blood, and physiological state is materially represented by a white cloth, known as *aso ibale* or *aso ayere* (virginity cloth), which is marked by the *ibale*-blood. Indeed, the inevitable mention of this cloth by older women suggests a quadruple conflation. If the *ibale* is present, there must be blood (*ibale*), which must be evidenced on a piece of white cloth (*aso ibale*), which serves as a surrogate for the virgin state—no stained white cloth, no virginity (*ibale*).

Other than that it should be white, there were no prescriptions for the type or size of cloth used as *aso ibale*. Some women described it as small, "like a handkerchief," while others described a cloth big enough to be used as a cover cloth for sleeping. It could be a commercially woven white cloth (one type, *teru*, was mentioned) or a handwoven one. A synecdoche for virginity, the journey of this cloth after its inscription with *ibale*-blood reveals another aspect of the Yoruba perception of virginity, which helps to explain its particular importance for older women.

After sexual intercourse between husband and wife had taken place, the bloodied cloth was publicly displayed to establish witnesses for the bride's virginal state. What happened to the cloth after that was described by one sixty-year-old woman:

My husband put the cloth inside a white calabash[4] to show to my parents. . . . [After that], my husband kept it in the house . . . for future reference.

Another woman in her sixties explained that keeping it in the house was a reminder of her virtuous behavior:

It was kept in the rafters of the woman's house after the cloth might have been shown to the mother and the father of the woman. This explains why there is nowhere that her husband will go that he will not have the love of his wife in his heart.

However, a few women mentioned another use for this cloth that hints at something quite different:

I used the cloth to carry my first child because we believe strongly that the cloth will serve to guard the child against any evil forces. And again, to show that the child is a good child and that the mother had passed [*iyege*].[5]

And:

We kept it in the house until I delivered my first child, then I took it and washed it and it was used as a spreading cloth for the child.

The association of a woman's first child with the blood-stained virginity cloth relates to the idea that an intact *ibale* confirmed that a woman had not "spoiled herself," that is, her fertility (see also Boddy 1989, 55; Hayes 1975). Several women mentioned the belief that if the *ibale* was present, they would immediately, on sexually meeting their husbands, become pregnant:

According to tradition, it was believed that any woman who was a virgin would get pregnant the first month. The belief was that she had not spoiled herself before moving to her husband's house.[6]

The presence of the *ibale* (virginity), then, was not simply a bodily state that indicated the fact of no prior intercourse and served as a point of pride for brides (Barber 1991, 114), husbands, and kin (Olusanya 1967, 15; Fadipe 1970, 66). Its loss was associated with immediate pregnancy, underscored by the use of the virginity cloth for carrying or covering the firstborn child.

The importance of the virginity, evidenced by the stained white virginity cloth, was related to ideas about the control of young women's bodies and about fertility. By restricting the movements of young women within and outside of houses, parents protected the integrity of the *ibale*, much as the *ibale* itself, that "internal security system," protected their daughters' future fertility from being "spoiled" or "broken."[7] The power of fathers to exert such control, and the consequences when this power was undermined during the period of British colonial rule, is evidenced in related shifts in imagery of the house and the female body. For, as Turner (1984, 2) has observed, there are "parallels between the idea of government of the body and the regime of a given society."

Hidden and Revealed Bodies and Knowledge

In Ekiti society, a father's authority over members of his house-compound—his wives and their children—was reinforced by an ideology of patrilineal descent and was represented in an everyday way by the power of the *baale* (literally "father of the house") over the passage of people through a central front door (*oju ile*), both controlling and protecting inhabitants on "the inside" from "the outside." Thus, a prospective suitor soliciting an arranged marriage would be "screened" by a young woman's father; the girl herself would be hidden in the house:[8]

> In the past if a girl was given to a man and the man came to greet her in the house, the girl would be hidden. If the girl was seeing him off, she would turn her back to him.

Once arrangements had been made between this man and the prospective bride's father, annual payments of yams (*isu obutan*) and labor (*owe* or *ebese*) were given to the father. This process culminated in the payment of bridewealth (*idano*), which was timed to take place after the appearance of menarche. The veiled bride would then be taken through the doorway of her father's house, outside, to her husband's house, where her entry was marked in various ritual ways.[9] Later in the evening, she was uncovered both literally and figuratively by her husband, after which the bloodied *aso ibale* cloth was publicly displayed. The cloth would then be taken to the bride's parents, marking the successful conclusion of their control. She was thereafter "covered" by members of her husband's household who awaited her first child, which was expected to arrive shortly.

The idea of the protected threshold-doorway of a house—referred to as the *oju ile*, literally "eye of the house"— is linguistically related to the vaginal threshold, the *oju ara*, "eye of the body," with its covering, the *ibale*, protecting the passageway[10] between the inside (*inu*, womb) and the outside (*aiye*, world). A house's front doorway represents the opening between inner domestic and outer public space, just as the vaginal opening distinguishes between inner and outer domains. The Yoruba phrase for womb, *ile omo* (house or room of the child), further reinforces this comparison of the house and the female body, both of which may be perceived as structures that protect those within from outside dangers.

This representation of protection and vulnerability associated with covered thresholds and with the inside and outside of houses and bodies corresponded with the power of fathers to regulate the passage between these two spaces. Their power to control these movements was reinforced not only by their status as heads of households, but also because they ritually controlled the passage of bodies between spiritual domains—at funerals and at childbirth.[11] However, with the incorporation of the Ekiti region within the boundaries of the Lagos Protectorate of colonial Nigeria, agreed upon in 1893, the power of the father-*baale* was undermined.

These changes in the basis of power were not felt immediately or uniformly throughout Ekiti. It was only after the formation of the Northeastern District (consisting of the Ijesha and Ekiti regions) in 1899, that the consequences of the British presence became tangible. For example, a sense of the presence of colonial officials (described from the British point of view) is evidenced in the comments of the "Travelling Commissioner" for the District, Major Reeve Tucker, who toured Ekiti in 1899:

> I have called in all the tributary villages to the capitals of the several Ekiti Kingdoms and have placed the Bales [*sic*; local quarter heads were also known as *baale*] securely under their Kings. The Bales who were endeavouring to make themselves independent, a lingering remnant of their old wars and disputes, I have effectively placed under their proper kings. At each capital I held a palaver and explained the Government policy to them. (de la Mothe 1921, 7)

The reality of British control was made more evident with the establishment of a separate Ekiti Division in 1913 (de la Mothe 1921) and the building of an administrative center in Ado-Ekiti in 1914 (Oguntuyi 1979). Despite the fact that British colonial officials instituted a form of governance known as "indirect rule," whereby traditional chiefs administered everyday local affairs, there was no doubt where the political buck stopped. British officers retained control of more important political decisions, underscoring the fact that a fundamental shift in the basis of power had occurred in colonial Nigeria (see Beidelman [1971] 1983; Chanock 1985).

The power of traditional chiefs was undermined economically and socially as well as politically. For example, by encouraging the growing of cash crops such as cocoa for sale to expatriate firms, the British created a demand for literate clerks who could negotiate with farmers and European buyers. By promoting the establishment of mission schools throughout Ekiti in the 1920s and 1930s to fill this need (Oguntuyi 1979), they encouraged a different basis for knowledge, and hence power, grounded on literacy and books. These developments favored the careers of a group of young literate men, consisting largely of clerks and schoolteachers, who associated the acquisition of power, wealth, and prestige in colonial Nigeria with Western-style education. Subscribing to the concept of what was referred to as *olaju*, "enlightenment" or "civilization" (Peel 1978), this group of newly educated young men challenged the authority of older, often nonliterate, chiefs, whose powers were based on what these younger men perceived to be outmoded traditional practices. What is more, in their promotion of *olaju* (enlightenment), they included a range of practices and tastes associated with Europeans—such as dress, hygiene, and bodily comportment (Mauss 1973)—to be part of their "civilizing" agenda. Ideas about marriage, love, and virginity fell under this rubric as well.

It is not my intention here to examine the complex intergenerational contests that developed over representations of "enlightened" and "traditional" authority and which have continued throughout this century.[12] Nor do I mean to suggest that the Yoruba concept of *olaju*, "civilization," is a new phenomenon, solely associated with Europeans. As Peel (1978, 146) has observed, the Yoruba idea of *olaju* refers both to a general appreciation of the relationship between knowledge and power as well as a particular association of knowledge with foreign practices, ideas, and things. Rather, I focus on a single part "of the body and the effects of power on it" (Foucault 1980, 58), examining how a shift in the perception of knowledge, reflected in the acclamation of *olaju*, and consequently power, is related to the representation and control of bodies during the colonial and post-colonial period in rural Ekiti. Further, the reading of a particular part of the body, the *ibale*-hymen and the concurrent evaluation of virginity and virginity cloths, did not simply reflect these changes in knowledge and the basis of power. They formed an integral part of this process. For it was through their representation of a "modern," enlightened body—the opposite of "traditional," virginal ones—that this shift in power relations, from the hands of the elderly chiefs to educated juniors, was quite literally embodied.

Enlightened Behavior: Attending Customary Court

It was not only ideas about "enlightened" behavior, education, and young men's access to independent income through clerical positions, teaching, and cash cropping that led to a reevaluation of women's bodies. One particular innovation introduced by the British served as the catalyst for this change, namely the introduction of procedures for divorce, which led to the demise of arranged marriage. On 1 March 1920, Ekiti *obas* (kings) meeting at Ado-Ekiti agreed to support the British initiative for the establishment of a system of Native Authority courts, which included the introduction of rules for divorce (Oguntuyi 1979, 130; see also Caldwell, Orubuloye, and Caldwell 1991; Renne 1992). As a result of this agreement, young women were able to extricate themselves from arranged marriages (Lloyd 1968). Thereafter, by repaying bridewealth (or a comparable sum for brideservice) to the original suitor who had made such payments, young Ekiti women and men were able to select spouses of their choice. During the 1930s and 1940s, many took advantage of this opportunity. For example, of the twenty-six Ekiti women aged fifty years or older whom I interviewed, twenty-one had arranged marriages and five of them had divorced their arranged-marriage husbands, marrying men whom they chose themselves (Renne 1993:123). However, other aspects of the marriage process remained the same during this period, at least in rural northeastern Ekiti. Once bridewealth had been returned to the "first husband" and permission to marry was granted by her father, traditional marriage rituals proceeded as if an arranged marriage were being performed, including the continued importance of virginity.

Several developments, particularly increased school attendance, altered these marriage procedures. Church-run primary schools were started throughout the Ekiti area in the 1930s[13] and in 1955, universal primary education was introduced in the Western Province, of which Ekiti was part. Many parents took advantage of this program, sending their daughters as well as their sons to school. As educated men preferred wives who could comport themselves in an "enlightened" fashion, many parents began to realize that their daughters' chances of marrying well, as well as acquiring white-collar employment, were enhanced by some education.[14] However, school attendance meant that young girls' physical movements were unmonitored. Also their exposure to new ideas and fashions in school, to "civilization," was believed to affect their behavior, as one sixty-year-old woman explained:

> Civilization has come and things have changed. Is it children who are fifteen years old who have become pregnant and go to their husbands' houses without taking anything from him [i.e., bridewealth] who will be virgins? All this was caused by schools because there girls are exposed to immoral acts. And they will say they are going to school, they will just detour off to their boyfriends' houses, which no one could do in the past.

Like their educated male counterparts, young women who attended school were likely to disparage certain practices associated with a parochial past, preferring modern, "enlightened" behavior instead. Hiding in the house—away from the eyes, let alone the arms, of men—came to be considered "antisocial" behavior (*suegbe*). Thus when young men pressed girlfriends and fiancées for premarital sexual relations, young women may have been inclined to concur not only for emotional reasons but in order to appear "enlightened," rather than traditionally chaste.

It is difficult to know how young girls felt about pressure from boyfriends or to what extent they themselves encouraged premarital sex. While some were clearly uncomfortable about their acquiescence (some said they were tricked,[15] others said they had not been "reborn" Christians at the time) and some may have felt they would lose their boyfriends' affection, others saw it as an opportunity for increased "enjoyment." Premarital sex had other benefits, as it was also used to ascertain the fertility of prospective spouses. Rather than trust in one's future wife's virginity to ensure fertility, the uncertainties of fertility and of getting and keeping a prospective wife (or husband) were alleviated by a woman's pregnancy.

In the northeastern Ekiti area, it was during the late 1960s and early 1970s that young women openly went outside of their fathers' houses (to schools, parties, etc.) to "meet" (a euphemism for sexual intercourse) prospective husbands. Some who got pregnant soon after followed these men to their houses as wives. It was also during this period that the importance of the vaginal covering—the *ibale*, perceived as sign of socially correct behavior as well as protection of the womb's fertility—diminished. What was once publicly proclaimed through the display of a bloodied white cloth came to be regarded as a private matter between husband, wife, and their immediate families. Indeed, this privacy was important, as a young woman who remained a virgin before marriage might be accused of being unenlightened (*suegbe*) and thus feel ashamed. The presence of the *ibale* no longer served as a sign of a controlled and fertile body but rather as a sign of a socially backward one, as one forty-five-year-old woman explained:

> During my own time, if a girl of twenty years had not lost her virginity, her age-mates and people around would be saying that she was not civilized, that she was not social.

Furthermore, for some, the continued presence of the *ibale* reflected not only antisocial behavior but also the possibility of a hidden disease, which would actually lead to infertility. The most frequently mentioned condition described to me was *akiriboto,* "no vagina," which led young women to run away from men.[16] Thus, changes in social practice in Ekiti were reflected in reassessments of reproductive health and in changing moral perceptions of virginity (Renne 1993).

Changing Perceptions of Virginity Reflected
in Bodies and Cloths

However, the importance of *ibale*-virginity has not disappeared entirely. Rather, the presence of the *ibale*-virginity is privately valued by some, despite the fact that other practices associated with marriage—such as the payment of *isu obutan* (marriage yams), the giving of virginity gifts to the bride, or the three-month observance of traditional marriage ritual (*gbe obutan*)—have been abandoned.

Some Ekiti women continue to perform a modified form of traditional marriage and go to their husbands' houses as virgins. But the importance of this state is not stressed, which the final destination of their bloodied virginity cloths makes graphically clear:

Were you given anything for being a virgin?
I was not given anything exactly, but everybody was happy about it and they were eating and dancing.

How do you know a woman is a virgin?
White cloth was given to me when I was coming to my husband's house and it was this white cloth that I used. When I slept with my husband, blood came out and stained the white cloth.

What happened to the cloth?
It was shown to my family. Later, I threw it away.

Or:

Yes, I was a virgin. A cloth was used; I took it, but later it got lost.

These images of discarded or lost virginity cloths reflect the decreasing importance of public displays of the *ibale*-hymen's presence. Among married women in their twenties, many were not virgins when they married, nor was white cloth used at first intercourse:

How do you know a woman is a virgin?
In the past, white cloth was used because of the importance they placed on being a virgin. But when I did my own, I did not use any white cloth but I saw blood on the bed.

The present insignificance of virginity has reached a point where some young women do not know what constitutes virginity at all, as indicated by this twenty-six-year-old woman's remark: "I do not know any sign if a lady is a virgin. I did not see any sign when I lost my virginity."[17] This woman and most others her age did not use the white *aso ibale* during their first sexual encounter.

Discussion

The decline in importance of the *ibale*-hymen cannot be said to have been caused simply by the introduction of divorce in colonial courts and the subsequent demise of arranged marriage in Ekiti. Rather, divorce was part of a process during a period when a shift in the basis of knowledge—from oral "traditions" to literate "enlightenment" (*olaju*)—and the focus of power—from local kingdoms to a bureaucratic state—was occurring in southwestern Nigeria. This shift undermined the power of traditional chief-kings who, despite British support of the policy of indirect rule, were politically superseded during the 1940s by younger, educated men (Peel 1978). Literacy and Western-style education came to be recognized as crucial to full participation in the economic and political opportunities of colonial society.

Thus it was schooling, rather than divorce or the demise of arranged marriage, that several older women associated with the decline of virginity. Some specifically mentioned the physical presence of girls and boys mixing at school. Others spoke more broadly of "civilization," of young girls being "exposed" at school, unlike the past when "we were not *open* to all the things that children of today are doing" [emphasis mine].

This exposure to the outside—to school, to different knowledge, to "civilization"—relates back to earlier ideas about the control and protection of bodies, hidden in houses, veiled and covered on their way to their husbands' house, and pregnant once opened. While these body techniques had worked in the past, they were no longer viewed as a viable means of acquiring power in a socioeconomic setting that depended on the development of new skills and on the open exchange of information, often in writing. Like the new forms of knowledge necessary for advancement in the modern political system, a young woman's marriage and employment potential, and consequently fertility, depended upon going outside the house (and sometimes community). It was unveiled, unvirginal bodies, without the *ibale*-hymen, that came to be regarded as a sign of *olaju*, of being civilized.[18]

Yet it might also be argued à la Foucault that *olaju*, while "opening up" women's bodies and seemingly liberating their sexuality, actually led to the application of further controls by submitting them to the "gaze" of colonial officials—in hospitals, maternity clinics, and schools. However, many Ekiti women and men would argue that practices associated with *olaju*, with the "lifting the veil from the world," have generally benefited individuals and society, as evidenced by better houses, easier transport, and lower infant mortality. This assessment does not mean that people have no reservations about these changes. They do, and they express them in remarks about empty family houses in home villages, about increased highway robbery, and about stubborn, disobedient children. While they long for change that they hope will improve their lives, many are aware of the dissonances and discontinuity that these changes have wrought. And some are more dissatisfied with this sense of discontinuity than others.

Thus, the positive associations of nonvirgins with openness and enlightenment are not shared by everyone, as evidenced by the term *olaju agbere*, corrupt enlightenment. Not everyone availed themselves of the options opened up by *olaju*, including some without the economic wherewithal to avail themselves of educational opportunities. Virginity practices have not changed uniformly among all groups in Ekiti society (see Ortner 1978, 30). While some young women say that it is not good to be a virgin because your husband might be afraid that something is wrong with you, others (a minority) have maintained more traditional attitudes toward virginity, saying their husbands have praised them for not "spoiling" themselves.[19] Those whose power has been eroded by changes attributed to *olaju* may nostalgically long for past practices, and to some extent continue them. One older woman expressed this sense of loss of a particular social order in terms of virginity, children, and virginity cloth:

> Being a virgin is good. . . . [It is because women are getting married without being virgins that] today's children are unruly. . . . Things were not like that [in the past]. . . . Now these children do not have roots, [they do not have a social] foundation. Unlike before when [girls remained virgins in the house after marriage and] the cloth [*aso ibale*] was kept somewhere.

In the past, she reports, children respected their parents, unlike nowadays when they are "stubborn," when "they will be thinking they know more than their parents." These children who go outside the house, to school, to university, and to live in urban centers, no longer have a foundation in their rural village homes, just as the white *aso ibale* cloth is no long used or kept in the house.

Conclusion

These interpretations and reinterpretations of a particular part of the female body, the protective *ibale*-hymen covering, and the mark of the *ibale*-blood on a piece of white cloth are part of a process in which ideas about what constitutes knowledge and subsequent relations of power have changed. Abandoning the public celebration of the *ibale*-hymen and the use of the *aso ibale* cloth have contributed to the process of what is considered "enlightened" or "civilized" behavior in contemporary Ekiti society. This discussion, then, touches upon questions raised by Elias (1978) in his analysis of "the civilizing process" in Europe, in particular questions about how changes in attitudes toward bodily behavior relate to changes in "the frontiers of shame and the threshold of repugnance" (139). However, a thorough examination of these ideas in the Yoruba context would require another essay. Instead, I have simply attempted to show how a shift in the basis of knowledge, characterized by the term *olaju* (civilization), is reflected in changing control over bodies with attention paid to one particular body part, the *ibale*-hymen, and the virginity cloths "that come next" (James 1890 [1950] 1:292).

Further, the reinterpretation of the *ibale*-hymen and its presence or loss may be viewed as reflecting the ways in which individuals may both materially embody and metaphorically make sense of these changes. The now largely forgotten images associated with the *ibale*-hymen—the "reddish plastic-film wrapping"; the "something like blood, very thick"; and the lost, "bloodied white cloth"—all relate to "greater truths that are impressionistically illustrated by certain features of the body" (Laqueur 1990, 33).

Notes

This study was conducted under the auspices of the Joint Research Project of the Faculty of the Social Sciences, Ondo State University, Ado-Ekiti, Nigeria, and the Health Transition Centre, The Australian National University, Canberra, with funding from the Mellon Foundation. I am grateful to Adenike Oso and to Comfort Ajayi for research assistance and to Wendy Cosford for editorial advice.

1   The Ekiti Yoruba are one subgroup of the Yoruba-speaking people of southwestern Nigeria. This study is based on interviews (conducted in Yoruba, later translated into colloquial English) with 95 women (ages 15–80+) and men from one rural Ekiti village in northeastern Ondo State, with supplementary information from the Nigerian National Archives in Ibadan. For a detailed description of the village and research methodology, see Renne 1993.

2   *Ibale,* defined as "virginity" by Abraham (1958, 87), is listed under the verb *ba,* to find. The word *ibale* might possibly be considered a compounding of the words *ba* and *ile,* meaning literally "found in the house."

3   The words *obo, abe,* and *oju ara* refer to women's genitalia in general and are sometimes translated as vagina. *Oju ara* is a polite way of saying *obo* or *abe* (the latter literally meaning "below"). I am not aware of words that refer to more specific anatomical parts such as the labia majora or the clitoris.

4   White calabashes are also used in an important village ritual, known as *Itale,* in which water carried by the king's wives is used in prayers for the future year (see Apter 1991).

5   A strip of handwoven cloth (*oja*) is often used by women to carry infants on their backs, although the use of the virginity cloth (*aso ibale*) is not common. However, a reddish stain on a white baby tie has carried certain associations, as in the saying *oja osun lo fi n hon pe a bi omo tuntun*—"when the baby tie is stained with [red] camwood, it means there is a newborn child" (Abraham 1958, 490).

6   This conflation of virginity and pregnancy is reflected in the proverb *Eni ti o fi ibale s'oyun, ko mo iva omo*—"Anyone who used their *ibale* to become pregnant, they don't know the suffering of children"—i.e., someone who is a virgin when she comes to her husband's house and immediately gets pregnant as a result does not know the suffering of childlessness.

7   The association of the calabash with infertility in women is reflected in the derogatory names given to nonvirgin brides, such as *aikaragba* (broken calabash) and *ajodi ikoko* (broken pot), which imply that they have broken or spoiled their fertility.

8   Among the Bunu Yoruba to the northeast, brides performing traditional marriage come to their husbands' houses with their heads covered with cloth, which both masks the bride's identity and protects her from malevolent glances.

9   In Ekiti, a bride's feet were washed before entering, and she was given a piece of broken calabash to step on, the number of resulting fragments indicating the number of her future children (Oguntuyi 1979, 19).

10   The birth canal is referred to (Buckley 1985, 71) by one Oyo Yoruba diviner-healer (*babalawo*) as *okun omo,* the pipe of the child; another *babalawo* translated this phrase as child's rope, which ties together the father's semen and the mother's remaining menstrual fluid. I have not heard this phrase used either way myself in Ekiti.

11   Prior to the introduction of maternity clinics and midwife deliveries, introduced by the British during the colonial period, male diviner-healers were likely to be present, particularly during difficult births.

12   See Peel (1983), Apter (1991), and Eades (1980) for detailed discussions of these contests.

13   Conversion to Christianity during the 1930s also played a part in changing marital practices. However, rather than reinforce the continuation of current virginity

practices, conversion to Christianity by the young further undermined the authority of elders.

14 A common theme in Nigerian popular market fiction depicted the upwardly mo-
bile, educated man married to an uneducated "bush wife," trying to dump her for a
more sophisticated spouse (Obiechina 1973).

15 One thirty-five-year-old woman who became pregnant before moving to her husband's house described her experience:

> I was going with a man and when I wanted to travel, he used a trick to invite
> me to his house so that he could test whether I was still a virgin . . . He used
> white cloth because he wanted to know whether I had been spoiled, but I did
> not know that he had used the white cloth. So, on the following day he came
> to my house to show me the white cloth, that what he thought I had done I
> hadn't done [i.e., had prior intercourse]. Because the cloth had been stained
> by blood (*ibale*).
>   *What happened to the cloth?*
>   I did not take it from him, so I did not know what he used it for.

She became pregnant soon after, and her father called the man to take her after
making a bridewealth payment—"That was how I married my husband"—no marriage ceremony was performed. Although she said she was "tricked" into going to
her fiancé's house, such behavior would have been considered scandalous in her
mother's time.

16 It is unclear whether this condition refers to *atresia vaginae,* closure of the vagina, a
condition that may result from an unbroken hymen or the growing together of the
vaginal walls (Kahn and Holt 1990, 32).

17 It should be noted that many of the 51 younger women interviewed did associate
blood with a loss of virginity. However, one woman said that while she saw blood,
not everyone did.

18 Similarly, the association of unveiling and opening up with enlightenment was also
carried over into the naming of new copper coins (*kobo*). Introduced in Ekiti in
1917, they were given the name Aiyelujara, "the veil over the world is removed"
(Oguntuyi 1979, 122), referring to the introduction of new things and a better life
that exposure to the wider world portended.

19 A few young women also mentioned conversion to one of the many Christian
fundamentalist churches as the reason for remaining a virgin. For these women,
virginity has more recently been reinterpreted as associated with Christianity
rather than with an older social order based on traditional religious practice.

2 "I DRESS IN THIS FASHION": TRANSFORMATIONS IN *SOTHO* DRESS AND WOMEN'S LIVES IN A SEKHUKHUNELAND VILLAGE, SOUTH AFRICA

Deborah James

Consciousness and its "colonization" have recently attracted some attention in the study of southern African societies (Comaroff and Comaroff 1989; Bozzoli with Nkotsoe 1991). Although not expressed in quite the same terms, the processes by which such colonization has been withstood have preoccupied scholars in southern Africa for somewhat longer (Mayer and Mayer 1971; Alverson 1978; McAllister 1980, 1991). While other writers have examined overt acts of resistance, anthropologists have concerned themselves with subtler means of defying domination, often through the reassertion of apparently traditional cultural forms, with effects sometimes perceptible no more widely than within local communities themselves.

Recent studies in this vein examine rural people's portrayal, through local knowledge, of their colonization and their incorporation as an industrial proletariat within the capitalist world. This knowledge is seen as both enabling people to conceptualize their own history as dominated but resilient subjects (Comaroff and Comaroff 1987, 193) and, in parallel, as facilitating the ongoing construction of group or individual identities by such people (Ferguson 1992; Thomas 1992). The production of this local knowledge often involves the invoking of tradition (Coplan 1987, 1991), and often counterposes this with images of modernity, resulting in sets of opposed dualities: town/country, townsman/ peasant, Christian/non-Christian, *setswana/segoa*[1] (Comaroff and Comaroff 1987; Roseberry 1989; Mayer and Mayer 1971).

Criticisms have been leveled at this writing. Spiegel, for example, disparages "dualist approaches" for the inappropriateness of their search "for persistences of a pre-industrial world view in the ways in which people order and perceive their contemporary relationships" (1990, 46). But the emerging contrast between, for example, *setswana* and *segoa*, was not "a confrontation between a primordial folk tradition and the modern world" (Comaroff and Comaroff

1987, 194–95). Rather, Tswana tradition came to be formulated largely through its complementary opposition to "the ways of the European." Indeed, the very images of a pre-industrial or pre-capitalist world that feed into the making of such dualities are products of people's encounter with the relationships and realities of the industrial or capitalist one (Roseberry 1989, 144, 201–3, passim).

An encounter of this kind has given rise, in northern Sotho- or Pedi-speaking communities of the northern Transvaal from which men migrate to work on the Witwatersrand, to a complementary opposition between *sesotho* (*sotho* ways) and its opposite *sekgowa* (white ways). *Sesotho* exists in dynamic interrelation with its opposite *sekgowa*. It is situational, lacks distinct boundaries, and has undergone substantive changes over the last few generations. The clothing of *sesotho*, with which I am primarily concerned here, has progressively incorporated elements from the clothing of *sekgowa* as well as from that of neighboring groups. The incorporation of these new elements has coincided with points of change in the life cycle, and was especially pronounced at the historical moment when significant numbers of children began attending school. Throughout this process of assimilating exotic or imported elements, however, *sesotho* has retained, or sharpened, the distinctiveness of its contrast with *sekgowa*.[2]

Although *sesotho* is not consistently identified with a particular group of people who subscribe to its tenets, it is sometimes thought of in association with distinct social categories. In some contexts it is used to describe the ways of those belonging to the social category "those of the nation" (*baditšhaba*) while *sekgowa* correlates with the category of those who converted to Lutheranism (*majekane*).[3] In other contexts it is women who are thought of in association with *sesotho*, while men appear to align with *sekgowa*. In yet other contexts the categorical oppositions of religion and gender that are dramatized by the *sesotho/sekgowa* opposition dissolve in the face of the particular domestic circumstances of specific men and women. The boundary between even these apparently highly distinct social categories is, then, fugitive and vague in practice.

But one context in which *sesotho* is very clearly identified with women is that of village-based musical performance, with clothing as one of the clearest visible markers of this identification. Here, the term *sesotho* qualifies an overarching genre, *mmino wa sesotho* (*sotho* dance/song),[4] of which the most popular expression is the style known as *kiba*, performed in urban areas by migrant men and women, but in rural areas only by groups of stay-at-home wives or sisters (James 1994).

The singing/dancing group whose members' experience I describe here is

Dithabaneng (those from the place of the mountain) from Nchabeleng village in Sekhukhune, the heartland of the former Pedi polity.[5] Dithabaneng was first constituted as a group in 1976, after its members had seen and been inspired by the new *kiba* style.[6] But many of them, and their mothers and grandmothers before them, had performed a series of earlier styles together before this group was formed.

Group members are linked by close ties of kinship, cooperation, and neighborhood. They do not, however, normally regard each other as equals. Even those as closely related as sisters are distinguished by their individual marriages, their differing levels of income, and their differing orientations to *sesotho*. They constitute an undifferentiated group only in the act of singing together, using a range of performative devices thought of as characteristically *sotho*. It is the dance and the dress that forms the group.

One of these unifying motifs is the invocation of "the lion" (*tau*). By virtue of marriage, if not of birth, all the women in the group—like most of the people in the village—hail each other as "lions,"[7] especially on occasions of heightened significance, or to assert a sense of overarching local unity when performing in front of people from other villages or places. Apart from the rhythmic coordination of voice and action, a further expression of group cohesion and uniformity is the clothing worn when singing. The entire performance, including song/dance (*mmino*) and clothing (*diaparo*) is characterized as *sotho*.

This essay describes how the details of *sotho* dress have changed substantially over about three generations. In parallel with innovations in the content of women's *sotho* dress, the means whereby girls acquire the clothes of adulthood have also changed, with older generations of women having been given money to buy them by fathers, brothers, or husbands, whereas their daughters spent short spells as farmworkers to earn the money themselves. These stints of independence were followed, for women remaining single as well as for those who married, by a return to the sphere of motherhood, household work, and farming. In contrast, the earlier and more consistent involvement of boys in the worlds of school and work have meant that their clothing, once they become adults, is invariably that of *sekgowa*.

However, although *sotho* clothing is worn by some singers every day, others, often due to the influence of their husbands, have switched to the clothing of *sekgowa*, saving *sotho* clothes for performance only. The opposition between male and female orientations and behaviors, as expressed in the outward and visible sign of clothing, is thus not consistently experienced or invoked. Indeed, in the context of particular women's domestic living circumstances with particular men, *sotho* dress may be absent altogether. It is on the occasion of

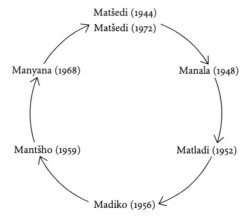

2.1 The cyclical succession of initiation regiments in Nchabeleng. Initiation dates shown here are for women, about two years later than those for men of the same regiments.

musical performance that *sesotho* is stressed—through singing, dance, dress, and the consumption of sorghum beer. Through these means, performance provides for a dramatization of a cohesive female identity phrased in terms of identification with customary ways, in opposition to men.

"I Dress in This Fashion"

It appears from ethnographic accounts that one of the important uses of clothing among the Pedi of Sekhukhuneland was in distinguishing between pre-initiates and initiates (Monnig 1967, 107, 123, 128; Vogel 1985, 81). At initiation, boys and girls were grouped separately into regiments of age-mates (*mephato*) (see fig. 2.1). In the approximately four-year cycle of initiation the formation of girls' regiments took place well after that of boys: the names of regiments derived in both cases from the names of the chief's sons who led the boys on each occasion (Monnig 1967, 120; Pitje 1950, 58). For people of both sexes, membership in these regiments provided an important point of reference in later life: it linked them in perpetuity to a group of age-mates, and gave them a chronological reference point, as I show further on. But initiation also served to distinguish boys from girls and immature children from mature pre-adults, partly through its teaching about the behavior appropriate to a gender-specific adult lifestyle. Dress was one of the ways in which this demarcation was signaled.

In a classically static ethnographic account of life in Sekhukhuneland, Mon-

Table 2.1. Pedi Clothing Demarcating Life-cycle Stages

	Life-cycle Stages	
Gender	Pre-initiate	Initiate
Female	*Lebole*: short string apron in front around loins	*Lebole*: short string apron in front around loins
	Ntepana: triangular skin apron to cover buttocks	*Ntepa*: long back apron of married women
	Semabejane: short cotton blouse just covering breasts	*Semabejane*: short cotton blouse just covering breasts
	Leetse: hair fashioned in long strings treated with fat and graphite	*Tlopo*: hairstyle of marriageable and married women
Male	*Lekgeswa*: skin loincloth	New loin skins
	Hair shaven close to the head	Hair reshaven

Source: Monnig 1967, 107, 123, 128.

nig discusses this role of clothing in demarcating the different phases of the life cycle from one another and in providing for a gradually deepening distinction between the sexes. But his account gives no sense of the flexibility or the variation of *sesotho*. He outlines the clothing worn by people in the first two major phases of life (summarized in table 2.1), but then comments:

> in practice, most [initiated] girls nowadays wear long, gaily-coloured cloths from their loins down to their feet, covering the traditional clothing, while very few women wear the traditional hair-style, usually covering their heads with a head-cloth instead. (1967, 128)

He also indicates that the short blouse worn by initiated and by older uninitiated girls (*semabejane*) "was introduced by missionaries, but has been adopted by all the Pedi, Christians and non-Christians alike" (128).

This account, like many of its kind, sets up an idealized version of the traditional life cycle with its accompanying clothing. If people adopt some Western clothes, they are seen as treading a one-way path from tradition to modernity. In fact, the semiotics of dress, and its social concomitants, are more complex.

The short, smocked, cotton garment Monnig calls *semabejane*—referred to by Dithabaneng women as *gempe* for initiates (from the Afrikaans *hemp*, shirt) or *gentswana* for noninitiates (little shirt)—is a good example of this complexity (fig. 2.2). By the mid-1950s these garments, although certainly deriving in style and material from European influence, were items of clothing indicating a thoroughly *sotho* orientation.[8] An orientation toward the paired opposite, *sekgowa,* was shown by wearing dresses (*diroko*) or pinafores (*dikhiba*). In the village, still cleft at the time by a deep social and geographical divide between Christians and non-Christians, it was mostly the former who wore the clothes of *sekgowa,* while the latter wore *sotho* clothing.[9] In this instance, then, adherence to one or other polarity of the *sesotho/sekgowa* duality was associated with membership in definable social categories.

But *sotho* dress,[10] like its opposite, was to undergo continual transformation. Although the *sotho* smocked shirt (*gempe*) and its accompanying string or leather apron (*lebole*) are still worn by returning initiates (fig. 2.3), in other contexts these garments have been supplanted by a new version of *sotho* dress.

2.2   Female *sotho* dress of Pedi, showing *semabejane* or *gempe* in its pre-initiate and initiate forms (Tyrell 1968, 67; Monnig 1967, 107, 123, 128).

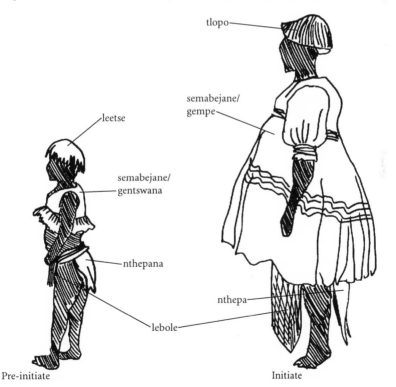

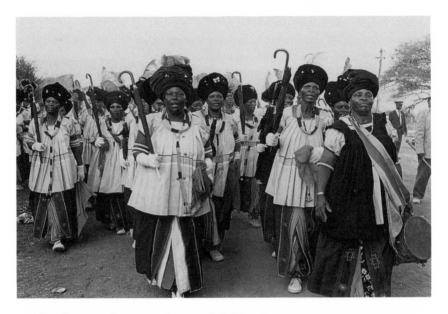

2.3   Rural women singers wearing smocked shirts, Mamone
village, Sekhukhuneland. Photo by S. Mofokeng.

This has three main identifying features: a length of cloth (*lešela* or *tuku;* from
the Afrikaans *doek*) wrapped around the waist: a headscarf consisting of a large
piece of fabric (*šeše*); and bangles (*maseka*). If these three elements are present,
the fourth element—a commercially made vest, cotton knit shirt, or overalls, or
another element such as a baseball cap—does not detract from the whole
ensemble, but indeed become a part of it (fig. 2.4). This ensemble of clothes
appears in various versions. For the performance of *kiba*, it is characterized by
the use of striking colors and of materials thought to be particularly attractive.
But in an everyday context, the materials used are often drab, and sometimes
old and tattered.[11]

It can be seen then that certain types of clothing deriving from mission
influence, and named with words deriving from *sekgowa*, were nevertheless
included within the definition of *sesotho*, and strongly contrasted with *sekgowa*,
throughout. The *sesotho/sekgowa* contrast thus coexists with an image of
change within the category of *sesotho*.

If, for these villagers, opposed polarities such as *sesotho/sekgowa* do enable a
conceptualization of historical change, as the Comaroffs claim (1987, 193), the
actual mechanism through which change occurs, and through which these

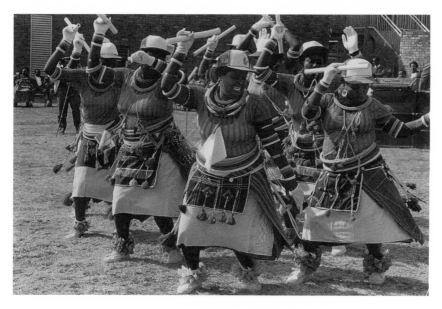

2.4   Migrant singers Ditshweu tsa Malebogo wearing waistcloths
(*dituku*) and cotton knit shirts. Photo by S. Mofokeng.

categories are continuously replenished with new elements, is through life-cycle
rituals, particularly initiation. The experience of successively initiated initiation
regiments orients these conceptions of change (Molepo 1984, 16–28). Apart
from ordering men and women into age groupings, enabling a rough calcula-
tion of age for people who do not know their precise date of birth, the cyclical
succession of regiments provides conceptual hooks that allow for a perception
of history in the absence of the linear time-plans of literacy. The life-cycle stages
that furnished an ethnographer like Monnig with his static view thus allow for a
more dynamic perception of society's changes, since each regiment has a different experience of these stages.

The transformation of clothing, and of the *sotho* lifestyle, was prompted
partly by a variety of what might crudely be called "culture contacts." These
included—for an older generation—the presence of trading stores and visits to
husbands in town and—for a younger generation, and far more influentially—
the proliferation of schools in the area after the 1950s. The means for purchasing the clothes defined as necessary to consecutive stages of the life cycle had to
be provided by wages earned beyond the domestic domain. For the older
generation of women, the present grandmothers in Dithabaneng, this money

was procured by men: by fathers and brothers in the case of initiates, and by husbands for their wives. A younger generation, Dithabaneng's present older mothers, followed the example of boys in leaving home to earn their own money on farms around the time of initiation. But in contrast to boys, who then went off to work in contract labor in the urban areas, these girls, having earned money to buy the clothes appropriate to their new status of initiates, then returned to the domestic sphere to raise children and keep house. There they came again to depend on male earnings for clothing and other basic necessities or, in some cases, were forced to subsist without these earnings.

For the village dwellers of Dithabaneng, then, the acquisition of clothing for different phases of life has necessitated links connecting them within their rural families to places of employment at the place of the whites (*makgoweng*). Although it became commonplace for women of an intermediate generation to make brief forays into employment at white farms (*mabaleng*, the place of the plains), these connecting links have been made mostly through fathers, brothers, and husbands.

Men's Earnings, Women's Clothes

For the oldest of the group's singers, like Mmakgolo wa Pine Khulwane,[12] who was born around 1930 and initiated around 1944 in Matšedi regiment, the money for the purchase of the clothes necessary to a proper *sotho* woman's lifestyle was earned by fathers, brothers, and husbands in contract employment. Worn by a married woman, these clothes served as outward and visible signs of her husband's wealth. The more material used in the extensive smocking of these, and the more garments worn one over the other, the richer the provider was seen to be.[13] The clothes were thus worn with pride on both a woman's own and her husband's behalf.

The lyrics of songs sung both by Dithabaneng and by older and now inactive singers reflect the dependence of this generation of women, and indeed of subsequent ones, on the earnings of men. In the song "Lebowa," women sing:

> *Lebowa la kgomo le motho*
> *Pula-medupe yana Mohlakeng*
> *Lebona ge ke te kapere*
> *Ke tšhonne ke hloboletse*
> *Ke setse ka dibesete*
> *Ke lebowa le kgomo le motho*

Pula ya mamehlaka e yetla
Nke be ke na le kgaetsedi
A nthekele onoroko
Re supa gore gare sa sila

Lebowa of cattle and people
Stormy rain.
Seeing me half-naked
I have no clothes to put on
Except a vest
It's Lebowa of cattle and people
A stormy rain is coming
I wish I had a brother
Who would buy me a petticoat.
We no longer grind our meal.[14]

The song can be understood, in one sense, as referring to the current performance context. In this sense, a member of the group is bewailing her lack of finery adequate to a good performance spectacle.[15] But the historical theme of dependence on male earnings for clothing, and of deprivation without these, can also be clearly heard. A similar theme occurs in the song "Marashiva," in which a woman again bemoans her husband's inability to provide her with dance regalia:

> *Ke reng ka hlaela pheta ye botse*
> I don't have a shiny necklace

This line evoked the following comment from a Dithabaneng member: "when other men have gone to town to work, [my husband] is always here at home not working, so I won't be able to dance, as I have nothing to put on."[16]

The dissatisfaction expressed here about men who have failed to provide new clothing might seem to indicate a greater desire for the fruits of an absent husband's labors than for his companionship in the household. However, rather than reflecting a callous desire for material gain, this theme coexists with others to suggest an ambiguity about one of the central paradoxes of migrancy in southern Africa—the fact that spouses have been forced to live apart in order to ensure the well-being of their families (see Murray 1981, 102).[17]

Siblings as well as spouses were separated in this way, as is shown in the song "Setimela" (steam train), which bewails the absence of a brother who has left for the city and never returned:

Setimela wa Mmamarwale
Nthshwanyama
Setimela nkabe se rwale buti bokgolwa
Buti e sa le a eya bokgolwa
Ngwana-mme o tla nwa ese ka mmona

Train of Mmamarwale
Black carrier
Train should carry my brother from *bokgolwa*
  [the state of being a migrant who never returns]
My brother home from *bokgolwa*
My mother's child would die without me seeing him

Songs thus express sadness not only about lazy men who had no employment but also about those whose employment took them away forever. On the other hand, the absence of a man who was working made room for his wife to have affairs with other men who were present in the area, and at times it was precisely those clothes bought by a woman's husband that she wore to make her look attractive to these other lovers.[18]

Wene o se nago lešira
Makolone a tlogo feta
Wene o se nago lešira
O wa hlaka
Makolone a tlo go feta

You who have no headscarf
Those from the Cape will pass you by
You who have no headscarf
You will suffer
Those from the Cape will pass you by

Those "from the Cape" to whom this song refers were men who came to the bus depot in nearby Apel as drivers of railway buses, and who would spend the night with local women. As single men who went home only once a year and who "saved all their money in a tin," they were seen as rich and therefore as desirable lovers.[19]

For the present grandmothers of Dithabaneng, sources of contact with *sekgowa* were fairly limited. Since all were from "the place of those of the nation" (*baditšhabeng*), none took any interest in church nor went to school. They dressed in *sotho* smocked shirts (*gempe*). Although this was a missionary innovation, by the 1940s and 1950s the garment already had long been re-garded as part of *sotho* apparel and was definitely not a part of the dress of Christians. These women paid visits to their husbands in town, but the visits were sporadic and of short duration. Sometimes the visits were made not only for the sake of general companionship but also for the specific purpose of falling pregnant.

When visiting town, the people these women met were not so much the white bearers of *sekgowa* as its black adherents from other parts of South Africa—an encounter for the most part equally alienating. For Mmakgolo wa Pine, the speech of the Christian Xhosa people she met while visiting her husband in Springs, where he worked as a compound policeman, sounded so incomprehensible that she thought they were asking her to fetch water when in fact they were praying. But more alienating still was her experience when she left her daughter with them for some hours while running an errand and returned to find that they had taken off the child's skin garments, cut her hair, and clothed her in a dress (*roko*).

> They took my child, undressed her and gave her a new style of dressing. I didn't like it, and as I didn't know what was going on, my husband found me crying. He asked me what the matter was and I told him that these people want to capture [*go thopa*] my child. They took away all that skin clothing and gave her a dress and had her hair cut. My husband told one old man about this, and he came and explained that they did this because they wanted the child to look like theirs and not to be different. Even if the children didn't understand each other, they should look the same. Upon realizing that I was against this, the old man called the others after a few days to come and apologize for the mistake they had made.[20]

In this rather dramatic narrative, the use of the word *go thopa*, normally used to denote the taking of captives in war, illustrates the strength of Mmakgolo wa Pine's fears that her daughter would be taken from her and from the nurturing bosom of *sesotho*, and lost to the world of *sekgowa* as represented by these Xhosa-speaking Christians.

At the time of the visit, around 1957, Mmakgolo wa Pine and other married women of her regiment Matšedi were still wearing the *sotho* smocked shirts and elaborately combed and greased hairstyles of Monnig's account. But by this time the most *sotho* of clothes were being reserved for occasions of greatest auspiciousness, like the time when Mmakgolo wa Pine had her photo taken for her passbook. Although she greased her hair for the photo, Mmakgolo wa Pine was at this stage putting on a headscarf (*šeše*) for everyday wear.

Women's Earnings, Women's Clothes

There were a number of things demarcating the experience of this older female regiment from those following it. One of these was that its members, while firmly believing that brothers and prospective husbands should go off to work on farms to prove their manhood, never worked on farms themselves, whereas most of the women from subsequent regiments did spend a period doing so.

For a number of male regiments, consisting of boys born from around the mid-1920s onward, farmwork was an expected part of the life cycle[21] and was seen almost as a second initiation, which proved a youth's adult male status and showed, especially to a prospective wife, his wage-earning potential:

> To show that you will work in future, you will first run away from home to the farms. This showed that you were a man, and you would work for yourself.[22]

But a more immediate consideration for boys themselves was the necessity to buy clothes.[23] This was also to be the main reason why girls in their turn began running away from home to work on farms. Those born around 1940 and initiated in Matladi regiment around 1954 were among the first to do this. A possible reason why they had not done so earlier, apart from the greater restrictions placed on girls generally, is that the arduous journey on foot from Sekhukhuneland to white farming centers such as Marble Hall and Roedtan was seen as more easily undertaken by boys. By the time girls began to undertake this journey, they did so in the trucks sent by farmers right into the reserve areas to recruit laborers.

For a variety of reasons, parents were mostly not in favor of their daughters' working on farms, so most of the girls who did so departed from their homes with stealth and subterfuge:

> We didn't ask for permission from our parents, we ran away whilst they were away at their fields . . . At times when they were around, you would just put your clothes and blankets over the wall of the yard without them seeing you.
> *If you asked for permission, wouldn't they allow you?*
> They would not allow us.
> *Were your parents and others upset about this?*
> In fact when we got on the truck, little boys would do so as well, but when the truck pulled off, they got off and we would ask them to tell our parents that we had left.[24]

Mmagopine Khulwane tells a similar story:

From my home, I met my father on the way . . . He asked me where I was going and I lied, saying I'm going to fetch water. It was when I was next to the truck that I showed him the blanket and said, I'm going to the farms. My father told my mother about this.[25]

But the reluctance of parents to let their daughters leave was in fact not always uniform: sometimes fathers were most strongly disapproving, while mothers were more ready to give permission, being unable to suggest any other means by which their daughters might acquire the clothes they wanted:

Sometimes, if you find your mother is at home, you say, I'm going to the farms: "Well, go, and buy yourself some clothes."[26]

For girls as for boys, then, the main spur to this phase of mild defiance against parents was the need for clothes appropriate to the status of an initiate. Mmagoshower Debeila emphasized the necessity of this, since "we would be thought naked if we continued to wear skins and greased hair."[27] She stressed that it was not her family's shortage of money that drove her to work at this stage, but rather the fact that she had seen older friends returning from work with clothes and was influenced by this, and by her coinitiates, to go. The departure for farms of Nchabeleng's adolescent girls, then, was similar to the phase spent working as domestics by young Phokeng girls aiming to buy their trousseaux (Bozzoli with Nkotsoe 1991): occurring at a phase of life when these women had not yet taken on broader familial responsibility, it was seen not as providing a contribution to general family finances but as facilitating the purchase of a specific set of goods for the girl herself.

A contract lasted three months, and at the end of the first of these a daughter like Mmagoshower brought her wages—a total of R18 in around 1960—back to her mother, who then used them to buy the vests and waist-cloths she needed. By the time a girl went off on her second three-month stint as a farm laborer, after a break of about a month, her parents no longer protested at her departure. And for most, the third or fourth contract was the last, since it was at around this time that most of them prepared for marriage—"we were being courted," as Mmagojunius Ramaila put it—and for building a home in the village.

While it is true, then, that running away to the place of the Boers (*go tšhaba maburung*) signified in some sense a rebellion by groups of age-mates against control by the parental generation, it is also true that the challenge to parental authority that this practice represented was soon coopted and transformed as its perpetrators in turn became stay-at-home women who took charge of the domestic domain and of the values and practices of *sesotho*.[28]

It must also be noted that the set of mores and practices rebelled against were based not on a monolithic and cohesive ideology, but on one deeply divided along gender lines. By the time the members of Mantšho regiment were undergoing initiation in around 1964, girls were rebelling not simply against the arduous duties defined as appropriate to them within the domestically defined boundaries of *sesotho*—child care, fetching water, weeding and chasing the birds away from the crops, and helping to repair the house—but also against the emergent modern definition of a girl's role as scholar. Parents were frequently divided over which behavior was most appropriate to a girl, and in some cases this division separated mothers as proponents of the conservative, domestic version of *sesotho* from fathers who, although not necessarily wishing to convert to Christianity, were keen to encourage their daughters to complete at least the primary levels of education and hence to engage in the world of *sekgowa* and civilization (*tlhabologo*). This was so in the case of Mmagopine:

> My mother said that I should leave school and stay at home. . . . If a girl could write a letter to her husband, that was just enough. . . . She said that I should repair the wall with mud and do weeding in the fields. So I ran away to the farms.
> *So you were running away from duties at home?*
> I also didn't like going to school. I knew that after stopping school for a week when my mother told me to do so, my father would order me back to school again. So I realized that if I ran away to the farms, I would spend three months there and during this time, the teachers would take me off the school registers, knowing that I had gone to the farms.[29]

For this girl, as for many others, the flight to the farms in order to escape conflicting sets of pressures from both parents nevertheless led her inexorably back home and back into the values and ways of *sesotho* when she returned to her mother's house to bear children and to become involved in domestic duties as a mother.

School, Clothes, and Women's Life Cycle

From around the 1960s it was school—whether attended or fled from—that people saw as playing a central role in transforming the attitudes, ways of dressing, and ways of behaving of men and women, and of older and younger people alike. Mmakgolo wa Pine gave an account of this process. Having wept at the efforts of Christian Xhosa to dress her daughter in the clothes of *sekgowa* in 1957, a decade later she and her contemporaries were to welcome the new dressing style seen as emanating from school. They came to feel that the necklaces, bangles, and many-layered smocked shirts of earlier *sotho* clothing had been heavy and uncomfortable. When their daughters were encouraged by teachers to wash out the grease and graphite of their pre-initiates' hairstyles, they eventually followed suit by washing out the grease of the married women's equivalent. Not wanting to be thought naked, however, they replaced this hairstyle with a small headscarf (*setlanyana*), "then I saw those wearing a bigger one, and copied them," until eventually the bulky headscarf of contemporary wear (*šeše*) became the norm.

The change in headdress is an example that demonstrates the full complexity of the transforming of *sotho* dress. A generation of non-Christian women whose resistance to the idea of school for their daughters was so strong that they actively encouraged them—in many cases, successfully—to leave school, nevertheless embraced some of the new stylistic trappings seen to accompany the activity of scholarship. Their incorporation of these trappings appears on the surface to have had something of the character of an acceptance of mission or colonial ideology.[30] From the point of view of the wearers, however, it represented on the one hand a wish to replace one kind of haircovering with another, and thus to continue to express the respect required of a woman by her in-laws and by men in general, but on the other it signified a moving beyond the discomfort and restrictiveness of statically defined rural dress and a pleasure in the attractiveness of rapidly changing styles.[31]

Although this liberation from unnecessarily restrictive ways was rejoiced in, there is a sense of ambivalence about some of the changes for which school was seen as responsible. The proverb used by Mmakgolo wa Pine to describe the older generation's imitation of their children in adopting new ways shows that this process was not viewed entirely in a positive light.

A cow will fall into a donga as it tries to follow its calf. This is the same with people. If your child is burning, you will go into the fire to fetch it out.[32]

School was seen by women of an older generation not only as having provided for changes in clothing styles, but also as having introduced transformations in behavior—and indeed in the *sotho* life cycle—which are viewed in a much more unambiguously negative light. Mmakgolo wa Pine offered the "pencil" and the ability to write as a monocausal explanation for the ability of youth nowadays to evade parental authority, and for the associated decline in sexual morals:

A boy may come and study with your daughter. The boy will take a pencil and write something for the girl to read. And if you as a parent suspect something and sit around with them to keep an eye on them, that wouldn't help. Because after the boy has written her something on the paper, she would also take her pencil and reply to him. All this happens in your presence, and when they do this, you will think that they are studying and that your daughter will pass at the end of the year because she has a friend who is helping her to study.[33]

Instead of engaging in diligent scholarship, however, the couple would be taking advantage of the mother's inability to read in order to plan a clandestine liaison, which would eventually lead to the pregnancy of the girl.

For some people, school and literacy appear jointly responsible for widening the generation gap between themselves and their children, and bring with them a range of related ills. According to such a view, it is because girls no longer mix with other girls but rather form friendships with boys in class that girls have begun to fall pregnant at a younger age. This has caused the age at which children are initiated to decrease (from mid-adolescence to the age of six or eight years). Previously, when "we had laws" (re be re na la malao), a girl would leave for the farms, return without yet having become pregnant, and become initiated thereafter. But now children must undergo this ritual earlier, as "we do not want to take a mother or father to be initiated." In this account, the virtual disappearance of the phase of childhood prior to initiation—bothumasha for girls, bošoboro for boys—is seen as having come about because of education.

Schooling thus had a range of significances: it allowed for an incorporation of new elements into the sotho lifestyle, but it also introduced lawlessness and indiscipline, seen as contrary to the principles of sesotho or, indeed, to any code of morality. From yet another perspective, schooling appeared as a harbinger of sekgowa. People's different orientations toward schooling were influenced by a range of factors. One was religious orientation—to Mmagomotala Mofele, who considers herself one of the nation or a non-Christian (moditšhaba), to go to school was foolishness: "as we grew up we only knew that those going to school were children of Christians [majekane]" while the latter in turn would mock them, saying "they're afraid of civilization."[34] Another factor was age: often older children did not attend school, or attended only for a few years, whereas their younger siblings acquired a fuller education, as the necessity for this became more generally accepted. Place in the order of siblings also played a part, since parents were sometimes able to send younger children to school once their older siblings had grown up and were contributing to the household finances. It was also sometimes the case that parents opposed to schooling for an older child had become accustomed to the idea by the time their younger children reached school-going age. A further factor was individual motivation. Mmagoviolet

Phakwago, a member of Matladi regiment, was so keen to be a scholar that her mother was persuaded to release her from the care of her younger siblings to attend school on every alternate day, in contrast to her younger sister who preferred to avoid school altogether by running away to the farms.

However, gender was perhaps the most important factor influencing which children were sent to school and which were not, before a time when it became accepted that all children should attend school as far as possible. According to the keen scholar referred to above, when she was a child and people "did not yet know the importance of education," mothers in non-Christian families thought it a waste to take a girl to school rather than having her come to help in the fields.[35] The perceived differential needs for education were expressed thus by another woman:

> A girl will always be at home, but a boy needs to go to school so that he will be able to find employment. If he finds that he does not know even a single "A," he will have to come back and stay at home.
> *So with a girl there is no problem [if she leaves school]?*
> No, there is no problem with a girl, because a man will come and marry her and she will get support from him. Now, with a boy, who will support him?[36]

It was therefore expected that boys would be more particularly exposed to *sekgowa*, first at school itself, and then through the careers that took them off to the farms and then to work at centers of industrial employment. This is reflected in the clothes worn by boys and men. Although Monnig's rather sketchy account of the differentiation of the male life cycle by clothing describes initiated boys as dressing in "a new loin skin," informants in Dithabaneng and elsewhere explained, in contrast, that from around the time of initiation—for an older generation, corresponding roughly with a boy's first trip to the farms; for a younger one, with the time of his first starting school—he ceased wearing a loinskin and began instead to put on trousers and shirts. In some cases, there was an intermediate phase in which short trousers were worn during school hours, then replaced with skins for the rest of the day.[37] But in general—in contrast to girls, whose clothing throughout the life cycle, although gradually acquiring new elements, was continually redefined as *sotho*—their brothers and cousins experienced a swift and decisive move from the *sotho* clothing of childhood to the clothing of *sekgowa*, which defined their adolescence and adulthood.

A similar differentiation of male and female clothing among reserve-dwellers is noted by Jean Comaroff in the case of the Tshidi Tswana:

... male hair and clothing styles have been more closely regulated by the idioms of discipline and production than have those of females, reflecting the greater engagement of men in the world of industrial capitalist production (Turner n.d.(a)). Women, on the other hand, remain closely associated with the domestic sphere. (1985, 224–25)

In Nchabeleng, the divide between the ways of *sesotho* and those of *sekgowa* was often thought of as aligning with that between two social groupings which, certainly for the first half of the twentieth century, were regarded as quite distinct: non-Christians (*baditšhaba*) and Christians (*majekane*). But from the evidence presented here it can be seen how even within the social category *baditšhaba*, and indeed even within a single family in that category, there are a number of further differentiating factors—age, place in the order of siblings, personal motivation, but especially gender—which align some members closer to one and some closer to the other side of the *sesotho/sekgowa* divide. To summarize: because the present members of Dithabaneng have since childhood been identified more closely with home and with the domestic than their brothers; have worked beyond the village only in rural employment and then only for short periods, while their brothers have spent years as laborers on the mines or in the city; and have had little or no exposure to schooling and always less than the male members of their families; it is easy to see how these women have had their role in the domestic domain identified closely with the idea of *sesotho*.

Women, Married and Unmarried

I suggested earlier that Dithabaneng's older members, as younger women, were dependent on male kin or affines to buy them the clothes necessary to the life of a proper *sotho* woman. As young married women, their adornment in heavy cotton smocking was an important means by which their husbands could display their wealth, derived both rurally and from contract employment. For the young women of later regiments, although their brief move into farm employment allowed them some independence and provided for the purchase of their own cloth, their return home was, ideally, a move toward economic dependence on a husband similar to that experienced by members of previous regiments. Indeed, it was the fact of "being courted" and of preparing for marriage that made further stints of farm labor inappropriate, since it was thought that a married woman should not work for money (*bereka*).

For members of these younger regiments, however, this ideal did not always correspond with reality. Almost half of Dithabaneng's members in this age group, who became marriageable from about 1960 onward, are now living their adult lives as unmarried mothers within their parents' or mothers' households and are dependent on the earnings of a brother or an uncle or on a mother's pension. For the other half of this generation the return from farm work did result in marriage: in most cases, to a cousin.[38]

Those members who are married and receiving regular remittances are dependent on their husbands for the purchase of clothes, among many other things. Such dependency also carries with it the obligation to listen to a husband's dictates about what to wear. Few husbands have much interest in influencing their wives' wish to wear the everyday contemporary *sotho* dress described earlier. But since husbands, even non-Christian ones, are often oriented more toward *sekgowa* than *sesotho,* wives' dependency on them sometimes entails a move toward a way of dressing, and of behaving, more in line with this orientation.

Such a change in style occurs, for some women, only on particular occasions. Mmagoshower Debeila, for example, was married in a conventional Western wedding dress, as a photograph on her wall testifies, and she wears dresses (*diroko*) when she spends some time staying in the location adjoining Premier Mine in order to visit her husband at his place of work.

For others, like Mmagoviolet Phakwago, the keen scholar mentioned earlier, her husband's preferences overlaying certain tendencies in her own background have effected her transformation from a girl wearing *sotho* dress along with female siblings and cousins to a woman dressed in the clothes of *sekgowa.* In both her own and her husband's family backgrounds there was a complex mixture of mission and anti-mission influences, and a series of physical movements between sections of the village designated as Christian and non-Christian, respectively. The couple has spent periods together in a Reef township, living in a house that they managed to acquire for the family: they thus enjoy a lifestyle in strong contrast to the more typical experience of some of Mmagoviolet's friends and relatives, in which a husband lives in compounded accommodation and makes weekend visits home, or is occasionally visited by his wife at his place of work.

What the case of Mmagoviolet and her husband shows is that membership in social categories, such as Christian or non-Christian, and affiliation to accompanying styles, such as those of *sekgowa* or *sesotho,* was neither static nor historically preordained. Within the life process of one family, different members could be oriented in a variety of ways, or the same members oriented differently over a period of years, with respect to these major social and conceptual divides.

Despite the ease of movement between these clearly distinguished and mutually exclusive categories, this family still displays the basic pattern in which women and the domestic domain belong to *sesotho* while men are seen to connect them to and even pull them toward *sekgowa*. Mmagoviolet, although she wore dresses as her husband wanted her to and went to town to be with and to keep house for him there, was far happier when she could return home, where she had the help and support of her mother-in-law and the companionship of her female neighbors. In this sense, the *sotho* style and *sotho* music of Dithabaneng's performance expresses an ideal of female cohesiveness to which group members aspire, even if they achieve it only momentarily.

Next I explore how—for Mmagoviolet as for her less "modern" sisters, cousins, and fellow singers—Dithabaneng's performances use the idiom of equality, subsistence agriculture, and female *sotho* identity to express this sense of cohesive female companionship and bonding, and to offset the economic factors that in material terms differentiate these women—married to different men or unmarried—from each other.

Women, Performance, and the Crops of Sesotho

For a period after Dithabaneng was formed in order to sing the new *kiba* style of music, the group was involved in a wide range of performance contexts. It took part in a number of local competitions and was very much in demand to perform at weddings for a fee of around "twenty pounds" (R40). More recently, however, their popularity has waned, and live performance has been replaced at weddings by taped music played on a hired hi-fi system. The range of possible performances has thus shrunk to one main type: "parties" held at the homes of individual members. These are ostensibly for enjoyment and pleasure alone, but in fact they entail an aspect of ancestral propitiation. A central feature of the parties held by Dithabaneng and similar groups is a "play" or dramatic tableau (*papadi*) involving two members of the group dressed up as policemen in khaki uniforms, peaked caps, and leather Sam Brownes.

> In August 1991 I attended one such party at the home of Mmagojane, one of the group's police. In an initial discussion between Mmagojane and her fellow group members on the one hand, and her husband on the other, he was informed that the group had designated her the host for the next of these parties. He expressed his surprise that this was the case and his reluctance to provide the food that he imagined would be required. He was assured that he would not be held liable for all costs but would be

asked to provide only a goat to be slaughtered and a tin of mealie meal. After some further protestations and expressions of dissatisfaction at not having been informed of this earlier, he finally agreed.

The next stage was for each member of the group to contribute a tin of sorghum from her year's crop, which was then made into beer by the hostess and some of her fellow members. Indeed, it was said that August was the best month for such a party, since it came in the time between harvesting and planting when there was still some sorghum left for making beer.

On the night before the party, the goat was slaughtered, leaving time for the meat to be cooked in black pots over a fire on the following day.

During the party itself, the sexes remained separate. The women of Dithabaneng performed in the open space in front of the yard, observed mostly by children and other women, who stood or sat on the ground in a circle around the dancers.

During breaks in the performance, singers and audience drank homemade sorghum beer from calabashes. Mmagojane's husband and other men who were home from town sat on chairs under a tree some distance away from the performers, and drank bottled beer out of glasses. Men and women, in these separate areas, had their food served to them by the women of the house.

Occasionally one of the "police" would approach the men in their separate circle and involve him in a mini-drama of mock arrest, with one of the "police" making as if to handcuff him, asking aggressively for his pass, and eventually fining him some money before agreeing to let him go.

At the very end of the party, the skin of the goat that had been slaughtered was spread on the back of the woman whom the group had agreed should host the next party. At the previous such event, held during December 1990 at the house of the other "policeman," Mmagolina Sebei, a similar laying on of the skin had signified that this present party would be held at Mmagojane's house: in their words, "We felt that, after one police, the other police should do the same thing." Proposed future celebrations will be held at the homes of the leader and of her deputy, since it is thought that officeholders in the group should host these events.

To understand the significance of the different foodstuffs served at this party, it is necessary to examine the practice of and the decline in agriculture in the village and in the broader area of the reserve in which it is situated. All Dithabaneng's married women acquired arable land from their in-laws when setting up house, and even its unmarried members work in the fields of their own parents. However, as in reserve areas throughout southern Africa, the significant factor influencing agricultural output is not the availability of land but rather the availability of cash.[39] The high cost of hiring traction makes it impossible to grow any food without an input from wages earned in urban employment. For married Dithabaneng women money for plowing comes from their husbands, while for unmarried women such funds may come from a mother's pension or from a brother. In economic terms, then, the greater amount of plowing money available to married women receiving regular and fairly good remittances certainly ensures a higher return on this investment: whereas unmarried Mathabathe Mokwale paid R50 to plow a section of her fields and reaped only one bag of sorghum worth R60, Raisibe Sebei paid R180 to plow a larger area and reaped five bags, worth about R300 in total.

Even for those households with a more secure access to male wages, however, their fields represent a supplementary rather than a primary source of food. This again is a common theme in studies of southern African reserve areas; indeed, seen from a more global view, it is the agricultural decline of these reserves that has caused reserve-dwellers' wholesale dependence on the sale of their labor to the industrial centers of the Republic. In this area specifically, unremitting drought has been a further major impediment to agriculture: people who a few years ago reaped a reasonable harvest have found the returns on whatever cash they do invest in plowing declining year after year. For some, the combination of a shortage of cash with the uncertainty of any return has led them to plow smaller and smaller sections of their fields in each successive year.

In this agriculturally poor area another factor that has led to the sense that field produce is supplementary rather than primary is the fact that the land here, while usable for growing sorghum, is incapable of sustaining the crop that has come to be regarded as a staple: maize or mealies. Maize must be bought directly with money remitted by men, without the intervention of female agricultural activity to make it available.

A song sung by young women during the 1950s shows clearly how, at that stage when sorghum was still a food eaten widely in the village as a whole, maize was becoming associated with migrant men, who both supplied it and demanded to be fed it:

Mararankodi, taba tša le sego
Moratiwa o tlile bošego ka tsoga kangwedi ka kgatla lehea
Mmamoratiwa o tlile bošego rrago-ngwanaka ka kgatla lehea
Ga a je mabele, ga a je leotša
Ke kgatla lehea

Mararankodi, news of laughter
My lover came at night, at the time of moonlight, and I woke to grind maize
My lover, the father of my child came in the night, I woke to grind maize
He doesn't eat sorghum, he doesn't eat millet
I grind maize.

This rejection of earlier subsistence crops in favor of bought maize has since become commonplace. The sorghum, which is still grown in varying amounts, having been assigned this marginal role, remains within women's sphere of control and is used mainly to make beer. Although this sorghum beer provides a small income to unmarried women in some poorer households, such as Mmagomotala Mofele, men's increasing rejection of sorghum beer in favor of the bottled variety makes such an income negligible in comparison with that earned, for example, by Mmagoshower from the sale of commercial brands at her informal bar.[40]

Thus, the main use of the beer made by Dithabaneng women from the sorghum they grow is for the ceremonial purposes associated with *sesotho*. The fact that all members—despite fairly wide disparities in income, deriving ultimately from differences in access to male earnings—can contribute some sorghum toward the beer which is to be drunk at a performance and then consume the resulting brew together, stresses the links binding them together as equal participants and as kinswomen, and de-emphasizes the economic differentiations that divide them and that link some to the ways of *sekgowa* through their links to particular wage-earning men.

Another aspect of the group's performance that dramatizes the sisterly communality of women and the division—even antagonism—between them and men is that of the "police" playact. Although police are not the only dramatis personae in *kiba*—Dithabaneng and other groups have a range of characters, including baboons and monkeys, *dingaka* (diviners), and doctors and nurses—the police act has most impact, since it involves members of the audience and even those outside the circle of onlookers. Its strong amusement value also derives from the fact that it involves transvestite dressing, and in this respect it is the reverse of some equally amusing pageants in male *kiba* groups in which men dress as women and engage in exaggeratedly female behavior, including kissing and mock lovemaking. Here, the relevant aspect of male behavior and dress is that of intimidating uniformed authority.

There is an element of genuine crowd control in the function of these figures: in men's *kiba*, for example, "police" do not dress in uniform, but are known merely for their use of a whip to keep extraneous people and onlookers from moving into the circle of dancers. For women's police, although they are thought of as having a similar controlling function, the limits on their authority, based partly on limited strength, have increased the playacting component of their role:

> Some men force their way through because we are women. When arrested, they will refuse to pay and just because we are women, we leave them.[41]

Mostly, then, women arrest unsuspecting men whom they suspect will comply with their demands for a fine, rather than genuine troublemakers:

> *Do they arrest men only?*
> Yes, they don't arrest women.
> *Do they arrest those men who have done something wrong?*
> It's a play—they just arrest them even if they haven't done anything wrong.[42]

Sometimes an element of secrecy is necessary so that the "police" can conceal her intentions from one of her innocent victims:

> As men are drinking there, we will go and arrest them. We will approach them as if we are dancing. . . . You can't arrest them in a group because, if you arrest one, the others will try to run away. . . . I will take him away and tell him, "Why did you come to the dancing without your jacket? It is against the law." He will take out some money, and then he is released. Whether he pays five cents or ten cents, there is no problem.[43]

But sometimes an arrested man might pay as much as R1. The fines are collected together and counted up at the end of the day:

> After eating, just before we go home, someone would tell us how much we have raised: "Lions, your money is so much."[44]

In these dramatic interludes, a range of elements are compressed, including an obvious component of social commentary and satire about the arbitrariness and frequency of police intervention in black people's lives within broader South African society. But an equally important aspect—albeit of symbolic rather than material significance—is that of concerted female action to wrest from returnee migrants an amount of money that can be put into the dancers' collective fund and "eaten" at a future party.

On a practical level, it would have been impossible to hold a party—despite the contributions in sorghum and female labor—without the pressure exerted by the collectivity of singers on Mmagojane's husband to donate a goat from his sphere of male-owned assets. In a similar vein, but in the domain of play, women police assuming the trappings of an authority normally denied them make inroads into a source of wealth within the possession of men—cash—and incorporate this under their collective control within the domain of *sotho* performance, dress, and celebration.

Women, the Domestic Domain, and Sesotho

Dithabaneng's stay-at-home wives and sisters are, then, associated with *sesotho* more strongly than are the men on whom they depend for a living. This association, while often invisible or minimal in nonperformative contexts, is foregrounded and dramatized especially through the use of *mmino wa sesotho* (*sotho* song/dance). To appreciate why this association should exist at all, we must look at the connections between the domestic domain and *sesotho*, and at how the assigning of women to the former often entails their cloaking in the guise of the latter.

The role of women in providing for the continuity or reproduction of the household or domestic sphere is a common theme in studies both of capitalism in the first world and of its intrusion into third world contexts. There is some ambiguity as to whether this role should be seen as a sign of subordination and oppression or as a source of social power, or perhaps as a mixture of both.

In some European peasant societies, for example, the domestic arena appears as a source of great influence to the women who occupy prime positions within it, while their menfolk, marginalized from power in the wider sociopolitical arena and denied any significant role in the family, are virtually without any influence at all (Rogers 1975, Gilmore 1980). In the case of southern African societies, there is a similar ambiguity about the assigning of women to the domestic sphere. It has been argued that the central dynamic of the pre-capitalist agricultural societies of the region arose from their ability to control women's productive and reproductive capacities within the homestead unit (Guy 1990). Later, the control of these capacities in turn lay at the basis of these societies' giving up of labor to the industrial centers of South Africa, while at the same time allowing them to escape full proletarianization (Bozzoli 1983, 151). Indeed, according to one viewpoint, South African capitalism depended upon and even purposefully enforced the conservation of families in the reserves as systems of support and reciprocity, in order to be able to exploit the labor power of their male members (Wolpe 1972, 108).

Some women were to escape from this realm of enforced and custom-bound domesticity, often under the rubric of alternative definitions of the domestic, provided by Christianity or colonial ideology (Delius 1983; Comaroff 1985, 150;

Bozzoli with Nkotsoe 1991, 15, 59–60). But those who remained as rural wives dependent on the earnings of male relatives continued to be seen as somehow responsible for the continuity of the household and the domestic domain. The ambiguity about the role of such women centers around whether this work has been assigned to them as unwitting dupes of the combined forces of pre-colonial patriarchal ideology and capitalism, or whether they have thereby derived some power previously denied them by actively retaining and augmenting their part in sustaining household and village life as partly autonomous domains.

A rephrasing of this issue in local terms reveals that women's keeping house amounts to doing the "work of custom" (Murray 1981, 150). In the absence of migrant men from Lesotho, it was mainly women who, although conceived of as inferior, played a major role in maintaining "the ideas and practices which are recognized as 'proper Sesotho'" and in using these to help "reproduce social relations, between the living and the dead, between men and women, and between the generations" (149).

The claim that women have become responsible for the "work of custom" does not derive only from the absence due to migrancy of males to do this work. In South Africa it has its genesis also in other dislocations of the public sociopolitical domain wrought by the apartheid regime. In an area northwest of Sekhukhuneland, Hofmeyr (1994) found that the genre of oral historical narrative, previously the domain of men and performed mainly in the central public space of a village, was unable to survive the destruction of this public space, which occurred with the forced relocations of Betterment planning, while traditions of female storytelling, situated in the household all along, did transplant successfully.

In Sekhukhuneland, as in Lesotho, what materialist approaches represent as women's role in reproduction translates in folk terms as women's role in enacting and behaving in the ways of *sesotho*. As with the more material tasks of reproduction, there is ambiguity concerning the status with which this role is endowed. On the one hand, some of the most *sotho* of the things that a woman does—such as sitting on the floor while men sit on chairs—are thought of as part of the respect she should normally show to her husband and parents-in-law in particular, but also to men in general. In such a case, her upkeep of *sesotho* is synonymous with deference and may appear demeaning. On the other hand, *sotho* performance as described above empowers women: even those as dependent on their husbands and brothers as the village singers of Dithabaneng. In song and dance, they dramatize their unity as women and their mock antagonism to men.

Conclusion

Clothing, together with the total musical performance of which it often is a part, is one of the most striking and visible markers of a *sotho* identity. In its differentiating of pre-initiates from initiates, men from women, and Christians from traditionalists, this clothing performs much the same signifying role as the Swazi dress discussed by Kuper in her seminal article "Costume and Identity" (1973a).

However, neither the statuses thus distinguished nor the clothing used to demarcate them are static and unchanging. Even in cases where *sotho* clothing delineates membership in distinct groups, as in its frequent association with "those of the nation" or non-Christians (*baditshaba*), other contexts prompt alternative uses and alignments, such as its link with women in contrast to the link of Western clothing with men. *Sotho* clothing does not, then, indicate a rigid adherence to the ways of the pre-colonial or primordial past any more than the clothing of *sekgowa* indicates a single-minded orientation toward modernity. Both are shifting markers: rather than describing the permanent orientations of bounded groups of people, they are used as templates to order experience in a variety of different settings.

Like these social identities, the clothes used to designate them are also undergoing continual change. Even those women who regard themselves as most strongly bound by custom and convention have found the rapid succession of changing styles appealing. The variations of fashion, albeit generated from beyond the local arena, have lent themselves to a more effective expression of local identities (Heath 1992), rather than supplanting this expression with a slavish devotion to fashion for its own sake, as in Kuper's account of the use of Western dress by the middle classes of Swaziland (1973a, 365).

If both the clothing that signifies and the statuses signified are undergoing transformation, there is a message that is nevertheless enunciated quite unambiguously. In women's performance contexts, *sotho* dress serves as an idiom of womanly equality and solidarity. As in the religious rituals described by Heath (1992, 26), dress underscores female sameness and reiterates that all women in the dance group are equally able to contribute to and benefit from the celebration, even if the circumstances of their everyday lives serve to stratify them.

In this case, as in others, women wear elaborate, distinctive, and allegedly "traditional" clothing in contrast to the standardized Western dress of men (Comaroff 1985, 224–25; Hendrickson 1994; Schapera 1949, 408). This makes a complex statement: it speaks on the one hand of the deference with which women confined within the domestic domain should behave toward male agnates and affines, while on the other it signals the authority of women's broader role as custodians of custom.

Notes

I gratefully acknowledge assistance from the University Research Committee, the Mellon Fund, and the Centre for Science Development, as well as the assistance and support of the African Studies Institute, University of the Witwatersrand. Thanks to the members of Dithabaneng singing group, to the sisters at Apel mission, to participants in the various seminars where earlier drafts of this essay were presented, and particularly to Patrick Pearson, Adam Kuper, Jim Kiernan, and Isabel Hofmeyr for helpful comments. Philip Mnisi, who gave me valuable help as interpreter, was senselessly killed on 5 July 1992. I dedicate this essay to his memory, with gratitude and sadness.

1   Literally, Tswana language and ways/white language and ways.
2   Where Sotho denotes a language or a set of musical or other features that have been attributed to a group of people by analysts, it is capitalized and not italicized. But where it denotes a state of being, a way of life, or a set of qualities that informants themselves have enunciated or commented upon, as the noun *sesotho* or as the adjective *sotho*, it is italicized and not capitalized. See Comaroff and Comaroff 1989 for a similar usage.
3   Substantial rifts were established, or newly conceptualized, within rural northern Transvaal communities around the pivotal feature of Christianity. The resulting social categories were named differently depending on the stance of the namer. Those proud to have affiliated themselves to the Christian way called themselves *bakriste* (Christians) and termed their opposites *babeitene* (heathens). Those aligning themselves with the chiefs called themselves *baditšhaba* (those of the nation) in opposition to the derogatorily named *majakane* or *majekane* (Christians). The geographical divide in many rural communities is named in a similar vein: *setšhabeng* is the place of those of the nation, and *majekaneng* is the place of the Christians. The paired terms *majakane/baditšhaba* and *bakriste/baheitene*, while orienting themselves by reference to a common dividing line, thus imply opposing moral views of the division.
4   Migrant singers, performing in an urban context, often refer to the same genre as *mmino wa setšo* (music of origin, or traditional music).
5   Sekhukhune was paramount chief of the Pedi when the polity was defeated by the British in 1878. His name was given to the reserve area that was allocated to his subjects in the wake of their defeat: Sekhukhuneland. The area, since augmented by the addition of "Trust" farms purchased from white owners by a government board established for the purpose, has subsequently become the magisterial district called Sekhukhune. *Sekhukhune* or *GaSekhukhune* is the local appellation, which does not

recognize the limits of this magisterial district but extends its boundaries to all parts of the northern Sotho homeland of Lebowa that are south of Pietersburg and even to much of the white farming area beyond.

6 This style is most commonly known by its rural practitioners as *mpepetloane* or *lebowa*, but its spread throughout the northern Transvaal countryside was part of the broader development of the migrant style of music, formerly exclusively male, known as *kiba*. See James 1994 for an account of the development of this style.

7 This sense of a unifying connection to a symbolic animal has been translated as "totemism" and described as involving membership of a "fairly loose association of agnatic kin" (Monnig 1967, 234). However, Kuper argues that these were not kinship groups or clans (1982, 46–48), and according to Hoernle, "there is no special native term" for such a grouping (1937, 91–92).

8 One version of the garment is called *sesothwana* (little *sesotho*). Hilda Kuper talks of a similar differentiation between Swazi and Western clothing, with "contrasted systems of clothing symbolising contrasting cultures" (1973a, 355–56), but it appears that these distinct cultures were not *within* Swazi society.

9 Members of Dithabaneng, recorded discussion with Deborah James and Philip Mnisi (hereafter DJ and PM, respectively) 20 July 1991, Nchabeleng. These women were mostly born into illiterate families and none knew her precise date or even year of birth. I have calculated dates according to when members of particular regiments were initiated.

10 Literally, "*sesotho* of wearing" (*sesotho sa go apara*); this is distinguished from "*sesotho* of speaking" (*sesotho sa go bolela*) and from various other forms of *sesotho*.

11 In similar vein, Hilda Kuper mentions that when new, Western, or trade-derived items were added to Swazi clothing, these were "peripheral . . . accretions to, not rejections of, Swazi-style dress" (1973a, 355).

12 Rural women singers address each other as "the mother of so-and-so" or "the grandmother of so-and-so," rather than by the names given to them at birth or at initiation. Thus, Makgolo wa Pine translates as "Pine's grandmother," Mmagopine as "Pine's mother," Mmagoviolet as "Violet's mother," and so on.

13 Mmagomathumasha Madibane, recorded discussion with DJ and Anna Madihlaba, Sephaku, 25 January 1989.

14 Mathabathe Mokwale, recorded discussion with PM, Nchabeleng, 29 December 1990.

15 Members of Dithabaneng, recorded discussion with DJ and PM, Nchabeleng, 14 July 1991. For more detail on the reinterpretation of lyrics as referring to the context of dance itself, see James 1994.

16 Mmakgolo wa Pine Khulwane, recorded discussion with DJ and PM, Nchabeleng, 28 July 1991.

17 Vail and White document a similar ambiguity by Tumbuka wives about labor migration, similarly expressed in terms of the clothes it can provide or the lack of clothes if a migrant neglects his duties to his far-off family (1991, 258–59).

18 In the Molepo district farther north, when male migrants began to use privately owned taxis rather than buses to return home, the taxis became known as *mmethisa [wa mathari]* (those which cause young married women to be beaten), since they brought husbands home at unexpected times and enabled them to walk in on their wives' illicit affairs (Molepo 1983, 77).

19 Song and comment recorded in writing during discussion with members of Dithabaneng, Nchabeleng, 28 July 1991.

20 Mmakgolo wa Pine Khulwane, recorded discussion with DJ and PM, Nchabeleng, 19 July 1991.

21 Lucas Sefoka, recorded discussion with DJ and Malete Thomas Nkadimeng, Johannesburg, 27 February 1990; Molepo (1984, 16); evidence presented to the Native Economic Commission (1930–32). Delius (1989, 595–96) claims that even traditionalist communities in Sekhukhune were changing their attitude toward education and beginning to send their sons to school from around the 1930s and that a number of "tribal schools" were established in the 1940s. However, judging from life histories of migrant men from Sekhukhune, it was only in the 1960s and 1970s that schooling for boys gained such wide acceptance, for non-Christians as much as for Christians, that it eclipsed or supplanted the period of work on the farms or displaced farmwork into the school holidays.

22 Mmagojane Kgalema, during recorded discussion with members of Dithabaneng, Nchabeleng, 19 July 1991.

23 This reason given by men for first leaving home to work is reflected in a number of other accounts from the Transvaal: Niehaus (1994), Molepo (1984, 16), Native Economic Commission (1930–32 [evidence of Neethling: 31, 50; Gilbertson: 50; Mareli: 333; Fuller: 412]).

24 Ramogohlo Diphofa, recorded discussion with PM, Mphanama, 20 December 1990.

25 Members of Dithabaneng, recorded discussion with DJ and PM, Nchabeleng, 19 July 1991.

26 Mmagojane Kgalema, recorded discussion with PM, Nchabeleng, 29 December 1990.

27 Mmagoshower Debeila, discussion with DJ and PM, Nchabeleng, 16 July 1991.

28 Rebelliousness followed by later conformity is of course a common theme of studies on youth. See, for example, Bozzoli and Nkotsoe's description of how in the successful peasant economy of Phokeng it was boys who had the greater desire to escape the strictures of society's patriarchal controls, but who were later to gain more rewards than women out of "accepting the system"—eventual independence and access to land (1991, 81).

29 Mmagopine Khulwane and Mmagojane Kgalema, in recorded discussion with members of Dithabaneng, Nchabeleng, 19 July 1991.

30 Comaroff suggests that "headscarves are widely worn by black women in South Africa and express the canons of mission modesty, which overlaid the elaborate code of hairdressing" (1985, 224).

31 Members of Dithabaneng, recorded discussion, Nchabeleng, 20 July 1991.

32 Ibid.

33 Members of Dithabaneng, recorded discussion with DJ and PM, Nchabeleng, 20 July 1991.

34 Mmagomotala Mofele, discussion with DJ and PM, Nchabeleng, 17 July 1991.

35 Mmagoviolet Phakwago, recorded discussion with DJ and PM, Nchabeleng, 17 July 1991.

36 Mmagojane Kgalema, recorded discussion with PM, Nchabeleng, 29 December 1990.

37 Salome and Andronica Machaba, discussion with DJ, Johannesburg, 19 October 1991.

38 Murray has indicated that most rural families undergo diverse temporal processes of change which may take them through several apparently discrete "types" within a single generation (1981, 100–107, 155). For example, after a period of virilocal residence as a wife in the absence of a husband, a woman might experience marital dissolution, work for some time as a migrant, and later return to rear children in a matrifocal household (155).

39 See, for example, Murray (1981, 76–85), James (1987, 76–78). As in the Lesotho villages studied by Murray, landholders in Sekhukhuneland who have no money for plowing frequently let out their land for sharecropping by people who have cash or own tractors (P. Delius, personal communication, 1991).

40 See Colson and Scudder (1988) for an account of the declining ability of women to produce an income from home-brew as men began to favor bottled beer. In Sekhukhune, the rejection of sorghum brew in favor of the bottled variety was fueled also by fears that women might bewitch men by concealing some poisonous substance in their home-brew (Sam Nchabeleng, personal communication, 1992).

41 Mathabathe Mokwale, recorded discussion with PM, Nchabeleng, 29 December 1990.

42 Raisibe Sebei, ibid.

43 Mmagojane Kgalema, recorded discussion with PM, Nchabeleng, 29 December 1990.

44 Ibid.

3 MEDIATING THREADS: CLOTHING AND THE TEXTURE OF SPIRIT/MEDIUM RELATIONS IN *BORI* (SOUTHERN NIGER)

Adeline Masquelier

Clothes, from the King's mantle downwards, are emblematic. . . . On the other hand, all Emblematic things are properly Clothes, thought-woven or hand-woven: *must not the Imagination weave Garments, visible Bodies, wherein the else invisible creations and inspirations of our Reason are, like Spirits, revealed*—Thomas Carlyle, *Sartor resartus* [emphasis added]

"Spirits Are Wrappers of Beauty": An Introduction

In Mawri communities of Arewa (southern Niger), devotees of the *bori* possession cult learn to identify the *iskoki* (spirits) who incarnate themselves in their mediums during *wasani* (possession ceremonies) primarily by observing the deities' respective stereotypical gestures and attitudes. While the Doguwa, a family of female spirits native to the area, emit characteristic screeching sounds, other deities, like the respected Muslim scholar Malam Zaki Sarki, remain silent and simply nod their heads pensively. Some of the Baboule, who imitate French colonials, walk stiffly as soldiers should, while Gurmunya, the lame sister of Zaki Sarki, can only sit with her legs under her and hop around by holding herself up on her hands (see fig. 3.1). Adama, the Doguwa who causes paralysis, is herself unable to move and simply lies on the ground, while her sisters and daughters are often recognizable because of the foot they keep behind themselves—toes pointed to the ground—even as they attempt to walk with the other. If the personalities of *bori* spirits are expressed in, and shaped by, the way they move their mediums' bodies and the sounds they utter, their identities also lie in the very fabric of the wrappers, robes and shirts they are dressed in during possession ceremonies. How those identities are given substance through clothing and what connections are woven through the medium of fabric is the subject of this essay.

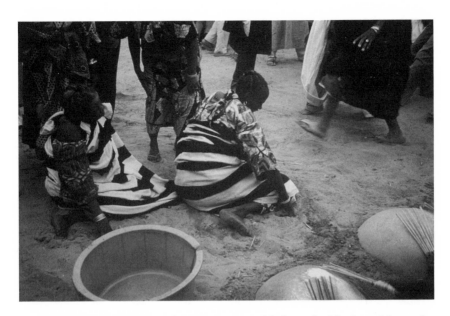

3.1   In front of the drummers beating overturned halves of calabashes with wooden sticks (foreground), two *bori* mediums are possessed by Gurmunya spirits during a ceremony. The mediums are wearing the characteristic black-and-white striped wrapper associated with the lame deities, and in their incarnations as Gurmunya they cannot walk. Photo by A. Masquelier.

As the Hausa proverb in the heading suggests, a spirit's beauty is represented by the clothing worn by adepts of the *bori* cult. This is how a Mawri man, with whom I was discussing the implications of the saying, explained what it meant: "If you leave in the morning with your wrapper of beauty, all the people in town, be they friend or foe, are going to admire your wrapper." Spirits are very beautiful, more so than regular humans, and they inspire endless fascination among people. They are thought to have fair complexions, big eyes, and straight, long hair that strokes their ankles. *Bori* devotees often depict the spirits who appear in their dreams as wide-eyed, smiling creatures whose smooth hair covers their entire bodies. Villagers who recall having met face to face with a spirit or having had visions of some deities in their sleep all say that these supernatural beings are irresistibly handsome. As I have shown elsewhere (Masquelier 1992, in press), Mawri discourse is fraught with cases of men who are seduced by extremely beautiful women who turn out to be flirtatious but dangerous female spirits hiding their evil intentions behind a seemingly innocent smile. There are, of course, ugly spirits, or rather—given that these creatures, by definition, have no carnal bodies—spirits who take on an unsightly appearance when making themselves visible to humans. Nevertheless, the *mutanen daji* ("people of the bush"), as spirits are sometimes referred to, are generally conceived as possessing a kind of beauty that very few humans exhibit.

Many of the *bori* deities are lovely and graceful in and of themselves, but their attraction also resides in the dazzling costumes worn by devotees of the *bori* cult during possession rituals. These garments are more than simple adornments whose color and shape vary from one spirit to the next. More than a mere piece of fabric or leather, and more than a uniform reflecting one's cultural, social, or religious status, the spirits' attire is the medium through which people create, and subsequently relate to, and communicate with, *bori* deities. As they are repeatedly worn by spirits incarnated in their human vessels during possession, the wrappers, robes, hats, and sashes that compose the deities' paraphernalia become extensions of their supernatural owners. This essay documents the use and abuse of spirits' garments in the *bori,* and shows how, for the Mawri, clothes convey meanings and embody memories in ways that mediate not only human relations in the community but relations between people and supernatural forces. As palpable, personal items through which identities and histories are expressed, constructed, and transmitted, clothes are "a medium for the transfer of essential substances" (Schneider and Weiner 1989, 18). They give contours and volume to amorphous beings and provide the connecting threads between distinct worlds of experience. It is this mediating dimension of clothing, its role in the making and recording of history and memory through its relationship with physical as well as ethereal bodies, that is the focus of this essay.

Clothing One's Spirit: The Making of a Relationship

Though they are commonly known as Mawri, the Hausa-speaking people who occupy the rural *arrondissement* of Dogondoutchi[1] do not constitute a homogenous group. Up until the 1889 French conquest and the subsequent colonization of what is now the Republic of Niger, Mawri society was built on a coexistence between two dominant groups: the Gubawa, an indigenous population of subsistence agriculturalists whose lineage elders claimed ritual ties to the land through their roles as priests and mediums of local deities; and the Arewa, whose ancestors had conquered the area in the seventeenth century and who were in charge of defense and political management. After the French established a colonial administration, the distinctions among the populations who had kept separate identities were progressively abolished while the spread of Islam intensified in a region that had long remained impermeable to the influence of the Muslim faith. Today, the various subgroups—who had mixed, inter-married, and fought each other in pre-colonial times—are indiscriminately referred to as Mawri. As farmers, they rely mainly on the sale of agricultural products (millet, sorghum, beans, and peanuts) to buy primary necessities such as clothing, food (meat, spices, corn meal, etc.), and medicine, although for many, secondary occupations such as petty trading, calabash carving, or tailor-ing also provide a substantial source of income.

Traditionally recognizable by their "ethnic" marks, a double scar that cuts the cheek from the corner of the mouth to the ear on either side,[2] Mawri villagers identify themselves with the Hausa, a large sedentary population that constitutes about 50 percent of the total population of Niger. Of these, 80 to 90 percent are estimated to be Muslims. The rest are primarily devotees and fol-lowers[3] of the *bori*, a possession cult that emerged from the indigenous cult of local deities and focuses on the management of spirit-induced afflictions and disruptions (see also Besmer 1983; Echard 1991a, 1991b; Monfouga-Nicolas 1972; Schmoll 1991; Tremearne 1914).[4] In Arewa, a Muslim is generally referred to as "the one who prays" (*mai salla*), while a spirit devotee will be known as "the one who sacrifices" (*mai yanka*).

Nevertheless, it is sometimes difficult to pinpoint what distinguishes a fol-lower of the Prophet from a *bori* medium. As has been pointed out elsewhere (Bernus 1969, 190; Masquelier 1993b, 1994; Nicolas 1975), the interaction be-tween Islamic and indigenous worldviews has been extensive and complex, and there can be much overlap between Muslim and non-Muslim identities. Be-cause Islam generally carries a higher status than "pagan" or "animist" prac-tices, even the most devoted spirit follower may ostentatiously accomplish the five daily prayers at the local mosque. Conversely, a respected *malam* (Muslim cleric) will confidently declare that he wants nothing to do with spirits even after allegedly visiting a *bori* healer in the deep of the night to find a cure for his wife's sudden illness. In contexts where donning Islamic attire does not neces-sarily mean one is a devout Muslim and going to Mecca on the hajj is not antithetical to sacrificing to one's favorite spirit, relying on religious affiliation as a means of identification becomes increasingly problematic. One thing re-mains certain, however: those who are chosen by spirits to become mediums cannot afford to ever sever their relationships to these superhuman creatures, especially once substantial ties have been created between them—to do so would only endanger their health, if not their lives.

People usually discover they have been selected to serve as mediators between spirits and humans when, after unsuccessfully trying several treatments to cure themselves, they are told that only after making an offering to the spirit sus-

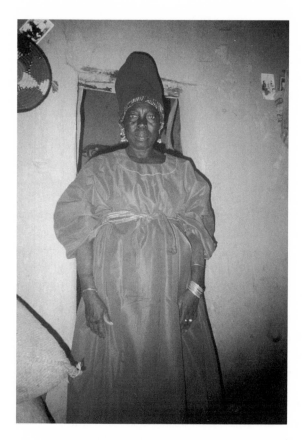

3.2   A medium of the fierce Kirai wearing the red robe, red sash, and red bonnet that make up the Zarma spirit's attire. Photo by A. Masquelier.

pected of having caused their illness will they regain their health—provided, of course, that they agree with the diagnosis offered by the *bori* healer they visited. Spirits send afflictions to those whom they want to possess or who have offended them. Once the spirit is placated and has agreed to forgive, the best way to remain healthy and prosperous is to undergo the expensive initiation ceremony (*gyara;* literally, "arrangement") that will officialize one's involvement in the cult and reveal to the attending devotees the identity of one's superhuman tormentor(s). Membership in the cult is open to all members of the society and transcends gender categories as well as social and economic boundaries, although women clearly outnumber men. Once duly initiated, and in exchange for the spirits' protection and help, mediums commit themselves to serving the spirits. This means agreeing to be the receptacle of the spirits and periodically undergoing possession during *wasani* (ceremonies). It also implies periodic offerings of sacrificial blood to the *iskoki*, since these primarily feed on animal blood. Finally, commitment to the spirits involves acquiring a set of clothing for each and every *iska* (spirit; singular of *iskoki*) a medium is possessed by. Each spirit of the *bori* cult has a specific set of clothes and attributes, which differentiate him or her from the other members of the pantheon during possession rituals. Thus, while Kirai, a powerful and cunning Zarma spirit, wears a red gown (*riga*), a red bonnet that looks like a phrygian cap (*hula*), and a red sash (*damara*) (see fig. 3.2) and brandishes a hatchet as an ominous symbol of his control over thunder and lightning, his younger brother Moussa owns a black gown, a red bonnet, and a red sash. Maria, the lascivious prostitute who takes such care of her appearance, wears a spotless white outfit which consists of a shirt, a wrapper, and a headscarf. In addition, she carries a mirror in which she endlessly looks at her smiling reflection.

Buying clothing for a spirit is the first step toward establishing a viable and enduring relationship with the supernatural. As a wordless message symbolizing trust and friendship, the gift tells the spirit that the gift giver is serious enough about securing the deity's protection that he or she is ready to make the financial sacrifices necessary to satisfy the spirit. Though they may be worn by the devotee outside of ceremonial circumstances, a spirit's clothes require special care. Ideally, they should be washed and pressed after each *bori* ceremony, particularly if the possessed devotees crawled on the ground and covered themselves with dirt, as mediums of Azane—an unusually strong deity of local origin who washes his body with dirt—are prone to do. If torn or damaged in any way, spirit clothing must be mended. Devotees are also responsible for periodically replacing any worn-out items in their spirits' wardrobe. Many take pride in displaying their collection of garments inside their house, while others carefully hide the spirits' paraphernalia inside trunks or baskets.

More than simple adornments that dazzle *bori* spectators with their loud colors and varied patterns, these clothes mediate people's relationships to the spiritual realm. As a material symbol of the fruitful harmony existing between a person and a spirit, they constitute a vital link with the sacred. Referring to the leather clothing worn by some spirits, Nicolas notes:

[the leather outfit] is above all a coating, a "second skin." It testifies to the alliance and the profound intimacy shared by members of the cult. The sacrificial victim's skin of which the garment is made is not a simple piece of leather; it belongs to the realm of "sacrifice." It is imbued with power, like the bark of trees to which it is likened . . . or like the skin of wild beasts which is used to make potent medicines. It is as if the man who wears the skin identified himself with the favorite animal of his hereditary spirit and proved through this identification his commitment to the deity. The animal emerges as a substitute for the person during the sacrificial act. . . . The skin he is wearing over his own body sets the individual in permanent communication with the spirits, and circumscribes him within a sacred field. (1975, 60–61; my translation)

While in the past, all spirit followers dressed in leather pants—and wore a bonnet and covered their torsos with a cotton blanket—nowadays the leather garment has become a strictly ceremonial outfit worn by the indigenous male spirit Azane (the husband of Doguwa deities). Adorned with mirrors—which connote vanity as well as the selfish dimension of unreciprocated transactions—and fringes, the garment will usually remain hanging in its owner's house until the proper moment, when ritual assistants carefully tie it around the devotee's hips as he or she incarnates one of the Azane spirits.

The Practice of Murfu

Anyone may own the garment of a particular spirit, regardless of the nature of his or her relationship to that deity. In fact, many villagers who have no direct link to the bori cult and who know little about spirits will readily admit having purchased a bori wrapper or keeping the one their father or mother owned. Such wrappers are readily available to anyone wishing to acquire one. Prospective buyers will usually visit a dan bori (bori devotee) who deals in spirits' clothing or who tailors them. Many of the wrappers—those of Doguwa spirits, for instance—are handwoven pieces of cotton that are hand dyed. Reflecting the more recent appearance of their owners on the bori scene, the clothes of the Zarma, Baboule, and Maria spirits are made of red, white, or black, mass-produced cloth, which is tailored according to the specifications of the buyer. Though the length, width, and pattern of bori garments vary slightly from one devotee to the next, the styles and colors are immutable. Thus the Doguwa Adama has always worn a white, handwoven wrapper, while the Zarma deity Kirai is invariably seen in a red robe tied with a red sash and wearing a red hat. The practice of keeping a spirit's garment or owning the favorite animal of a spirit is called murfu. Often that particular spirit is an ancestral deity who is attached to a specific lineage and whose protection has been sought by generations of villagers eager to secure the health and prosperity of their families. In many cases, the last devotee of that spirit has died leaving no descendants to serve as the deity's receptacle during bori ceremonies; yet, someone among the children or grandchildren of the deceased may have kept the spirit's wardrobe out of respect for his or her heritage (*gado*) or out of fear of supernatural retaliation.

Though critics of *bori* would never admit to practicing *murfu,* it is widely believed that they secretly keep the garments of their ancestors' spirit and that among the handful of goats their wives or mothers own, one could recognize that deity's favorite animal. Nevertheless, because many villagers nowadays tend to neglect "traditional" religious obligations pertaining to the care of spirits, some deities slowly fall into oblivion. They are never forgotten forever, though; when one business venture after another fails, or when their children become afflicted with mysterious and incurable diseases, people are suddenly reminded that they once gave away or burnt the lineage spirit's clothing or that for years they have neglected to make the annual sacrifice to the deity. Clothes shape spirits who, after all, lack physical contours by creating a virtual body for them. They delineate the space that itself defines the outlines of their personae, extending these personae in space and time. In this manner, clothes are directly implicated in the configuration of their wearers' identities.

I was told once that a Dogondoutchi woman who never practiced *bori* but regularly visited *bori* healers saw her son almost die before her eyes. He had suddenly taken ill and was entirely paralyzed. All the cures had been tried in vain and his health was rapidly deteriorating when a *bori* healer told the mother that she needed to purchase a white wrapper for the spirit Adama. Adama, the healer claimed, was responsible for the child's state of health. Reputed for causing paralysis in her victims, Adama is a fearful and impatient spirit who belongs to the Doguwa family. When possessed, her devotees lose their ability to walk and lie on the ground, wrapped in a white[5] cotton cloth. Upon hearing the healer's diagnosis, an old neighbor who used to know the child's deceased maternal grandmother remembered that the dead woman had been a devotee of Adama, whom she regularly propitiated. After her death, no one had shown signs of inheriting the spirit, and the Muslim members of the family had pressured the others into dropping this "*bori* business." Years had gone by and everyone had forgotten about the spirit. It had taken a major crisis such as the critical condition of her young child to remind a woman of her responsibility toward her ancestral spirit. As soon as she brought a white wrapper home with her, the child started to recover. A few days later, he was able to sit on his mat, and soon he was out playing and running with his friends again. He recovered the full ability of his limbs except for his right hand, which remained paralyzed, an ominous reminder of the Adama's revengeful temper and fierce power.

Owning the wrapper or the robe of a spirit enables one to communicate with this spirit without seeking the services of a *bori* healer who would act as an intermediary between the natural and the supernatural. As a palpable sign of the deity's presence, which people can hold and wear, the garment mediates human and spirit relationships by giving "body" to an immaterial being. One might say that clothes concretize the conversation between humans and spirits by literally providing the connecting threads through which they can relate to each other. Mawri talk to, and through, the cloth in order to address a spirit whose help, intervention, or protection they seek at one moment or another. Holding the cloth in their hands or laying it out on a mat, they pray to the spiritual owner of the garment, knowing that she or he will listen to their plea for help. The garment recreates the physicality of a being no longer present, thereby objectifying the spiritual tie connecting the deity and the villager in need of superhuman assistance. Just as people needing a spirit's guidance or help often concretize their prayers and make them more effective by shedding sacrificial blood on that deity's altar, the individual who makes use of an *iska*'s clothes to elicit that spirit's attention transmits through, and inscribes into, the very fibers of the garment the words he is directing at the ethereal creature. Through such means, one's "conversation" with the spirits can be carried out in the privacy of one's home, and without anyone else knowing about it. A Christian woman I knew admitted to owning clothes for various spirits and occasionally displaying the garments the way she had seen her mother do to seek supernatural assistance. She had entrusted a friend with the money necessary to purchase several wrappers because she herself knew very little about spirits. She explained:

> When I have problems, I sometimes ask for a spirit's help. I have seen how you do it. I do it in the room, in my room . . . I just set the clothes on a mat. I just follow my ancestors' traditions. Sometimes, you get good results, sometimes not.

There are other ways of communicating with the supernatural, but for many who do not wish to publicize their gesture, "talking to the cloth" remains a discreet, expedient, and relatively inexpensive way to achieve results. Many Muslims who readily condemn any form of dealing with *iskoki* are widely suspected of secretly resorting to such unobtrusive means of gaining access to the supernatural. Though they may have burnt or gotten rid of their parents' *bori* paraphernalia in a public display of Islamic piety, rumors have it that they have all been painfully reminded of their obligations to their ancestral *iska* at one time or another, and that they now keep the "things of the spirits" (*kayan iskoki*), although they pretend otherwise for the sake of respectability.

Though one of the first duties of an individual plagued by a spirit is to buy the clothing of this deity, *bori* followers sometimes delay the purchase because they cannot afford it or because they need to settle some pressing debts in priority. If proper apologies are made to the spirits, they usually will be patient and wait to have clothing until their devotee saves up enough money or receives a monetary gift from a wealthier kin. Though often lenient, most spirits will become angered if, for whatever reason, a devotee abuses their trust and never presents them with any gift. A sudden relapse of illness is a clear sign that a neglected spirit is pressuring her adept into fulfilling his part of the bargain. A young woman who had postponed acquiring the garments of her spirit Zanzana after she had been initiated into the *bori* soon found out how Zanzana punished those who neglected her. Zanzana—her name means "smallpox"—gives pimples and stomach aches and provokes skin rashes and eye sores. When a woman offends her, she makes her hemorrhage. If a man insults her in any way, she renders him impotent. When incarnated by one of her horses—mediums are referred to as "horses" mounted by their spirits—Zanzana continuously scratches herself as if "her" skin were itching.

Zanzana gave the young adept who had neglected to purchase her wardrobe a painful vaginal wart. The wart receded only after the girl bought Zanzana her wrappers—a white one with thin red stripes referred to as *mai gorori* and a smaller black wrapper with white stripes known as *kyan kyandi*, both hand-woven—with money she borrowed from her mother. After this unfortunate experience, this adept never trifled with her spirits' demands for new clothes and always made sure each of her *iskoki* was well provided. She claimed to receive orders from her spirits in dreams. One night, she dreamt that she pierced her foot with a spear, a vision that she interpreted a sign that her Doguwa, a fierce warrior spirit named Rankasso, wanted to own a spear. Like other spirit devotees, she came to take pride in her spirits' extensive wardrobe, and enjoyed displaying it to her *bori* acquaintances when they came to visit.

Wearing and Tying Clothing in Mawri Society

Both Mawri men and women love clothes, have an elaborate conception of what it means to be fashionable or richly dressed, and spend comparatively vast sums of money to periodically replenish their wardrobe. Cloth is the most important household expense after food and housing. Men are responsible for annually providing new sets of clothing for their wives and children. Wives and children usually eagerly await the Muslim festival of Babbar Sallah ("the great festival," Id-el Kebir, performed on the tenth of the Muslim month of Zulhaji) because this is when they will receive new clothes. Though displaying an impressive array of clothing and parading in expensive looking outfits are primary indicators of a person's wealth, impoverished people who may not own even a thatched hut may outshine others when it comes to showing off their richest gowns. In fact, women are sometimes accused of ruining their husbands or going heavily in debt to satisfy their lust for rich cloth and compete with colleagues who wear only expensive imported fabric—such as Dutch wax-printed cloth,[6] referred to locally as "wax"—because of its prestigious status (see Mamamane 1982). Every social event, from a naming ceremony to a market day to a *bori* ritual, is an occasion to dress up. While women wear gay, cotton, custom-made blouses adorned with flounces, puffed-out sleeves, elaborate collars, or rows of brightly colored buttons and wrappers of the same fabric,[7] the majority of men don the voluminous *babban riga* ("large robe"; plural, *riguna*) of brightly colored and embroidered brocade—an ample robe worn over a matching loose shirt and drawstring pants, which is associated with an Islamic status. As Nicolas (1976, 61) stresses, the *babban riga* is above all adornment, whose prohibitive cost is not justified by the need to protect oneself from the cold, the sun, or the rain. With its large sleeves and cumbersome layers, it hampers its owner and is easily soiled. Yet it gives poise and respectability to its wearer, and that is why even *bori* adepts have adopted the Muslim dress on market day, on holidays, or whenever they need to dress up. Thus, even if the *babban riga* is, by definition, Muslim attire, it has become the garment of choice for any man—regardless of his religious affiliations—who wants to look elegant and dignified or who needs to assert his ethnic origins at an official function. Non-Muslims, especially, increasingly tend to adopt such "uniforms" in their efforts to dissociate themselves from the backwardness and rusticity often attributed to "animists." As early as 1975, Nicolas noted that in the Hausa-speaking Maradi region (east of Arewa) there was not a single Azna (non-Muslim, usually translated as "animist") who did not have at least one Muslim robe to wear on formal occasions (1975, 32).

There are *riguna* and *riguna*, of course. As with women's clothing, the wide variety of cloth types and stylistic treatments—the material, silk or cotton, used in embroidery, the extent of embroidered ornamentation—say a lot, according to Renne (1986, 54), about the value of the robe, and hence about the status imparted to the wearer. Thus, it is not simply through their clothing but also through the quality, style, colors, and feel of the very fabric out of which their garments are made that people express something about who they are and the amount of money they can afford to spend on refining their appearances.

Putting on different layers of cloth is not so much a matter of modesty as of dignity. Padding the body with cloth denotes prestige (Darrah 1980, 123), and the more voluminous the clothed body, the better. In contrast, nakedness—that is, a state in which certain bodily parts (in the case of women, legs, thighs, breasts, buttocks, or the abdomen) are not covered with cloth as they should be—or even being scantily clad, connotes deprivation, madness, and other forms of social deviancy. Thus, if women of child-bearing age occasionally remain bare-breasted, wearing only a wrapper tied around their hips within the walls of their compound, they would never step out of their homes without being properly clad. In addition to a blouse and a matching wrapper covering one's legs and ankles, proper attire includes a headscarf and a second wrapper folded in two and tied around one's waist. For women, covering one's head connotes modesty, a quality that is very prized in women. Hence, going out without a headscarf usually implies sexual promiscuity and prostitution, which in itself is a form of social deviancy—although *karuwanci* (prostitution, courtesanship) does not always carry the stigma associated with prostitution in the West and sometimes provides an acceptable, short-term alternative to marriage for women looking for economic independence.

Other marginal individuals can also be identified through their clothing. For instance, young Koranic scholars (*almajirai*) who must rely on the generosity of other villagers for their daily sustenance—by begging, they learn humility—wear tattered, secondhand clothes. And *bori* devotees who suffered from temporary insanity at the hands of their spirits often recall wandering in the bush, feeding on roots and berries, and wearing dirty rags. Initiation into the *bori* often concludes this liminal stage and reinstates the individual as a full member of the community. Another example of social deviancy that is expressed through the state of one's clothes is provided by witchcraft. Once they have been convicted of dealing with evil spirits and have been neutralized (Masquelier 1993a), Mawri *mayu* (witches) are thought to spend their days picking rags on the ground. Inoffensive, yet insane and unable to lead productive lives, they collect the refuse and debris of those who were once their friends or victims. In a maddening attempt to patch their lives together, they turn their attention to these shreds of cloth, whose decaying state—ironically—appears to speak to the vulnerability and transience of human existence. Thus, clothing lends itself to manipulation and distortion when it comes to constructing or altering the persona one presents in public. The very texture of clothing, its layers and folds, its density or lack thereof communicate substantial information about one's social and economic status.

The style, color, and lavishness of clothes also connote religious affiliation and educational background. Hence, educated civil servants characteristically dress in tight-fitting European pants and multi-pocketed shirts of dull colors and go hatless, while Muslim traders wear brightly colored, voluminous *riguna* (the three-piece attire) made of heavy brocade and colorful, finely embroidered hats and/or large turbans. Male *bori* practitioners can usually be spotted in crowds because they often don red and black clothes—*bori* colors—and the distinctive red or black bonnet of *bori* devotees. Yet they are also known to adopt the Muslim *riga,* which spells prestige and sophistication. If clothing shapes identities, it also lends itself to creative manipulation and inscriptions. Since the elections held in 1993, women can be seen wearing the "uniform" of the political parties they voted for: the fabric of their outfits colorfully advertises the parties' respective slogans in French while displaying the faces of the presidential candidates as large cameos.[8] Let me add that making the medium into the message is not a new practice in Niger: printed cloth has long been used to advertise the virtues of breast-feeding or the benefits of fertilizer.

Clothing speaks not only of status, wealth, and beauty; its very manufacture and usage metaphorically reenact—or at least, used to reenact—the processes through which the social fabric is woven. Hence, the basket and the spindle used in spinning cotton respectively symbolized the male and female genitals in their productive coupling (Darrah 1980, 125). In Mawri society, women used to spin while men wove (and dyed cotton threads). Husbands provided women with the raw materials for cotton spinning, an activity women undertook when they gathered together after the evening meal. The thread produced would then be sold. Or it would be brought to a professional dyer and then to a weaver (Cooper 1991). The rise of a market economy, which made imported cloth readily available during the colonial period, led to the demise of local cotton production.[9] It was precisely the availability of imported cotton cloth in the context of intensified monetary transactions promoted by the production and sale of peanuts for cash that contributed to the gradual disappearance of local textile manufacture, according to Cooper (1991, 5). Today, everyone wears clothes made out of mass-produced fabric. Locally woven cotton fabric is used only to design clothes for certain *bori* spirits such as the Doguwa, or to manufacture the bright and multi-colored blankets that are given as wedding presents and which, together with the bright enamel pots that are prominently displayed in large glass-door cabinets, constitute women's most prized possessions.

Going back to the sexual symbolism woven into the very fabric of cloth itself, the verb *darme* (to tie), which describes the action of putting one's clothes on, is also used to refer to the process of contracting a marriage (*darmen arme:* to tie a marriage) (see also Darrah 1980). Tying one's clothing originally referred to the action of tying one's wrapper around one's waist or over one's torso (for women) and tying one's leather pants around one's waist and in between one's legs. Today, men actually tie something only when they wear the loose-fitting trousers that are secured around the waist by a string. Clothing the spirits during a possession ceremony is also referred to as a tying, because female spirits wear wrappers—tied around their waist or under their armpits and across their chests—and male spirits wear sashes around their waists or turbans which must be wrapped tightly around their heads. Frobenius (1913, 563–64) noted the importance of tying and of belts in his description of a *wasa* among the Hausa of northern Nigeria:

> The Bori folk gather for the dance in the afternoon about two hours before sundown . . . Then the Magadja [*bori* priestess] rises to her feet. She wears two girdles of cloth (called Damara), in which the amulets are sewn, knotted together over her breasts and hips and in her hand she holds a slender rod of bronze. . . . While all this is going on the Adjingi [*bori* priest] stands aside unmoved. But now his body is suddenly convulsed, he snatches at the air with cramped up fingers and stammers words without meaning. . . . The attack is soon over and the Adjingi begins to put on his garments.

Chest and body are covered with cloths and several "Damara" are knotted over them. Although the scene described by Frobenius took place at the turn of the century, it is comparable to what goes on today during a *bori* possession ritual in Arewa. After a spirit shows signs of wanting to remain a while in the body of his devotee, the medium is dressed, wrappers are fastened tightly around waists, sashes (*damara*) are knotted over robes, and scarves are bound around female medium's waists over their wrappers to prevent the spirit from inadvertently untying and discarding some of her layers of clothes (see fig. 3.3). Apart from securing the spirits' clothes on the mediums' bodies, tying the body with belts, scarves, and wrappers is a way of physically enclosing the spirits within a shell of cloth and thereby creating the contours of the deities' physical substance. The possessing spirit is literally tied, strapped to her human vessel and bound within the layer of fabric that covers the devotee's frame. Clothing thus underscores the coming together of human and superhuman forces by binding the amorphous spirit within the corporeal structure of a *bori* medium.

If the act of weaving cloth or tying clothing has conjugal and reproductive connotations, the act of giving clothing to someone creates a relationship between the gift giver and the recipient. In fact, clothing plays an important role in making or unmaking relationships within society and between the world of people and the world of spirits (see Feeley-Harnik 1989 for a description of the active role of clothing during the second burial, which makes ancestors in Madagascar). I have noted how providing clothing for one's spirit is a crucial

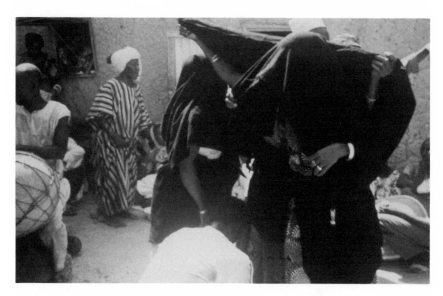

3.3   The tying of the spirits during a possession ceremony. While an assistant is tying a wrapper around the waist of a medium possessed by a Doguwa spirit, another helper is fitting leather shoes on the medium's feet. Photo by A. Masquelier.

step in establishing a viable bond with that spirit, and in cementing the alliance between the human and the supernatural worlds. In the past, according to a colonial report,[10] a gift of clothing would create a filial bond between a man and a child. If a man wanted to adopt a boy, he would dress him in new clothes in the presence of his matrikin and patrikin and say: "I now consider you as my son." Clothing establishes new statuses and connotes new identities in several rites of passage. When a new village chief or king is installed, the first step and one of the most crucial moments of the ceremony consists in tying a turban around that individual's head. Conducted by the king's bodyguard, the turbaning (*nadin rawani*) is a long, careful, and ostentatious process whose unfolding is continually interrupted by the loud praises of loquacious singers and the monetary contributions of villagers eager to help defray the cost of the installment ritual.

Untying: The Breaking of a Relationship Through Clothing

Except for marriage, which is seen as a contract that can be broken any time one of the spouses becomes dissatisfied, the relationships that have been woven through the use and exchange of clothes are supposed to endure until one of the parties dies. For instance, no one can terminate a relationship with a spirit for whatever reasons may be invoked. Only the spirit has the authority to decide she no longer wants to possess or help her horse. Yet, every villager knows of one person who tried—usually unsuccessfully—to sever his bond with the *bori*. To break away from *bori*, dissatisfied adepts destroy the most tangible sign of their involvement with spirits, the deities' clothing. As can be expected, such actions do not meet with the *iskoki*'s approval and are greeted with fierce reprisals.

A Mawri villager I heard of had once decided to abandon his spirits because he was being ostracized by the Muslim community of which he longed to be a respectable member. He knew his friends and neighbors did not approve of his ties to the *bori*. He prayed and wanted to be recognized by other Muslims for his religious commitment. The day he held the naming ceremony (*suna*) of his newborn son, his Muslim neighbors and acquaintances did not show up to share his new happiness and attend the festivities. The new father had been profoundly hurt by this contemptuous gesture and he thus decided to get rid of all the spirits' clothing that he kept with him in order to totally commit himself to Islam. He was a devotee of Malam Alhaji, a quiet and contemplative Muslim deity who usually wears a white *riga* and turban and teaches his horses how to write in Arabic script (see fig. 3.4). He gave Malam Alhaji's walking stick and gown to a *malam* (Muslim scholar/healer) who had offered to destroy the stick for him. After he broke the stick in two, the *malam* felt his hand swell. He became sick and suffered a high fever for a long time. And he lost the use of his hand. The unfaithful *bori* devotee himself was extremely ill until he decided to hold a *wasa* (ceremony) for his spirit in order to apologize for his behavior and beg his forgiveness. He felt compelled to keep on doing *bori* in spite of his aspirations to become a pious follower of the Prophet.

This testimony particularly exemplifies how *'yan bori* and Muslim attitudes differ with regard to the treatment of bothersome spirits. These attitudes are themselves revealing of the differing conceptions of personhood, health, and the cosmos held by *bori* devotees and Muslims. Though most, if not all, Mawri see themselves as enmeshed in intricate webs of visible and invisible forces that must be controlled or kept at bay by whatever means available, *bori* and Islam stand opposed when it comes to dealing with the spirits that occasionally plague people. Islam, along with *bori*, recognizes that there exist spirits (known as *djinns* in the Koran) who form an invisible society in parallel to the human world, but it condemns the coupling of humans and spirits through possession on the grounds that it contradicts fundamental Muslim values based on bodily

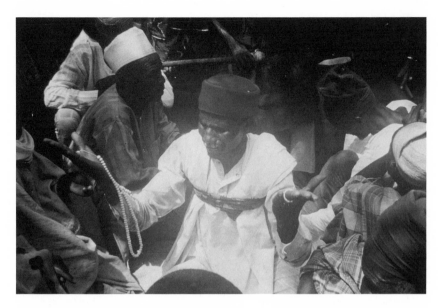

3.4 Zaki Sarki, the contemplative Muslim deity, has possessed one of his mediums, who is now dressed in a white robe and red hat and holding a set of prayer beads. Photo by A. Masquelier.

closure and self-control. Muslim rituals strive to produce self-contained individuals who do not easily let external forces control them and impinge on their bodiliness. Thus intruding spirits must be exorcised, not tamed. That Islamic practices seek, to a certain extent, to free the self from the environment explains why Muslims—that is, those who wish to become, or consider themselves to be, Muslims—would destroy the last tangible remnants of their involvement with a deity. Moreover, anything that emphasizes one's devotion to the spirits, from amulets to *bori* clothes to stone altars,[11] only prevent a person from placing his full trust in his creator and directing his prayers to God only, Muslims say.

Devotees who feel burdened by their religious obligations or aspire to free themselves from what they conceive as an enslaving relationship often attempt to burn their *iskoki*'s clothing. Others simply abandon them on a pile of rubbish. *Iskoki* resent such destructive actions not simply because they signify the rupture of the spirit-devotee bond, but also because the very objects that have been destroyed or desecrated have come to stand for the spirits themselves. For this reason, careless treatment of a deity's wardrobe, even if unintentional, may bear dire consequences for the *iska*'s devotee, as the following examples demonstrate. A man from the village of Ligido sold all the clothes of his very powerful Doguwa spirit—whom he had inherited—to play cards. "Before he spoiled everything," as my informants put it, "he could accomplish extraordinary things because he had the full support of his spirit." If someone gave him raw cotton when he was possessed by the Doguwa, he would put it in his mouth. A few instants later, he would pull cotton threads out. "Now," people said, "he cannot do anything because he did not treat his spirit right." Note that raw cotton was commonly offered to Doguwa spirits when they possessed their devotees. To this day, 'yan bori welcome Doguwa mediums mounted by the deities with a faifai (circular handwoven mat used for covering vessels) covered with cotton. Though Mawri do not, to my knowledge, make an explicit connection between speech and weaving, it is relevant to recall how, most notably in the case of the Dogon (Griaule 1965, 27–29), a relation is established between cloth and word so that to weave cloth is in effect to weave words together in a tight and meaningful fabric.

As I was discussing bori matters with a friend one day, she told me what had allegedly happened a few years ago to her neighbor, a man who had spirits but "fooled around too much." One day, she recalled, he took the wrapper belonging to one of his spirits, and slept on it with a prostitute (karuwa) he had picked up. He used the garment as if it were a vulgar tabarma (mat). During a bori ceremony he attended several weeks later, his spirit mounted him and said: "Why did you take my wrapper to lay down on it with a karuwa? You'll see, it is I who is going to kill you." A few days later he was dead. Aside from pointing to the dangers of misusing and desecrating what belongs to the spirit, this story reminds Mawri that spirits hate seeing their devotees engaging in extramarital affairs or having sex with prostitutes, even though it is common practice among mediums (see Masquelier 1993a). Having committed a double offense against the spirit to whom he owed respect and faithfulness in all things, the man had paid with his own life for his negligent and inconsiderate action.

Clothes need not be destroyed to actualize the severance of a relationship. When a death occurs, the clothes of the deceased are not kept by the surviving kin, but are given away. For instance, a mother who has lost a baby must give away the child's clothes lest they constantly remind her of the deceased when her thoughts and attention should be directed at her other children—the living as well as the yet-to-be-born. Mawri women—as well as men—must remain firm and stoic in the face of such tragic losses, and everything must be done to prevent them from despairing. They must not be left alone to grieve. Rather they must be entertained by the idle chatter of their female kin, friends, and neighbors so that they may soon forget their pain and go on leading productive and happy lives. The deceased's clothes are distributed among his cousins, especially if they took care of him before he died—or if he was sick—and among those who prepared and washed the corpse before burial. If the dead was a grown man, his children should not wear his clothes because they will remind his wife of her late spouse and aggravate her grief instead of helping her to overcome it. Thus, we can begin to discern the structural logic behind the gesture of the grieving mother getting rid of her dead child's garments. The deceased kin now belongs to the dead, whose realm must be kept separate from that of the living in order for the human community to survive and to prosper. By relinquishing personal items of clothing suffused with a child's or spouse's essence, the surviving kin actualize the deceased's new identity as a soul devoid of a body—and which therefore has no need of clothes—while reinforcing the boundaries between the living and the dead.

Women I knew complained that nowadays people were greedy, did not care and did not respect such traditions; sons would thus wear their dead father's clothes if they found items that fit them. Fathers, on the other hand, complained bitterly that their grieving wives had repeatedly given away their deceased children's perfectly good clothing to cousins instead of wisely keeping them for the children to come. They thought everyone should do away with a tradition that was so costly to household heads already faced with the heavy burden of renewing their children's wardrobe on an annual basis.

By giving away a deceased's wardrobe, Mawri acknowledge that the dead individual is no longer among the living, and that anything evoking the dead must be eliminated from the survivors' daily surroundings. It is not that haunting might occur if the deceased's possessions are left among the living kin. I heard of only one instance of the ghost of a dead woman visiting her surviving brother's household, and this ghost was not claiming her belongings. Though those who have died in abnormal circumstances (i.e., in childbirth) had to be buried outside of the village periphery with all their belongings to discourage their spirits from haunting the living, these practices have been progressively eroded by the wave of Islamic fervor that has swept Arewa communities in the last thirty years (see Masquelier in press). Thus, if, in the past, getting rid of the clothes that had belonged to a recently deceased child or spouse was a way of dealing with uprooted souls, haunting is no longer invoked to justify a practice that husbands and fathers would gladly give up. Clothes are such an intimate part of an individual's social persona and presentation of self that they preserve the memory of their owner even when this person is dead. As a tangible evocation of their owner, clothes are in effect extensions of one's body.

This is also suggested by the use of cloth in sorcery. One way to harm someone is to bury a charm (*biso*) made with the hair or pieces of a wrapper belonging to the intended victim. Imbued with malevolent and even deadly power after the proper formula has been uttered, the *biso* will be buried in the victim's compound or field to provoke misfortunes or cause dissension. A fragment of someone's worn garment is as much part of a person's bodiliness as her hair, and like hair, it can be used in manipulations that require a parcel of an individual's social and biological essence. There, clothing no longer creates boundedness or social cohesion. As the metonymic extension of the body, clothes provide the means for destruction itself. Rather than concretizing alliance and reproduction, it captures the frailty and finitude of human lives and enterprises.

The Role and Properties of Clothing in Bori

While most people have to buy the garments that their *bori* deities traditionally wear in order to insure the spirits' satisfaction (and such a wardrobe constitutes a considerable investment for many who have little cash left once they have attended to their primary needs), some individuals are allegedly fortunate enough to find their spirits' garments in the bush. They usually recall that as they were walking, they just stumbled upon a pile of clothes that was just lying there. Though such occurrences are rare, they are commonly interpreted as a sign of deep love from the spirits. Because they are truly attached to these individuals—whom nothing differentiates a priori from the rest of the *bori* community—the spirits do not want them to suffer any hardship or to sacrifice their well-being in order to afford their deity's clothes. "Those who are not loved by the spirits, they must suffer in order to buy spirits' clothing," *'yan bori* commonly say.[12]

Once *'yan bori* have acquired *bori* garments, they have an obligation to bring them to each and every possession ceremony that they will attend. This means that ideally each individual possessed during a ritual will have the proper attire in which ritual assistants will dress the spirit in due course. Getting the spirits appropriately dressed during a ritual is a crucial and delicate operation, which separates the two phases of the *wasa*. Phase one is considered "play" and entails a re-creative performance during which *'yan bori* dance, "warm the place up," and promote the cheerful and enthusiastic mood that will induce the spirits' possession of their human vessels. Play, in this sense, is "work" in that through their dancing and merrymaking, devotees work to bring about the state of receptivity that is prerequisite to any encounter between flesh and spirit. Phase two is about "work," that is, the transformative processes that the spirits control and provoke while they inhabit the bodies of their mediums.[13]

Though spirits—as well as people—are supposed to enjoy the party that has been thrown for them in the first half of the ceremony, once they have enjoyed themselves, they must accomplish whatever is required of them. "Work" (*aiki*) starts with the dressing up of the possessed devotees, a process that entails the shaping of amorphous spiritual entities into virtual bodies. Work then usually entails listening to people's complaints or demands for help and providing adequate counseling. It may also involve healing[14] and a variety of other ritual procedures. At what particular moment in the *wasa* the ritual assistants are to dress the spirits is often the object of considerable debate among the *bori* community. Old devotees often accuse the younger generation of being impatient and of speeding up the entire process so that they can get it over fast. "While work is important, so is play. Nothing should be rushed. The spirits should be allowed to have some fun," one of the old guard told me.

Many people do not bring their spirits' paraphernalia when they attend a *wasa*, either because they do not own any *bori* clothes or because they never suspect that one of their spirits will choose to possess them that day. To remedy such situations, the ritual specialists in charge of the ceremony bring with them several sets of clothing for the various members of the *bori* pantheon. *Bori* healers usually own a vast array of ritual clothes, which they conspicuously display in their homes for visitors and patients to see. They often take the garments throughout their traveling, as much to impress prospective clients as to lend them to devotees whose possessing spirit has no attire.

Some spirits are seriously offended when their horse neglects to bring their gowns or wrappers to a *wasa*. They resent the humiliation of having to borrow clothing in order to make an appearance in the world of humans. Upset and mortified by their devotees' lack of consideration, they might decide to punish them by giving away their clothing to the musicians who by their chants invoke the deities and invite them to possess their human receptacles. While some *'yan bori* see such actions as simply signs of generosity on the part of the spirits, most agree that it is the *iskoki*'s way of making their adepts "suffer" because the gift to the musicians means that another set of clothing will have to be purchased sooner or later.[15] To avoid such unwelcome expenses, one must also keep ritual garments neat and clean. This is especially recommended to the horses of Maria, the coquette prostitute who spends so much time admiring her own reflection in the mirror she keeps at hand. Because Maria dislikes dirt in all its forms—she is often seen sweeping flecks of dust off her immaculate white wrapper—she cannot allow anyone to dress her in soiled attire.[16]

Once it has been given to a particular spirit, a piece of clothing is no longer an ordinary garment that anybody may seize or wear.[17] It is imbued with a power that might prove potentially harmful, even lethal, to the individual who uses the attire in an inappropriate manner or abuses the deity's trust. For many villagers, simply touching the garment of a spirit to whom they have no connection is enough to trigger the deity's anger and cause them to fall ill.[18] As illustrated by the following incident recalled to me by a *bori* healer, *bori* clothing sometimes becomes an accessible and readily manipulable substitute for its supernatural owner. Having been worn by the spirit at countless possession ceremonies, it is forever saturated with that deity's essence in the same way that a person's clothes are suffused by his bodiliness.

An old man came from the region of Tibiri, in the south, to attend a *wasa* in Dogondoutchi. When he arrived at the site of the ceremony, he sat next to a woman whom I shall name Rakya to preserve her anonymity. Rakya wanted to dance as women usually do before the spirits take hold of their horses' bodies to converse with humans, receive offerings of blood and money, and help those in need of divine intervention. Dancing is part of the fun of attending a *wasa,* but it is also necessary to "heat up" the place so that possession may take place. As she got up to dance in the middle of the crowd assembled in a circle, Rakya grabbed her neighbor's black wrapper. Holding the wrapper with both hands extended into the air like graceful wings, she glided over the sandy arena. As her bare feet rhythmically stomped the ground, raising a cloud of dust, she probably smiled as admirers stood to praise her performance by showering her with money. Male and female dancers customarily receive coins, and more rarely banknotes, from members of the audience who enjoy rewarding performers by ostentatiously sticking money on their foreheads—one coin at a time. Upon finishing their performance, dancers usually throw the money to the musicians as a token of their appreciation for the good music they danced to. When her dancing was over, Rakya looked for the stranger from whom she had borrowed the wrapper in a moment of enthusiasm, but he was nowhere to be found. Nobody had seen him leave, nor did anyone know where he had gone. He had been just another man in the faceless crowd of *'yan bori* and cult sympathizers who attended large possession ceremonies in Dogondoutchi. When she enquired as to his identity, Rakya found out from some acquaintances that the person she was looking for was a man whom no one trusted.

Unable to find the stranger whose wrapper she had borrowed, Rakya kept it, not suspecting that in doing so she would become the victim of a carefully planned scheme and that her life would be irremediably changed. No one in Dogondoutchi apparently knew what was wrong with the stranger with the wrapper, or else they might have warned Rakya before it was too late. Thus it was only after the tragedy had started unfolding that it became known that the man from Tibiri had a mean spirit, a Doguwa who, though helpful in the past, had been getting greedier and less manageable as time went by. Determined to get rid of the deity once and for all, the man had consulted a healer who suggested that he go to the distant region of Arewa with the Doguwa's wrapper. "Sometimes, at a *wasa*, people get excited and they want to dance. They borrow anybody's wrapper without paying attention to whom the wrapper's owner might be," said the *bori* adept who was recounting the story to me. Together with the wrapper, the unfortunate Rakya had inherited the old man's spirit. Soon afterwards, the ferocious Doguwa started harming and killing people in Rakya's family circle. A ceremony was held to placate the spirit but to no avail. Within a few years, nearly all of Rakya's children and grandchildren were dead. Two sons, Dade and Dauda, survived the ordeal. One of Dade's sons, whom I shall name Tahirou, later inherited the evil spirit after his grandmother died. "If one borrows the Doguwa's wrapper, only God can protect him against the spirit's attacks. And if Doguwa attacks him but does not choose him as her horse, then she wants to kill him," my storyteller had concluded.

Such a way of becoming a spirit's horse is highly unusual in Mawri society. People most commonly become members of the *bori* by inheriting one or several spirits from a deceased agnate or cognate. Hence, a woman may inherit one spirit from her maternal grandmother and another from her father. Other individuals become members of the *bori* after they are "caught" by a spirit with whom they crossed paths while in the bush, at the market, or on the road. In both cases, the spirit is said to have chosen her devotee because she loved him, even if such love first translates itself as misfortune and affliction for the human vessel. The devotee, who is considered a victim until he succeeds in obtaining the deity's forgiveness and protection, and in achieving a cure, has no control over the situation and cannot prevent spirits from setting their hearts on him. In Rakya's case, in contrast, no feeling of attraction guided the Doguwa's actions. It was not the Doguwa who decided to abandon her previous horse, but rather he who successfully managed to get rid of his troublesome spirit. And it was not the deity who chose Rakya as her new vessel, but rather Rakya herself who unknowingly invited the Doguwa to follow her when she picked up the spirit's wrapper. As she grabbed the wrapper to dance to the sound of the one-stringed violin and calabashes, Rakya irremediably changed her fate and that of her family.

In Rakya's innocent gesture[19] is condensed all the powers attributed to clothing. Clothes may not only bring back disturbing memories of their deceased owner for surviving kin or transmit an individual's message to the world of spirits; they can actually force their spiritual owner to relinquish one human vessel for another. Though the incident recounted is an isolated case, it suggests that clothing are never to be considered neutral elements, insulated from the multiplicity of forces, spiritual and material, that are part of the Mawri universe. Porous and permeable, clothes become so saturated with the personality of their wearer that they become part and parcel of the wearer's essence.[20] So much was clothing a part of the Doguwa's being that the spirit could not let go of it. She had to go wherever the wrapper went, even if it meant relinquishing her hold on a human devotee before he died.

Conclusion

In the way that it shapes, encloses, exposes, and interacts with the body, clothing plays a crucial role in defining and expressing social, economic and moral identities. In the context of *bori* possession, this role becomes even more preponderant as spirits' clothes give shape, volume, color, and texture to ethereal beings. Clothes take on a life of their own in actively mediating relations between deities and people and binding an amorphous spirit within the confines of a human body. Because clothing provides a tangible medium through which to reach out to the spirits wherever they are, it is, like music and words, an essential tool for constructing and physically inscribing in the very fiber of the cloth one's relation to a spirit. In other words, clothes offer a space in which spirits can become, in a tenuous and temporary way, substantial entities. Part of the power of spirits' clothing resides in their ability to transcend the world of mortals, connecting it to the spirit world. The data I have presented also underscore the absorbent quality of clothing, which soaks up words and prayers; imbibes material, moral, and spiritual substances; and absorbs personal identities.

Qualities, relations, and configurations are created, transformed, and exchanged through the clothes that *bori* devotees keep and wear to objectify their bond with supernatural entities. Long after spirits have abandoned their human vessels, their clothes remain as evidence not simply of possession but of all the communication and transactions that have taken place between them and the people with whom they interacted. The clothing of a spirit not only sets its present owner or wearer in a privileged field of relationships, it also absorbs all the moral and material essences and processes that define one's relationship to a spirit. Thus onto each *bori* wrapper or robe are inscribed the stories and histories of a spirit and her human devotees or victims. Yet, such inscription is impermanent because clothing, like mortals who age, wither and die, wears out and turns into rags. As Renne (1991, 714) points out, on the one hand, such impermanence constitutes a poignant expression of the recycling of mediums, whose bodies are transient vessels that must be replaced as they wear out. On the other hand, Renne notes, the ephemerality of old clothing, which disintegrates and turns to shreds, entails its replacement with new clothes, thereby contributing to a sense of continuity. It is such constancy that *bori* stresses through its injunctions that cult members constantly replenish their spirits' wardrobe.

By focusing on clothing, I have stressed how deeply the spirit world and the realm of humans intersect. *Bori* devotees meet the spirits on the possession grounds, but they are also in constant contact with them thanks to the clothes that they may be wearing or keeping in a trunk—as residues, folded contours of tenuous "bodies" that give spirits life. As such, the practice of keeping a spirit's wardrobe also exemplifies the rootedness of *bori* in mundane settings and daily life. *Bori* does not come alive solely in the arena of trance when spiritual forces take possession of their human vessels in the context of ritually circumscribed events. By the same token, engaging in a fruitful relationship with a deity of the cult does not simply mean attending noisy ceremonies and theatrical parades of colorful costumes. For *bori* is part and parcel of one's everyday experience, and its meanings and conventions help shape Mawri lived realities as much as enduring Mawri values inform *bori* constructions of the world. Indeed, *bori* is so rooted in the fabric of quotidian life that it cannot be circumscribed as a discrete sphere of knowledge or as a separate form of practice. The spirits themselves continually intervene in human affairs. Though they belong to a mysterious and distant realm, they are intimately part of people's daily lives thanks in part to the *bori* clothing, whose very fabrics provide the strands that link distinct worlds of experience on a quotidian basis.

Notes

This article is based on research conducted in southern Niger in 1988–1989. I am grateful for the support of the National Science Foundation, the National Institute of Mental Health, and the Wenner-Gren Foundation for Anthropological Research. Jean Comaroff, Nancy Munn, Misty Bastian, Brad Weiss, and Hildi Hendrickson provided helpful critiques of earlier versions of this essay. I also thank William Fisher for his invaluable editorial assistance.

1   An *arrondissement* is the administrative division within the *département,* the latter corresponding roughly to the notion of county. Dogondoutchi, which counts about 20,000 inhabitants, is the administrative seat of the *arrondissement* and the town where I conducted a large part of my fieldwork.

2   Today children are generally no longer scarred, and only individuals who are over age twenty exhibit these marks of their cultural "heritage" (*gado*).

3   The audience at *bori* rituals is composed largely of mediums, but there are also those who regularly attend *wasani* (ceremonies) without ever being possessed. They might come to the ceremonies to ask for a spirit's help or advice or simply for the sheer enjoyment of watching people dance, meeting friends, or finding romance (see Masquelier 1993a).

4   Christians account for 1 percent of the population, of which the majority live in Niamey, the capital, and is made up of expatriates. A small minority of villagers are also referred to as *Azna:* they descend from the Gubawa who first settled in the area and still claim ritual ties to the land through their worship of local deities.

5   White is Adama's color, which is why she is called "white Doguwa" (*fara Doguwa*) or "the owner of a white wrapper" (*mai farin zane*).

6   Wax cloth is produced by first spreading onto bleached cotton fabric a thin resin or wax resist in a repeating pattern. When the resin has dried, the cloth is first crinkled (to leave thin cracks in the resin) and then submerged in a dye bath to color the areas that are free of resin. Thin veins of color are left on the cloth as the dye seeps through the cracks in the resin. These veins are what identify factory-produced wax cloth (Bickford 1994, 7).

7   *Zane* (Hausa) or *pagne* (French), which we commonly translate as "wrapper," are the designated terms used to refer to a standard measure by which factory-produced cloth is sold (2 meters by 1.6 meters). Such cloth, generally destined to outfit women, is sold by units of three *pagnes*.

8   For an interesting account of the shrewd and creative use of textile imagery in Ivoirian politics to elicit widespread support, incite feelings of loyalty, or resurrect the flagging popularity of a party, see Bickford 1994.

9   For a fascinating account of how the nineteenth- and twentieth-century Euro-African textile trade shattered mercantile Europe's distorting lens of preconceptions and later refined this continent's image of Africa, see Steiner 1984.

10 Monographie de la Subdivision de Doutchi (c. 1936–1940), Documents 6.1.6. Niamey: Archives Nationales du Niger.

11 Mediums shed the blood of their spirits' favorite animal on a stone (*doutchi*) that has been ritually erected in a place chosen by the deities. Each spirit has a stone that in some cases is considered a home and to which any villager may come when in need of the *iska*'s help.

12 Many *bori* devotees to whom I spoke insisted that it was the spirits themselves who made sure their mediums had enough resources to buy the paraphernalia they required (by bringing to their human receptacles "clients" who needed the mediums' assistance in securing supernatural advice or protection, and who would later reward them for their services). Nonetheless, it is clear that having a spirit one must "clothe" and "feed" is a financial burden on most cult members.

13 As Drewal (1992, 15) has put it in reference to Yoruba ritual, "Performing ritual is at once 'hard work' and 'playing.'" This implies that, not unlike the Mawri concept of *wasa*, the Yoruba notion of play is not opposed to "work" but rather that it

must be understood as a re-creative process (i.e., a process at once diverting and transformative).

14   Though each *wasa* (possession ceremony) that is held, and financed, by a particular medium or initiate—in contrast to community-sponsored rituals—focuses on the particular problems and ailments of this individual, it also caters to the needs of all those who seek to resolve and make sense of conflict-laden experience. Though it ostensibly deals with the reconstruction of one individual's life, the *wasa* simultaneously addresses the renewal of the community at large.

15   More often than not, the garments are purchased from the musicians to whom they were given by the spirit in the first place. The devotee pays the musicians a sum of money referred to as *hansa riga*. It is not a monetary equivalent to the actual value of the wrapper or robe given away, but rather a compensation given to the musicians so that they agree to let the garment go. It usually amounts to whatever the devotee is willing to give.

16   At one *wasa* I attended, a devotee possessed by Maria got up from the mat where she was sitting to reveal a conspicuous blood stain on the back of her white wrapper. Everyone in the audience shuddered before an old woman rushed to tie a wrapper on the woman's hip and pull her out of the *bori* ring. Aside from having deeply offended Maria's sense of cleanliness and propriety, the devotee had committed an abomination by participating in a possession ritual while she was menstruating. I left the field too soon after the incident to witness any form of supernatural retaliation on the part of the spirit. Nevertheless, *bori* adepts whom I talked to were convinced that Maria's punishment was imminent.

17   Spirits' clothes do not burn like ordinary garments when they come in contact with fire. An informant once told me that the spirits burnt her house down because they did not want her to engage in trading. She had stocked some bags of flour in her room. One day, a fire started in there. The flour was burnt. My informant lost her own seven outfits, but none of the spirits' clothes or paraphernalia were damaged.

18   According to Rheinhardt (1979, 263), the costumes worn by members of Mende secret societies who impersonate spirits are equally suffused with the dangerous power associated with these superhuman forces. Hence, "all the spirits have medicine as part of their accoutrement. It is the medicine which activates the costume as a spirit and makes it very wonderful and dangerous at the same time." Rheinhardt also notes that when the costumes are worn by Sande women,

> there are also other attendants, one of whose jobs it is to pick up even the very smallest pieces of rafia that may fall from the costume. The reason given for this is that if a man unknowingly should step on such a strand of the sacred costume he will contract genital elephantiasis. (1979, 244)

19   Rakya's gesture was innocent insofar as she knew nothing of the devilish scheme masterminded by the wrapper's owner. It is possible, of course, that borrowing the piece of clothing from this total stranger was Rakya's way of teasing the man or, at

least, of catching his attention before she went on to show how graceful a dancer she was. *Bori* ceremonies are known to be the scene of numerous romantic encounters and attempts at seduction, and this is why married men who fear for their wives' virtue forbid their spouses to attend possession rituals.

20   The following incident also illustrates how clothing becomes identified with its owners. A villager had once been accused of being a *maye* (witch) and of killing half a dozen people. Rumors had it that he had made a contract with a Doguwa spirit who helped him become rich in exchange for which he designated human victims to the bloodthirsty deity (see Masquelier 1993a). When the man died, no one had wanted any of his clothing. People were afraid that if they took some of his clothes, they would be followed by the evil spirit who had followed her master like a shadow.

II CHALLENGING AUTHORITY

4 FEMALE *"ALHAJIS"* AND ENTREPRENEURIAL FASHIONS: FLEXIBLE IDENTITIES IN SOUTHEASTERN NIGERIAN CLOTHING PRACTICE

Misty L. Bastian

Introduction: Western, Consumption-based Theories
of Fashion and Identity

In her definitive, historical work on cloth, clothing, and the practice of revealing and concealing the human body in Western art, Anne Hollander (1975, 452–53) observes:

> When people put clothes on their bodies, they are primarily engaged in making pictures of themselves to suit their own eyes, out of the completed combination of clothing and body. The people who do this most readily are those living in civilizations in which the naturalistic image of man is the cornerstone of art, and the pictures they make when they dress are directly connected to the pictures they ordinarily see and accept as real.

Writing during that ancient era of the 1970s, before theories of representation emerged from the province of the art historian and engaged social scientists as well as humanists, Hollander tied her own theorizing of bodily figuration and clothing practice to a belief that the fixed image was required for bodies to be made as stylish as the objects that adorned them. This image-centered notion of bodily styles is important, because the images that surround us in the print and electronic media certainly do influence our notion of "proper" bodily presentation. Because of what we see when we peer through the lens of popular media, we have (sometimes quite peculiar) ideas about how ordinary people dress and look—from the constantly attenuating female form, to spandex exercise gear color-coordinated with one's Rollerblades and even one's portable stereo equipment, to skin tones that both suggest and deny the significance of racial difference for music video and Benetton sportswear.

Until very recently, it has also been fashionable in Western cultural theorizing to suggest that these images oppress the clothing consumer, rather than to argue for the radical, subversive possibilities inherent in dress.[1] As an example of one form of image oppression, Hollander's work on body-based representation and clothing-based bodies was taken up by Kaja Silverman (1986, 145–46) and pressed into service for an argument about woman-as-spectacle, the object of an increasingly self-conscious male gaze. In Silverman's essay, women's bodies in clothing became objects for (visual as well as material) consumption, along with being represented as objects of sexual desire. She maintains the basic premise of passivity in women's dressing, even while noting its transformative qualities:

> The endless transformation within female clothing constructs female sexuality and subjectivity in ways that are at least profoundly disruptive, both of gender and of the symbolic order, which is predicated upon continuity and coherence. However, by freezing the male body into phallic rigidity, the uniform of orthodox male dress makes it a rock against which the waves of female fashion crash in vain. (Silverman 1986, 148)

Although agreeing that men are often fascinated by the intricacies of female dress in Western society, Silverman disallows any lasting effect from men's experience of women's clothing practice. In so doing, she disallows men an active clothing practice: they are represented by Silverman as frozen, rigid, rock-like, and phallic in their relations to clothing and subsequently in their relations to women.[2] The only salvation that Silverman sees in contemporary Western clothing practice comes from harvesting the not-quite-fully-consumed use value of secondhand clothing, making an intimate connection both to past fashion practices and to the bodies of men and women who once wore those clothes.

Silverman's argument made an immediate impact on Western theorists of subculture, style, and fashion. For example, Angela McRobbie (1989) took up and elaborated Silverman's point about used clothing in her essay "Second-Hand Dresses and the Role of the Ragmarket." McRobbie demonstrates how young women in Britain took up "retro" clothing by searching it out, buying it, restoring or altering it, and combining it with elements from mainstream dress in a bricolage that marked retro consumers as fashionably different and as part of a potential fashion avant-garde. The mixing of gender and other identities played an important role in the experiments of McRobbie's youthful clothing practitioners, these mixtures allowing young women[3] to express their perceived disconnection from mainstream cultural constructions as well as their sense of how those constructions must be reordered.

Irony and the ethos of masquerade were at work as women effected male style and appropriated ill-fitting male dress: this attire "imposed a masculine frame on what was still unmistakably a female form. All sorts of softening devices were added to achieve this effect—diamante brooches, lop-sided berets, provocatively red lipstick and so on" (McRobbie 1989, 44). This was a far, resistant cry from the so-called "success dressing" of the 1970s and early 1980s, which required businesswomen to take on the classic "rigidity" of Western male clothing referred to by Silverman above—liberating the retro-dressers, as Susan Faludi (1991, 176) notes, "from fashion-victim status" and, more to the point, from a need to constantly reinvest in their wardrobes. By appropriating aspects of male style without necessarily seeking to infiltrate the male-dominated world of capitalist business, McRobbie suggests that British female youth were able to take an ironic position toward and even to make implicit critical statements about gender privilege in their society through their clothing practice.

The notion of a clothing practice, rather than the more abstract concept of style, arises out of the work of scholars like Hollander, Silverman, and McRobbie—although none of these theorists, to my knowledge, use that term. By invoking practice when discussing how people dress themselves, within and outside the limitations set by their society's conventions, I also want to invoke Bourdieu's stricture on practical logic.[4] It is possible to take our understanding of Western consumption and clothing practice and apply it too widely to what may appear to be a similar phenomenon. Even if so-called non-Western societies now use popular media images to convey a sense of the fashionable to their "populace," for instance, how can we be sure that non-Western readers/listeners/viewers are receiving these media messages and are proceeding to practice an exactly parallel or purely Western-style consumerism because of them? The idea of consumption itself needs to be problematized, and only studies that take very specific notice of local practice(s) give us the space to construct such a problematic. My discipline, anthropology, has not been lax in looking at specific practices associated with clothing—but there still remains a tendency to focus on the production of clothing's raw materials or to analyze clothing practice strictly in Western, theoretical terms.[5] One of the best recent collections of anthropological essays on cloth can serve as a case in point.

In their introduction to *Cloth and Human Experience,* Jane Schneider and Annette B. Weiner (1989, 1) suggest the importance of cloth to the making and transformation of political and social meanings in human societies. My difficulty with their formulation is that their emphasis on cloth tends to make clothing, and clothing practice, seem a secondary construction—sometimes even a superstructural form, masking the more important reality of material production. (Here I am purposefully using the term superstructure in a way that would be greatly disapproved by Raymond Williams [1980, 31–49].) I do not discount the important work done by the contributors to *Cloth and Human Experience,* but I do want to go beyond a notion of the importance of cloth itself to discuss what may seem a more commonsense problem: what it means to be clothed, to experience clothing on one's body, and to clothe others—in short, what might constitute the embodied practice(s) of clothing.

Clothing is not discussed here as an *artifact* of Nigerian society so much as an expressive cultural form—what might once have been called *artifice.* Taking my cue from Hollander and her followers, I am especially interested in how memory, history, and identity adhere to and exist in the very seams and folds of clothing: how clothing shapes bodies and even, in some cases, gives form to amorphous bodies and calls up temporary and tenuous but nonetheless embodied, historically specific identities. This means I want to talk about the relationships between bodies and clothing, and how a knowledge of gender, history, and the powers of a wider world can be physically transmitted through the textures, shapes, smells, and understood aesthetic judgments embodied in clothing.[6]

One of the purposes of this essay, then, is to think about clothing as "a medium for the transfer of essential substances" (Schneider and Weiner 1989, 18), but without defining too strictly what might constitute such substances—whether material, spiritual, moral, or any combination of the three. I do not argue, however, for the primacy of any one substance, unless that substance be the constructed quality of the body itself. Clothing is not only cloth or even a combination of cloth and accessories. Clothing is also constructed from the bodies that are purposefully concealed and revealed by cloth and other forms of adornment. The purposeful quality and practice of clothing is my main concern, and therefore the interplay of images of clothing and observed clothing practice within Nigeria constitute my data.

The "Alhaji" Look: Gender, Class, and Ethnic Identities through Clothing Practice

"Mr & Mrs": cross-dressing on the cartoon page

In an early essay on the history of "Western" dress among Luo-speakers, Margaret Jean Hay (1989, 14–15) poses several very salient questions about the importation and reception of Westernized clothing in colonial Kenya. One of those questions has to do with the moral system encoded in the clothing that mission Christianity considered appropriate for girls and women to wear, and

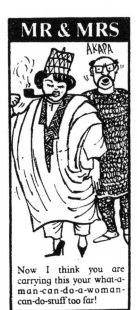

4.1   Cartoon from *The Vanguard* (Lagos), 23 July 1987.

the other deals with how clothing practice can challenge "older forms of status and authority" (Hay 1989, 14). The first question is fully implicated in the second: it seems clear from Hay's analysis that moral systems as well as status hierarchies were at risk in Luo women's (and young men's) adaptation of Westernized clothing. Men found it difficult to exercise control over women who covered their bodies from neck to ankles with missionary-designed dresses, and male elders experienced a distinct lack of respect and tolerance from young men who took on fashions similar to those being worn by colonial officials.

In this section of the chapter, I trace how similar moral and hierarchical dilemmas are at work in contemporary Nigerian clothing practice, as indigenous peoples experiment with combinations of Westernized and local dress (now considered "traditional," even though historically quite recent in its introduction and popularity) and particularly as women experiment with dress generally associated with men and male-dominated business.[7] As several Africanist historians and ethnographers of clothing (Wass 1979; Michelman and Erekosima 1992) demonstrate, what seems most "traditional" about Nigerian traditional clothing practices is their constant experimentation and co-option of outside forms and objects.

Images of dress and gender are often conflated in popular media, making explicit just this sort of experimental practice. Figure 4.1 is a cartoon clipped from the Nigerian daily newspaper, *The Vanguard,* during my fieldwork in 1987–88. "Mr & Mrs" by Akapa appeared regularly; as probably can be surmised from the content of this strip, the series depicted a Nigerian, comic version of the "battle between the sexes." In "Mr & Mrs," Akapa took on both men and women as culprits in this war—sometimes showing men caught lying about their infidelities or sending women up for their extravagant tastes. It always showed two figures in conversation or dispute, a man and a woman dressed in some variation of contemporary Nigerian style. In 1987–88 *The Vanguard* was the only daily to offer a comics page in every edition, and this, according to my Nigerian friends, was one of the reasons for the newspaper's success. "Mr & Mrs" seemed to appeal most to the well-educated, slightly younger urban audience whose tastes, experiences in relationships, and images it monitored and reflected.

In figure 4.1, the female figure effectively dominates the strip by having been placed in the foreground, overshadowing her male counterpart with the (as we shall see) manufactured height and width of her body. Behind this female power figure—signified even more clearly by the "muscleman" gesture she makes with her right arm—is an annoyed male figure. He is ostensibly telling off his female companion, but is actually talking to the back of her head. The woman is shown with a pipe clenched between her teeth, wearing trousers, a flowing, embroidered overtunic, high heels, and a tall, patterned hat. In contrast, the male figure wears a much simpler dress, consisting only of a uniformly patterned long shirt over a pair of trousers, with very neat but plain sandals on his feet. Besides the obvious sight joke consisting of the relative disparity between their physical sizes and positioning in the strip, the cartoonist's humor depends on a very elaborate understanding of Nigerian fashion practice and its recent transformations among his readers / viewers.

Most of the woman's garb is encoded as "male"—furthermore, as a form of male dress associated with well-to-do, Muslim men from the north, the so-called "Hausa" or "*Alhaji*" style. Only her shoes and hairstyle are "female" or "feminine" in their orientation. The man's dress is also encoded as "male," but it is very much the uniform of the average Nigerian man—suitable for everyday wear and made fashionable only by the fashionability of its *agbada* print.[8] The woman's expropriation of the prerogatives associated with male dress is made explicit in the text, where the man says, "Now I think you are carrying this your what-a-man-can-do-a-woman-can-do-stuff too far!" As Marjorie Garber (1992, 28) so sufficiently points out, "Excess, that which overflows a boundary, is the space of the transvestite." Akapa's cartoon seems to suggest that having political and / or economic equality is all right, to a point. The boundary that should not be transgressed is a symbolic, representational one; the space created by cross-dress practice is the space that takes women "too far." Our own question must be: Too far from what?

Issues of gender and class are called on in this cartoon to make the point that women are attempting to place themselves (wrongly) out of category, and that men's "true" gender identities are suffering thereby. By wearing the *"Alhaji"* style dress most associated with Hausa—or well-to-do, northern—businessmen, the cartoon woman associates herself with the fast-paced, highly public world of both men and Westernized business. Her dress is also much richer than that of her male counterpart, an ostentatious arrangement of cloth and embroidery that usually is equated with extreme wealth throughout Nigeria. This oppressively ornate attire closely affiliates the female figure in Akapa's drawing with a minute and elite (male-dominated) class who are believed to control most of the nation's wealth, including money administered for the public. Very like this renegade class, the cartoon woman pays no attention to the voice of male, Nigerian reason. She displays her strength and power heedlessly, not deigning to notice the strictures addressed by the man who is trailing her. The "Mrs" of figure 4.1 has thus adopted a problematic male frame for her new persona/style. Even the few "feminine" articles of clothing or adornment in her outfit are threatening or out-of-category in another sense; her shoes are all dangerous points and angles, and her hairstyle is determinedly "relaxed" and western in its cut.[9]

There is something ludicrous about the woman's attire, however, that adds to the comedy while undercutting "Mrs's" gender and class pretensions. Her female body is obscured by the ballooning folds of her overtunic—she bulges at the abdominal area rather than at the hips or breasts. Although women's protruding stomachs can be considered attractive in southern Nigerian societies, this undifferentiated curve from neck to thighs is not how a womanly stomach would ordinarily be presented: it is as if she had become all stomach, able to consume everything she surveys.[10] The rakish tilt of her tall cap—associated indelibly in the minds of many southern Nigerians with the excesses of the last republic—and her large, awkward pipe, add to the overall feeling of oddity at the same time they give her added height and width, allowing her to dominate the frame. Although she does not appear uncomfortable in this dress, an implicit contrast is quite literally drawn between the modest, appropriate neatness of the man's attire and the overwhelming volume of her costume. By the combination of his eyeglasses, nicely groomed mustache, and generalized dress, "Mr" is shown to be a solid, middle-class, Nigerian everyman—a (male) person of some but moderate substance. The appropriate quality of his power/knowledge (in a Foucauldian sense) is therefore played against "Mrs's" broken social and gender boundaries, to her detriment; she is excessive; she has gone "too far."

The visual-rhetorical device of the mannish woman and the womanish man is ancient in Western comedic discourse; it is now a cliché. And, while many of the Nigerian readers of the *Vanguard* newspaper in 1987 were certainly aware of this cliché, they also knew that the cartoon rested upon what was a current fact of southern Nigerian clothing practice: that some (mostly urban) women actually were beginning to take on male dress as part of their everyday wear.[11] It was also commonly recognized, at least among my urban friends in the southeast, that the power of this usage lay very much in women's symbolic association of male dress with the prerogatives of men. Women who took on a feminized variation of the outfit that Akapa satirizes in figure 4.1 wanted to make a public statement about transformations in gender, education, and economic status that they had already experienced or that they considered the obvious next step in "development" for their country.[12]

"Alhaji" looks: playing with bodily, gendered, and class stereotypes
While doing fieldwork in Onitsha, Nigeria, I was witness to women's business and leisure dressing that played upon the very contradictions in understood gender status and clothing practice that exercised Akapa's pen in figure 4.1.[13] I saw outfits being constructed that were quite similar to the one shown in Akapa's cartoon—with the exception of the tall, "Hausa-style" hat. Among Igbo-speaking women of the elite classes in Onitsha—women whose economic position usually came from their ties, through men, to the professions and lineage ownership of expensive rental properties—it was fashionable to buy expensive, finely woven cotton brocade to be made into local variations of the classic wrapper and blouse, elaborate party frocks, and other Western-inspired fashions, as well as the daring, new *"alhaji"* outfits. Guinea brocade was a cloth imported from and always associated with the northern regions of Nigeria, where it was the fabric of choice for all rich attire.[14] However, we should note that the brocade cloth's provenance only begins to suggest the complexity of political, social, and economic interactions being referred to in the *"alhaji"* style. It is especially important for a non-Nigerian audience to understand exactly whose dress southern women were modifying and affecting in this fashion, as well as how they modified or affected it.

The term *"alhaji"*—a man who has made the *hajj*, the pilgrimage to Mecca—was used as an honorific in Nigerian Muslim circles, but during the late 1980s, this honorific was taken up in the Christianized south, with more satiric intent, to imply a certain clannishness, class exclusivity, and signs of (both overt and covert) overindulgence among socially prominent followers of the Prophet. The stereotypic image of a "rich *alhaji*," for my southern Nigerian friends, consisted of a sleek, fat-stomached man wearing a voluminous overtunic, long shirt, and drawstring trousers, elaborately embroidered at the neck and along the trousers' edges. His hat should be colorful and tall, perched on top of his well-cut hair, his shoes either foreign-made (and highly polished) or locally produced creations decorated with carvings and dyework. To complete the picture, he should wear costly, dark sunglasses—preferably Ray-Bans or designer glasses—and carry a Western-style briefcase or some other type of leather bag.

Interestingly, this was *the* Nigerian male image of the 1970s oil boom. The "Hausa style," or *agbada* (a Yoruba term), was taken up by most politicians and businessmen—who abandoned the three-piece, European suit in its favor—as a symbol of national pride and unity after the 1960s civil war. Outside the country's boundaries the "Hausa style" was used, by prosperous male elites who traveled abroad in search of lucrative private deals as well as trade and aid packages, to signify a badge of committed Nigerian nationalism to a world that was skeptical about the continuing effects of Nigerian "tribalism" on business relations.[15] It should be remembered that the Nigerian civil war (aka the Biafran civil war) was a major media event in the West, one of the first African tragedies to establish what is now a televisual staple: the image of the emaciated, swollen-bellied child staring directly into the camera lens and Western living room. The new Nigerian male style of the 1970s, signified by the free-flowing *agbada* and signifying a freewheeling, laissez-faire approach to capitalism, gradually replaced Biafra in Western media consciousness. Within Nigeria itself, the practice of dressing in *agbada* or "Hausa" was firmly associated with the high life, the art of the deal (which included "kola" or "express," the judicious use of gratuities and bribes), and with sanctimonious public oratory (e.g., President Shagari's "ethical revolution") that covered, like the folds of the *agbada* overtunic, a multitude of sins.

Paradoxically, the negative stereotypes attached to "Hausa style" did not serve to make it less attractive or popular in male Nigerian clothing practice— except sporadically—throughout the years. Even the collapse of the oil boom and the Second Republic did not signal the collapse of the *agbada;* although it did go into a slight remission, with overtunics trimmed down from fifteen yards (or more) of expensive brocade to seven or even five yards and embroidery made more discreet for everyday wear. For younger men, the overtunic was often discarded altogether in favor of the simpler shirt and drawstring trousers represented in the Akapa cartoon.[16] Nonetheless, the full *agbada* look was still available and still worn by men at parties, book launchings, and other appropriate social events. Although young men would wear the *agbada,* many no longer saw it as the definitive Nigerian male style, even for brocade dressing. New (male and female) designers, often university friends of the young elite, were busy exploring the dramatic possibilities of cutting, tucking, and silhouette reconstruction for men's brocade clothing based on *agbada* and other local attires.

It was southern women, in the late 1980s, who threatened to reconstitute the full *agbada* as a popular Nigerian fashion; particularly young southern women who wanted to design clothing for themselves that would be extravagant but not constrictive. This was partially a response to several decades of Nigerian women's (Westernized) dress practice that stipulated tight skirts, nipped-in waists, low-cut necklines, and increasingly elaborate sleeves, collars, and peplums. Arising out of a continuing—several decades long—sensibility that "frocks" should strongly emphasize the rounded bosom and hips, this hyper-feminine clothing practice required a body shape that most women could achieve only with artificial enhancement, "pushup" brassieres or padding and pinching waistbands or girdles being the most common ones.[17]

Since the 1970s, some southern, urban women had also worn trousers, especially tight jeans with T-shirts or variously styled blouses. This was not as much a departure from their frocks as one might think, because the midsection of their bodies was just as surely emphasized in these garments—the waist could be even more securely cinched in by encircling waistbands and belts, and the stomach was flattened, thrusting out the hips. The shape of the frock and of other Nigerian women's westernized garb thus tended to foreshorten their bodies, making them appear shorter than they really were. Most young women would alleviate this—particularly in the case of the frock—by wearing high-heeled shoes or sandals and a small hat or discreet, matching headtie.

The other preferred form of female attire during 1987–88 has been referred to already: the wrapper and blouse combination. This consisted of a loosely constructed blouse, usually with short or no sleeves and a low back and neckline, and a three- to five-yard piece of unconstructed (or little constructed) fabric that was wrapped and folded securely at the natural waistline. Southeastern women wore this in many combinations, using matching fabrics like that shown for the man in figure 4.1 or contrasting ones. In the case of wealthy women's richest finery, the latter might consist of a "lace" (*broderie anglais*) blouse and two bottom wrappers made of "george" (an expensive, embroidered and/or painted cloth from South India). Like the frocks discussed above, blouse and wrapper tended to emphasize the body's midsection with its low-cut bodice and purposeful thickness between the waist and hip.[18]

Hip size was even more accentuated by the wearing of the "Igbo style" of double wrapping—when the smaller, top wrapper was unraveled, pulled out from the waist, and rewrapped in an emphatic and common gesture, it could create the illusion that the lower body was greatly extended out into space. In the Igbo blouse and wrapper style women also could display a protruding stomach simply by pushing the front waist of their overwrapper down, under the belly's swell. The female bodily aesthetic based on the rounded torso was still supported, and even augmented, by this display: a slightly protruding stomach could mean either a well-nourished, "wet" woman (fat female bodies were aesthetically pleasing, especially to older people) or a newly pregnant one.[19] Neither of these stomach displays were, like the drawing in figure 4.1, threatening because they were part of a complete mid-section, sexualized bodily emphasis. (However, it should be said that, among Onitsha Igbo-speaking people, really large women who dressed richly and had reputations as powerful people in the town were potentially threatening—and such women could use the display of their bodies in clothing to intimidate men as well as other women.) By deflecting the focus of internal preoccupations and external gazes from the midsection of their bodies, southern Nigerian women's espousal of the "alhaji" look offered a new and contradictory view of female body aesthetics that intersected with more overt issues of gender, class, and power.

Before addressing these issues more directly, we should pause to examine exactly what the "alhaji" look consisted of, particularly since it was not the exact duplicate of agbada men's wear—including pipe smoking—implied by Akapa. Some young women did have embroidered overtunics made for themselves, but they were not the enormous Second Republic variety. One woman of my acquaintance had a less bulky overtunic constructed that opened down the front, rather like a long vest. Like the agbada, she wore this on top of a simply cut, knee-length shirt and drawstring trousers. The frontal opening of the tunic allowed for an elaborate and continuous embroidery that was different in appearance from that of "traditional" Hausa-style. The effect, as she told me in English, was "to slim me down, and to let me be comfortable." She wore her "male attire" with modest high heels or extremely delicate, "feminine" flats and a matching handbag. Although she commissioned both a small, round cap and a headtie of the same brocade fabric, she rarely ventured to wear the cap.

Other women were more daring in their co-option of the agbada costume and wore both a recognizable overtunic (although generally cut out of five yards of cloth, like a wrapper) and a cap, rakishly planted on the tops of their heads. Some women added sunglasses for dramatic effect, as well as for practical reasons. The female "alhaji" look was completed with heavy makeup, gold necklaces, bracelets, and earrings (if the wearer owned such riches), and noticeable perfume. Hair could be arranged in a Western, relaxed style or in braided "attachments."

Men were not overwhelming in their support of the new look—even young, urban men who liked women to wear jeans and Western styles. Resistance against the "*alhaji*" look came from several male quarters. When some of the young Onitsha women of my acquaintance heard about the style (from friends in the Nigerian metropole, Lagos) and wanted to adopt it, they went first to the market to procure the necessary guinea brocade. Male traders were happy to sell the expensive cloth and to give advice about how much was needed to construct a "Hausa" outfit (as many as fifteen or twenty yards, in their hopeful, commercially based imaginations)—so long as they thought the women were buying for their husbands, fathers, or brothers. Upon hearing that the women wanted the material for their own use, some traders tried to convince their customers that it was "impossible" for them to wear such a dress. One Igbo-speaking trader went so far as to refuse to sell women the necessary yardage in a single piece; he would sell them only enough to make a wrapper or frock. (The women, who were his regular customers and who liked his prices, simply sent other female friends to Main Market the next day, and these friends bought the rest of the fabric needed.) Other, more pragmatic traders sold the cloth, but prefaced its purchase with moral instruction: "Women shouldn't look like men. Our fathers never heard of that, and it isn't in the Bible."

The young woman whose "*alhaji*" outfit I described above also had difficulty finding a northern tailor who would make the attire for her. Like the traders, these nonindigenous residents of the town depended on the custom of women like my friend to make a living, but they actively resisted the idea of making menswear for women. After considering how much trouble it would be to force "one of those Hausa" to sew her outfit, she took her innovative design and the brocade to an Igbo-speaking seamstress, who quickly cut out the pieces. Then she took the pieces that needed embroidery back to one of the northern tailors and convinced him to do the detail work. The garment was actually put together, after sections were embroidered, by the seamstress. The compromise solution proved to be an excellent one: the tailor did not have to make men's garb for a woman, but he still had some skilled work for which he was paid, the seamstress not only had work but learned how to make the new style, and my friend finally had her "*alhaji*" outfit. Other young Onitsha women had similar difficulties and similar stories to tell.

The attire's critical reception among men and some women was extremely mixed. Although younger men tended to take the new style in stride and even to celebrate it as a good fashion joke, some older men were less amused. After seeing an "*alhaji*" at a social event, the successful, well-educated, middle-aged father of one of my friends forbade her to own such a "disgraceful" costume. (This was just one in a long succession of generational battles in their household.) She confided in me that it was too late; she was already having it constructed: "I'll just wear it when I go to Lagos for parties." Her mother, engaged in her own domestic disputes, paid for the expensive brocade. As in the case of the northern tailor, above, a circumlocution defused active resistance to the dress, which enabled its wearer to both have her clothing gesture and keep the issue from becoming the subject of outright familial confrontation. At the same time, the attire was covertly endorsed by a woman who intended to make her husband pay, however indirectly, for the cross-gender clothing practice he wanted to control.[20]

Not all older women were as supportive of the new fashion as my friend's mother. An Onitsha female elder told me, after seeing the "*alhaji*" look on one of her youthful relations, that—if women still had the power of her mother's day—this would be stopped. When I asked why the attire so offended her, she remarked that it was not good, maybe even an abomination against the earth goddess, for women to look the same as men. I persisted, asking what was wrong with women wearing men's dress, and the elder clearly was incredulous: "Do you want to be a man and have a thing hang between your legs? In that cloth you cannot see her breasts. Are women now going to be men? *Ana onicha* [earth of Onitsha] forbid that bad thing."

At the time, I (like the young women to whom I related the story) put this down to the conservatism of age, but I now wonder if the elder was not making a more complex argument about bodies and difference. By turning the implication of my question back on me, and asking if I wanted to undergo bodily change—to become a man in a very physical sense—she was inquiring about my image of my (womanly) body/self. Did I not like the contours and physical equipment of my own gender and sexuality? Why would I want to mask them and pretend an affinity with what is often viewed, in Igbo-speaking female discourse, as an alien set of beings? The call to the (female) earth as well as the reference to female ancestral forces and powers pointed to a view of women's knowledges and practices—encoded in their very bodies—being subsumed by those of men.[21]

However, it also seems clear that young women were playing with more than the bodily, powerful boundaries separating men and women in their "*alhaji*" fashion, and this went largely unspoken—except, perhaps, by northern tailors who absolutely refused to construct the outfits—in local discourses about the fashion. Young women were also using the *agbada* to establish some connection between their persons and the ethnically, regionally, and religiously based politics of the wider Nigerian context. Indeed, they could not fail to call all these important issues into mind when they donned permutations of the garb most associated with Nigeria's north, Islam, and a major failure in civilian rule. By wearing this attire, young, well-educated, urban, Christian, and southern women drew uncomfortable attention to the continuing importance of a set of Nigerian values generated most explicitly by *people they were not:* senior, Muslim men who effectively controlled both public resources and public political discourse in the country.

It is possible that some of the southern, Igbo-speaking men I knew who tolerated the *"alhaji"* look did so because of the possibility of satire and parody inherent in this contradiction. Southern men could hold the *"alhaji"* as a stereotypic figure to scorn very effectively by supporting a carnivalesque image of gender misrule: the female *"alhaji,"* a figure of (cartoon) fun. And it was quite evident to me that women took on this particular male dress because they realized that they were more likely to get away with expropriating the power costume of a despised and problematic outsider elite than in trying to use more familiar, explicitly southern dress markers of male seniority—notably chieftaincy caps, long woolen overshirts, and certain objects like staffs. The most general male outrage surrounding the *"alhaji"* related to women wearing caps, a feature of male clothing that tended to look more southern (and hence more dangerous) than "Hausa style." By 1988, most of the women who had *"alhaji"* outfits tended to wear small headties or to leave their hair unadorned in a compromise response to the male dislike of their caps. Changes adopted in the *"alhaji"* style during the limited time I could observe southeastern Nigerian women's fashion thus came both from inside the style (in how its women practitioners modified it to their current taste) and from outside (men's opinions and influence).[22]

For a particular moment in Nigerian fashion history, the *"alhaji"* look seemed to have a satiric or ironic intent, both for the young women who co-opted it and for some male observers who gave it their (covert) approval. For others, the "shock of the not-so-new" translated into denunciations of the shameful transgressions of social and/or bodily boundaries involved—a response that itself suggests the power of cross-dressing, even for those who disapproved of it. At this late 1980s moment and with this particular look, young women's clothing practice therefore showed how it was possible to use clothing to make subtle, contested, but effective sociopolitical statements as well as high style. In the next section, I consider the clothing practice of young men during the same period and look at how generational status hierarchies in Igbo patrilineages were explicated and experimented with in men's dressing. This discussion also points to significant differences in the experience of style and the social use of coded (or stylized) hierarchies between the young men and women of Onitsha's elite.

Designs for (Young) Living:
Junior Men and Senior Fashions

Let's try to imagine a not imaginary situation. A firm produces polo shirts with an alligator on them and it advertises them (a traditional phenomenon). A generation begins to wear the polo shirts. Each consumer of the polo shirt advertises, via the alligator on his chest, this brand of polo shirt (just as every owner of a Toyota is an advertiser, unpaid and paying, of the Toyota line and the model he drives). A TV broadcast, to be faithful to reality, shows some young people wearing the alligator polo shirt. The young (and the old) see the TV broadcast and buy more alligator polo shirts because they have "the young look." . . . [A]t this point who is sending the message? The manufacturer of the polo shirt? its wearer? the person who talks about it on the TV screen? Who is the producer of ideology? . . . There is no longer Authority, all on its own. . . . All are in it, and all are outside it: Power is elusive, and there is no longer any telling where the "plan" comes from. (Eco 1986, 148–49)

Understanding the need for the shoes:
youthful consumption and styles of masculinity
Material on young Nigerian men's late-1980s fashion requires us to construct a slightly different imaginary out of a "not imaginary situation" than the one posited above by Umberto Eco. In the present imaginary, young southeastern Nigerian men—jural juniors within (largely) patrilineal situations—began to wear both variations on the "traditional" dress of their lineage elders and on the "modern" dress of their professional superiors. In neither case did young men exactly mimic the clothing practice of those senior to them. In both cases, discrete elements of elder men's dress (e.g., fabric, cut, and/or drapery) were changed or subverted to establish a fashionable, and perhaps ironic, distance between the new clothing's models and its current incarnations. The "New Look" in Nigerian young men's fashion was, however, as firmly based in older silhouettes and dress ideologies—ideas of (male) empowerment instantiated in and around the body—as Dior's postwar and profeminine "New Look."[23]

Throughout the southeast, the clothing practice of so-called traditional elders has been defined—at least since colonial times—by large amounts of cloth, swathed generously about the body, and by special items of regalia like red felt caps, expensive coral or ivory necklaces, various types of fans, and staffs connoting authority and power. Senior men without the wealth and resources derived from urban properties and trade might wear a less expensive quality of cloth, carry a straw fan rather than one made of rare cowhide, wear beads of polished red clay rather than coral, bone instead of ivory, and bind their *ofo* (staffs) with twine instead of brass, but the basic uniform of generational power remained intact across boundaries we might define as those of class. This basic uniform was maintained through admission to title-taking societies, where redistribution of middle-aged men's wealth was rewarded with increased social prominence and responsibility as well as items of specialized clothing, and through sumptuary rules that forbade young men from taking on the garments and accessories of authority. Men who dressed as though they were wealthy or senior were expected to produce communal tokens of their wealth and seniority.[24]

Although we do not know what subversions of these sumptuary rules were possible (and very likely occurred) prior to the colonial period, it is clear that young men soon took advantage of new colonial models of dress—in Nigeria and elsewhere in Africa—to represent the generational *difference* of their everyday experience (see, e.g., Hay 1989). In colonial Onitsha it was certainly no oddity—except, perhaps, in her colonial imagination—for Sylvia Leith-Ross (1943, 20) to view "white-trousered clerks gravely debating together on their way home from factory or office, or shouting curious oddments of English slang amid a great waving of helmets and smart grey felt hats."

The command over a kind of idiomatic English and the command over an eclectic European-based style were actually two sides of the same cultural coin. Youthful, indoctrinated into colonial/mission social norms and practices, and professionalizing, the newly emergent "educated class" of Onitsha men were distancing themselves from their fathers and searching out new standards of masculinity in the early decades of this century. From the recollections of elderly Onitsha men some fifty years later, this was a heady time. After viewing a photograph showing one elder in his late 1930s finery—which consisted of a rakishly tilted derby, a woolen Western suit, and highly polished leather shoes— I was told how proud his entire family was of this outfit and all that it signified about their son's (clerical) success. I then asked the elder what his father thought of such dressing: "He thought it was too expensive, especially the shoes. My father didn't understand the need for the shoes."[25]

Understanding the need for the shoes—feeling the pinch of Western fashion commodities—was only one thing that separated the everyday experience of colonial Igbo-speaking fathers and sons, but it was an important marker of their increasing separation. Young nationalists like Nnamdi Azikiwe did not return from sojourns overseas or colonial postings in the first half of this century wearing "African" dress and espousing a return to "tradition."[26] They returned in the at-home uniforms of the male colonialists, adopting the clothing of Western patriarchal power so as to be taken seriously in Western power arenas. In the late 1980s, many of these former male fashion iconoclasts—including Azikiwe—had reestablished the preeminence of local power dress and wore flowing robes, chieftaincy caps, corals, tooled leather sandals, and ankle-strings based upon those of their remembered (and now important ancestral) fathers.

The sons of Azikiwe's generation came into their fashion own during the early years of the First Nigerian Republic—or during the subsequent military interregnums—when they opted for the Westernized khaki garb of the army, the three-piece European suit, or the modified "national" dress, the *agbada*, already discussed above. By the time of the 1970s Second Republic, their generational style settled on the *agbada*—modifying it to suit the general expansiveness of that era by bringing in new, rich fabrics, fabulous embroideries, and adding expensive accessories. Even former military rulers could be photographed at their leisure wearing this patriotic costume, and it became de rigueur for diplomats, male media personalities, and other public figures. Professional men might still appear in other, Western-style male uniforms: lawyers maintained their sartorial ties with the British legal tradition by wearing horsehair wigs and dark, scholarly robes over somber wool suiting; medical practitioners continued to wear white coats over their mufti. But it seemed that a renewed nationalist commitment following the Biafran civil war, as well as an increased awareness of 1960s Western Black Power philosophy, dictated the interest in returning to local silhouettes.

By the late 1980s, the sons of the founders of the Second Republic were coming out of university and facing a very different social and professional situation than that known to their fathers and grandfathers. The 1970s oil boom had most emphatically gone bust, the FMG (Federal Military Government) was embarking on a period of austerity and structural adjustment that eliminated many of the civil service positions that educated men once took as the prerogative of their class, and private entrepreneurship was becoming the buzzword of the day. Without much of a "national cake" to cut into, young Nigerian elites looked to entrepreneurial capitalism to restore their fortunes, and society parties hummed with talk of "seed money" and the price of opening commercial showrooms in major urban centers like Lagos, Kano, or Port Harcourt. Under the telescoping length of Major-General Babangida's administration, there looked to be little hope of immediate national political work for the graduates—and the military was not considered a viable career by many young, educated southeasterners.[27] The result of these social transformations was that young men often found themselves drifting between school and employment, trying to decide whether further education—preferably abroad—offered any palliative for their malaise. While deciding, they looked for opportunities to enter into a business that would afford them stimulation in the form of the travel and access to luxury goods to which their fathers' relative prosperity had accustomed them.

The modernization of the agbada: entrepreneurial dress and dressing entrepreneurs

One young man I knew well, who came from a privileged lineal background in the town of Nri,[28] settled upon men's fashion design as a means for establishing himself in the local business world. This does not mean that he went out, borrowed start-up capital from a bank, and opened a shop in Lagos; quite the contrary. Instead, he began to call upon his university friends—both male and female—and tried to interest them in purchasing cloth for the construction of new, exciting garments. When I first met this would-be fashion entrepreneur, whom I will call Ifeanyi, he did not even have a set of sketches to show his prospective clients—nor had he arranged for a particular tailor to assist him in the actual cutting and sewing of his commissions.

What Ifeanyi did have was a reputation for "creativity," an ability to market himself, and a series of connections among the Igbo-speaking young elite—many of whom had disposable income that Ifeanyi himself could not match. By dint of sheer persuasiveness, Ifeanyi soon had several commissions in the form of expensive brocade fabrics and very generalized client instructions that the new garments be "different" and "something new." Interestingly, none of these clients were female—although several young women were enamored of Ifeanyi for other reasons, they chose to design their own frocks and trouser outfits. Among fashion-conscious young men, however, Ifeanyi had found a willing market.

The new entrepreneur's market consisted of young, mostly single men who were accumulating their own wealth or using that of their parents to accumulate more and who perceived themselves as being too busy, or too important, to spend time tracking down tailors. Looking "smart," however, was key both to their self-image and to the image of success they needed to project for prospective clients—often their social peers. Prior to Ifeanyi's arrival on the scene, these young men were generally dependent on their mothers, sisters, or girlfriends for fashion advice—as well as for such practicalities as finding cloth, taking it to seamstresses, and arranging fittings. It should be noted, however, that some of these men's favorite clothing came from overseas shops and owed little to a *Nigerian* female-dominated taste culture.

While studying abroad or vacationing, these young men experienced shopping for themselves and buying—in the less stressful environment of the department store or mall—Western clothing that appealed to them personally. Ifeanyi, who shared similar life experiences and tastes—as well as a gender—with his clients, looked to provide an alternative vision of men's "African" dress that duplicated the lack of stress and satisfaction of a Western, male-oriented pattern of clothing consumption. Ifeanyi's "attires" (a Nigerian English term for complete, accessorized outfits) would be locally produced, using popular Nigerian or imported fabrics, but they would reflect the *lifestyle* of youthful Nigerian capitalists—very much a thing of shared male companionship, helped along by drinking parties and frequent, all-male business meetings in private homes. The exclusion of women from the new male fashion process—except as passive admirers of the end result—was, I argue, quite significant for several reasons.

Primarily, excluding women from the process of men's fashion offered a challenge to certain gender stereotypes and hierarchies that supported other, powerful hierarchical relations within the Igbo-speaking southeast. Although men historically owned their own cloth and stockpiled it as a form of wealth, it was not as important as a foundation for men's socially recognized accumulation as stockpiles of yams, slaves, or other imported goods (e.g., "hot drink" [liquor], kola nuts, guns and ammunition). Indeed, it appears that cloth formed part of an engendered reciprocity throughout the southeast from the earliest days of European colonial and mercantile contact: men would borrow rich wrappers and scarves from their female relations—especially mothers, aunts (father's sisters), and sisters—in order to make stylistic displays at feasts or other social events, or well-to-do women would gift male relations with the appropriate cloth(s) for important occasions.[29] Conversely, men were expected to give cloth to their wives regularly—but especially at defining moments in their relationships, such as their weddings, the birth of children, or to mark the wives' success in trade. Since a goodly portion of any Igbo-speaking woman's wealth consisted of cloth, she served as a sort of repository, for her male relations, of both cloth itself and a specialized knowledge concerning cloth and style. (It seems clear, from what we know about the female-dominated market system of the southeast in the pre-colonial period, that men who were not traders themselves would be less likely to be aware of fashions than the women who moved from local periodic market to periodic market.)

More senior women tended to support more men—both junior and senior—out of their accumulated cloth-wealth than did junior women, for obvious reasons. Partially because of this, senior women served as a valuable conduit for mediating male-male relations. An intelligent older woman might therefore withhold her best cloth from her son and lend it instead to a man who could be a useful contact for her son—like a powerful mother's brother in preferentially endogamous Onitsha.

Kept by sumptuary rules from assuming title regalia, younger men were also often prevented—by older, cloth-accumulating women—from using sartorial capital for local politics as well. The professionalizing classes of the 1930s may have signaled the first real challenge to women's specialized clothing knowledge, as those men took their models of dress from male colonial officials and European traders—establishing within the urban southeast a true gender dichotomy in what could be worn (and borrowed)—but even they were still dependent on indigenous women's specialization and clothing mediation for "traditional" events. The radical quality of Ifeanyi's 1980s entrepreneurship lay in an ability to unhook young men both from senior women's wrapper-ends and from their mediating role in local, male clothing practice and politics. A new type of style wars was suddenly possible.

From the beginning, Ifeanyi's fashion creations were based on the Nigerian male power dress, the *agbada,* which had been somewhat discredited by its previous association with the excesses of the 1970s oil boom. Trying to make this look more acceptable to late-1980s, Western-educated consumers, Ifeanyi stripped away the voluminous overtunic and concentrated on the long undershirt that was an everyday staple of the local male wardrobe.[30] Bringing that Westernized sensibility of the beauty of weightlessness to a dress that had previously emphasized the weighty quality both of cloth and the body within the cloth was Ifeanyi's most difficult problem and reflected what I would consider the essentially "modern" slant of Ifeanyi's designs. As Stuart Ewen (1988, 183) notes, this perceived need to eliminate bulk in fashion is a matter of "form follow[ing] value" in the world(s) of modernity:

> It speaks for a life that claims to live beyond the consequences of nature. It reflects the pure logic of abstract value—the economy of thin air—transported and implanted within the inner realm of the human sub-

ject. . . . the ideal body is one that no longer materially exists, one that has been reduced to an abstract representation of a person: a line, a contour, an attitude, skinned from its biological imperatives. Regardless of the shape one's body takes, whatever flesh remains is *too much;* image must be freed from the liabilities of substance.

Unsurprisingly, then, Ifeanyi began to refine the image of youthful, elite, male Nigerians by emphasizing their height and thereby opposing it to their width—their bodies' bulk—and he showed a reluctance to take on initial commissions from men who were not tall or slender. (His own body shape may have been influential in this as well; Ifeanyi was both taller than most of his peers and quite thin.) By keeping the designs' shirts long, making hips, waist, and legs one continuous line, and by using dark colored brocades (black, indigo, and deep burgundy), Ifeanyi actually reshaped young men's bodies into apparently flat, abstracted planes.

In keeping with this new, uncluttered *agbada* attitude, most of the baroque embroidery was stripped away as well. The occulted, monochromatic designs woven into the brocade either served as sole ornament, or else a small neckline embroidery was permitted. In a couple of cases, these embroideries were placed on the shoulder and consisted, suggestively enough, of three abstract bird shapes—ready to fly off the fabric. Ifeanyi completed his look with a cap made of the same fabric, generally without contrasting embroidery, and a pair of dark shoes; on a tall, dark-skinned man like himself, the effect was something of a large, moving shadow.[31] The wearer stood out, like Beau Brummel and his late Georgian imitators, by the very dearth he seemed to represent; only close scrutiny would disclose the luxuriousness of the fabric and the detailing of the cut of a yoke or sleeve.

Not everyone could afford Ifeanyi's services, and not everyone approved of his designs—particularly his elders. Some older women commented to me that his choice of colors was inappropriate; they were offended by his use of dark blue and black. Since at least the early colonial period, Onitsha Igbo-speaking peoples have used unpatterned indigo or black cloth to signify mourning.[32] The invasion of a late-1980s Western color standard—the fashion of dressing in deepest black from head to toe—seemed, to their perplexed elders, suddenly ready to plunge a whole, elite generation into mourning. As one women acerbically inquired of me after hearing that I liked black: "What do you have to be sad about?" It was an interesting question, and I relayed it to Ifeanyi and some of his peers. Ifeanyi told me that black and other dark colors were strong colors, and he liked his clothing to "show strength." A young man and woman of our mutual acquaintance agreed and told me that they liked wearing black for several reasons: it made them look taller; it was the "most beautiful brocade"; and they saw lots of black clothes in London the last time they visited there, so they knew it was fashionable. Mourning, or sadness, supposedly had nothing to do with the choice of color.

It seems to me, however, that the senior Onitsha woman's comment was insightful, and that the beauty of black (or dark blue) brocade was an ambiguous beauty, partially tied to local, antisocial associations of mourning and unhappiness—and to the experience of colonized clothing practice. Ifeanyi's customers, by taking up his color aesthetic, were subverting part of the "traditional attire" aesthetic of their parents and grandparents. These senior people—most of whom lived under colonial domination and experienced the headiness of the early days of independence—tended to keep local and Western clothing practices separate. (This, in turn, reflected the compartmentalization of their everyday professional lives from what was increasingly the evening and weekend's business of "village politics" and indigenous ritual activity.) Although drab colors like black, dark blue, and greys in men's Western dress were perfectly acceptable to—even required by—senior people, the elders' local clothing practice remained firmly oppositional to the puritanical aesthetic and emphasized pattern, bright hues, and ornamentation.

Bringing the colors of Western suiting, but not the Western suits, into the heretofore protected arenas of dance group outings, wine-carryings (weddings), and title-taking ceremonies showed a dangerous mixing of categories and possibly a lack of respect for the local value of these events. Western clothes were certainly worn at these events before Ifeanyi's designs made fashion inroads, and men—young and old—had appeared in Western suits as a (barely) acceptable substitute for expensive local dress. The key was that the Western suits remained determinedly *Western*, markers of an acceptably differentiated attachment to modernity. They did not presuppose an absolute melding of modernity and tradition within the person representing himself, and therefore they offered no real affront; although men wearing such suits would invariably be offered the loan of a wrapper if they intended to participate in dance or the sharing of blessings (kola and liquor). Even though pieces of Western clothing—notably suit coats—were used by dance ensembles and other "cultural" groups to enhance the dignity of privileged members or to lend comic effect during performance, the clothing's usefulness came from its lack of real incorporation into a "completed" outfit; its ability to make boundaries on the body that spoke to the boundaries that people experienced in their own lives. For elders, the sight of young men rejecting the carefully constructed divide between their Westernized business lives and their deep, local obligations and enjoyments was profoundly disturbing. It may even have appeared as a rejection of the elders' historical experience and an outright embrace of what Mbembe (1992) calls the "postcolony."

A tacit rejection of one generation's historical experience does not necessarily constitute an ability to transcend historical processes, however. The melding of "traditional" clothing forms—modified but recognizable—with the sleek surfaces of modernity actually spoke, with an eloquence made more poignant by being unacknowledged, to the difficulties of contemporary Nigerian life. Young Igbo-speaking men demonstrated how much they valued local structures by seeking a kind of recognition in them, through the difference expressed in their clothing practice. Unlike the case of the regendering of the *agbada*, above, this use of the attire did not subvert it as a power costume—quite the contrary. By attempting to alter the *agbada* just enough to show an embodied understanding of changed social and political circumstances, Ifeanyi and his customers both reaffirmed the importance of access to male-dominated, relational hierarchies and challenged the generational means by which these hierarchies functioned. This "New Look" was new only in that it suggested how "traditional" the terms of modernity could be.[33]

As Ewen (1988, 77) notes, while considering the perceived consolations of style for nineteenth-century American immigrants: "A central appeal of style [is] its ability to create an illusory transcendence of class or background." By trying to represent a new model of Nigerian masculinity to their elders through clothing practice, young men received, at worst, disapprobation, and at best, a most unsatisfactory lack of acknowledgment. Interestingly, no male elder tried to keep the young men from experimenting with their clothing practice so long as it involved the *agbada* alone—as occurred in the case of the young women, above. As part of the status hierarchy by virtue of their gender, there may even have been an expectation that men would experiment, no matter what. Changing (male) *agbada* styles simply did not constitute the threat that women wearing "men's attire" did.

If the story of Nigerian men's late-1980s fashion experimentation ended there, we could comfortably conclude that young men were simply replicating, in a more contemporary guise, the clothing practice of their grandfathers. We might also predict that these young men would eventually find their own place in the patrilineal hierarchy and abandon—or peripheralize—their earlier experiences in favor of "tradition." Finally, we might suggest that the most subversive clothing practitioners described in this essay were the cross-dressing women elites. Nothing so neat and potentially satisfying, however, is possible regarding the clothing practice I witnessed during the period of my field studies, because Ifeanyi and his peers were not content simply to modify the *agbada* and go on about their business. Instead, they took on an even more activist posture and began to reconsider the use of ornament and accessory in male dressing.

"It isn't a chieftaincy cap!": representing seniority
Although young, elite women seemed to approve of their brothers' and men friends' new fashions—and did not seem to mind that they had been displaced in their clothing responsibilities by the entrepreneurial Ifeanyi—the young men themselves seemed unready to rest on their fashion laurels. I should add here that Ifeanyi soon was joined by other young men and even a couple of women in his entrepreneurship. Tailors around Enugu, Onitsha, and Port Harcourt also began to turn out attires similar to those commissioned by Ifeanyi and his patrons, and brocade cloth traders laid in better stocks of dark-colored fabric to meet the increased demand. In a classically progressive case of fashion consumption, Ifeanyi and his friends were therefore under pressure to maintain their hard-won style status in a few, short months after the first outfits were debuted.[34] Rather than seek out newer and more outré cuts or new silhouettes, Ifeanyi's group next gave its attention to the creation of a more complete ensemble—including caps, some jewelry, Italian shoes, and other ornamentation. As it turned out, the putting together of ensemble wear, with all its possibilities for extravagance and parody, did concern the elders.

Young southeastern entrepreneurs were already looked on with suspicion by the older generations in late-1980s Onitsha. Rumors were circulating wildly relating to entrepreneurial involvement in smuggling of drugs and other banned import goods (see Bastian 1992, 184–91). The consumption of luxurious brocade fabrics, the use of a (male) designer from the same social stratum as his patrons, and the wearing of gold chains and expensive wristwatches all pointed to a dangerous and unrestrained accumulation of young men's wealth. Some such young men in Onitsha were also investing their expendable income in attempting to take titles, usually under their fathers' aegis—at an age when the men in the two previous generations were barely beginning their professional careers and families.[35] During a time when most of the elite population was experiencing a downturn in its fortunes, the emergence of a seemingly prosperous young male group may have appeared as even more of a potential threat to the generationally based hierarchy than usual. (And it is certainly the case that struggles between young men and their elders were already very much a part of the history of towns like Onitsha.) This eternal, generational struggle burst out, during 1987–88, around young men's use of certain accessories that seemed to co-opt symbols of political and lineage power associated with their elders.

As noted above, "traditional" authority is encoded in most Igbo-speaking areas by items of regalia like red felt caps and bound staffs. The caps (and some of the staffs) are a residuum from Nigeria's colonial past: they were used by colonial officials to mark out the infamous warrant chiefs, local men chosen by the colonizers to act as their representatives in towns and village-groups all around the southeast (Afigbo 1972, 105). The so-called "Red Cap Chiefs" in contemporary Onitsha are invariably *ozo*-title holders (which suggests age, wealth, and political prowess), and only patrilineage elders are permitted to carry the *ofo* bundle or staff that signifies ready access to ancestral forces and power over lineage mates.

Untitled men are permitted to wear caps, but they must not be red or carry too much embroidery or other ornamentation—specifically feathers, since certain feathers connote movement within the ranks of the *ozo*-title society and the *ndichie*.[36] They may not carry staffs, fans, or horse tails except while serving as principal mourners or celebrants at certain events.[37] Younger men may also wear caps, but elders frown upon the use of felt or velvet of any sort for those caps—since these fabrics are used in the making of senior men's headgear. They are certainly not expected to carry staffs or use any fans—except, possibly, fans belonging to their dancing mothers—on their own behalf, although they might be called on, as a mark of favor, to hold their fathers' or other male relatives' regalia.

In the face of this long-held, elder clothing practice, Ifeanyi and his patrons began to add caps to their ensembles. Ifeanyi's first caps were nonthreatening, made from cloth that matched that of the attire as a whole. As such, they were well within the sumptuary bounds established for young men's wear, although some of the caps sported delicate embroidery that raised a few senior eyebrows. Difficulties mainly arose after Ifeanyi suggested to one young man that he wear a velvet cap, as well as a modified velvet shirt, for a close relative's title-taking.

These velvet caps were readily available in Onitsha's markets, and older men who could not yet take a title often wore them at special events, strictly at the sufferance of more senior, titled men. The velvet shirt also was problematic: although black, it was embossed with various designs that brought to mind the chieftaincy attire of southern Igbo-speaking groups.[38] By itself, the shirt would pass; the addition of a velvet cap made too close a mimicry of chieftaincy attire for senior comfort. Although some elder women seemed to admire the young man's audacity in claiming the clothing practice of his social superiors—or, perhaps, enjoyed seeing senior men with their noses out of joint—male elders attending the ceremony sent word that the "youth" should bring them kola and *mai oku* ("hot drink," liquor) to atone for his transgression. Besides paying what amounted to a sumptuary fine, the young man was capless when he returned to his friends. I was told later that the elders decided to confiscate the cap as a lesson to other would-be young fashionables.

Ifeanyi's group was disgusted by what it perceived to be an undue expression of the power of seniority in this episode. The man who was fined and who lost his costly cap in the process explained that he pleaded his case on the basis that the cap was not really a chieftaincy cap: it was neither red, felt, nor decorated with bird feathers. This argument evidently was unsatisfactory; he still had to buy kola and drinks for the offended elders and was told that he should not question the judgment of people senior to him. In the view of one of his friends, this last was sheer oppression—and an oppression specifically targeted toward the young business class: "They always choose to pressure us, because they know we can afford it." The pressure in this case, however, did not serve to stop the sartorial subversion; if anything, it caused the entrepreneurs to take the next step in co-optation.

Having been unsuccessful in taking over the meager cap privileges of older, untitled men—and in fully invading the "traditional" realm of seniority dressing—some junior businessmen turned their attention back to the Western suit. Images of early forms of "Afrocentric" dressing were beginning to filter back from the United States and Britain, and these images—in videos, magazines, and on musical recordings—suggested a different strategy. Although the young businessmen did not want to wear *kente* cloth strips on their clothing, they were intrigued by the idea of bringing a Nigerian quality to their Western attire. The Nigerian fashion industry had not yet geared up, as it would in the early years of the 1990s, to produce suits and casual, Western-style men's wear in local fabrics. (In 1987–88, Ifeanyi's entrepreneurship was more the exception than the rule.) One elegant possibility that was experimented with was the use of a locally produced walking stick, carried along when wearing a well-tailored suit. These suits, I would hasten to add, were modeled more on the lines of American basketball players' wear than on the conservative Western suiting favored by their professional fathers.

Young elite men who effected this look were immediately taken to task for aping their seniors—using walking sticks in imitation of older men's staffs, or, in some formulations, in imitation of the English upper classes. The connection between the elders and the former colonial authorities was not as strained as it might appear: formerly colonized Nigerians often recognize the power of their colonizers by still referring to them as "the colonial masters." (And we should not forget that British colonial officials gave out staffs to designate their own approved "elders.") Yet there was a difference in response to the walking sticks, partially because they were used with Western suits rather than "traditional" outfits. The elders grumbled, but they did not impose fines; syncretizing Western menswear did not constitute the same threat to their localized power. They had done much the same in their own day, and they said they did not take it seriously.

But I would also argue that the senior men did not feel that they had the same authority over the use of Western garments that they could impose on any more local clothing practice. By wearing suits, the juniors armored themselves in another respected power—an *appropriate* (and appropriated) modernity—one that elders had felt the transcendence of firsthand. The rules of local clothing practice were different from the rules attached to international consumption; elders did not try to fight Eddie Murphy or Hakeem Olajuwon and Michael Jordan. Such a battle would not only have been inappropriate to their dignity as senior patriclan members, it would have to be waged in an arena where their powers held little sway—that of internationally sanctioned media-style. Presumably, just as the ancestors "do not speak English," neither can they impose severe sanctions against the material stuff of the world that does.

Some Conclusions

Dandyism was thus acceptable in Onitsha so long as it did not impinge too closely upon the boundaries that separated local (male) powers and authorities from the larger, more difficult-to-contain world of international style. And elite men's power was never seriously disputed during the small battles over young men's use of color, caps, and canes—even though the generations engaged in a contestation around clothing practice. For southeastern Nigerians, at least, Eco's notion that "All are in it, and all are outside it: Power is elusive, and there is no longer any telling where the 'plan' comes from," must be mediated. All are in it and outside of it in relation to the encompassing, exteriorized universe of styles, images, and commodities generated by international capital—but some, in Nigeria and elsewhere, are more "in it" than others.

In the case of the female "*alhajis*," young Nigerian women sought to represent themselves as powerful (wealthy, interesting) by allying themselves in their clothing practice with a group of people they could never really be. If we extend Matory's notion (1994), that cross-dressing is more than theatricality, we might suggest that they were attempting to become something closer to what they could not be.[39] Although possibly subversive in intent, we must recognize that the use of men's dress to signify power showed the young women to be realistic in their reading of *content*. Young women, just as involved in schemes of modernity as their brothers, did not attempt to take on women's "traditional" clothing practice—even though senior southeastern women have their own power costumes that could be mimicked and transformed. For young women, power is perceived as residing outside the boundaries of their gender—and it can be reached for only in attenuated, masked gestures.

Senior Igbo-speaking women are not as reticent in their common interests as more junior women are, but they have invested their lives in a system that weighs men's authority more heavily than their own. Since, in many ways, women's authority depends on that of men, senior women since colonial times have accepted one seemingly small defeat after another in the attempt to keep men's local authority intact. The fact that one more means of women's power was eroded during the men's late-1980s fashion skirmishes went largely unnoticed and completely unremarked upon. This did not mean that women were unaware of the narrowing of women's power/knowledge under conditions of increasing patriarchal control. When I asked one extremely sophisticated young woman what she thought about Ifeanyi and his clothing machinations, she laughed: "Before you know it, these men will want to be hairdressers and chefs. And, like you say in the States, they will be the best. No one will want to eat women's food again."

The most general point I would like the reader to take away from this analysis has to do with the connections between bodies, clothing, and power. Clothing practices, like other forms of practice, are plainly about the embodiment of power—whether through the construction of conventional attractiveness or through the transgression of boundaries and setting up of alternative social/ gendered/political spaces for people to occupy. How much transgression is made possible and even probable—as we see in the very different cases of elite young men and women in late-1980s Onitsha—is relative to the practitioners' previous peripheralization in their society. Bodies and persons that are already somewhat askew to (generally senior, generally male) Igbo orthodox notions of the appropriate may chart a wider course: no young women were fined or otherwise publicly remonstrated with for dressing "*alhaji*"; young men did not think to appropriate their mothers' headties and wrappers, even though women were once firmly in control of Onitsha's huge markets. The embodied histories that interested both young men and women in the late 1980s were gendered male; history had been represented as a male province (like economics and politics) in their education and experienced as a male province in their everyday lives. Whether cross-dressing male or senior male, the Nigerian reality of modernity that underlies these practices should be recognized for what it is: a thoroughly patriarchal one with decreasing space for female participation and a decreasing respect for female value. The dress of men is seen as *the* dress of power in southeastern Nigeria, whether mediated by generation, class, or ethnicity, and clothing practices that are based in a desire for power— as most modernist clothing practices seem to be—must take this fact into account.

Notes

1   See, for example, Barthes 1983. The position for a more subversive rhetoric of fashion is adroitly presented by Wilson (1992, 8–9) in her reconsideration of fashion and postmodernism: "Dress could play a part, for example, either to glue the false identity together on the surface, or to lend a theatrical and play-acting aspect to the hallucinatory experience of the contemporary world; we become actors, inventing our costumes for each successive appearance, disguising the recalcitrant body we can never entirely transform."

2   The problem with this type of psychosexual rhetoric immediately presents itself to anyone with basic knowledge of the male body: being phallic does not always equate to rigidity. The male body adapts itself to softness as well as to hardness. The dichotomous idea of sexuality that Silverman and other similarly influenced theorists do not question tends to give their own pronouncements a quality of rigidity I think they would recognize as patriarchal.

3   Strangely, McRobbie is silent on the "retro" clothing practice of young men in the last two decades—even though the subcultural style of British male youth has traditionally been marked by extreme differences in modes of attire. Discussing late-1950s male style, for instance, Dick Hebdige (1979, 51) notes that "the teds' shamelessly fabricated aesthetic—an aggressive combination of sartorial exotica (suede shoes, velvet and moleskin collars, and bootlace ties)—existed in stark contrast to the beatniks' 'natural' blend of dufflecoats, sandals and the C.N.D." Both the teds and the (male) beatniks were originally retro practitioners whose fashions gradually found their way into the more mainstream marketplace, much as McRobbie suggests women's retro fashion practice of the 1970s and 1980s affected mainstream clothing design (McRobbie 1989, 48).

4   Bourdieu (1977, 109) writes, "One thus has to acknowledge that practice has a logic which is not that of logic, if one is to avoid asking of it more logic than it can give, thereby condemning oneself either to wring incoherences out of it or to thrust upon it a forced coherence."

5   See Heath 1992. Although the Senegambians she studied have an elaborated conception of "dressing well" (*sañse*), Heath presents more about Bakhtin's ideas on

heteroglossia than about what Senegambians mean by *sañse*. Heath is so sure that fashion must be discussed in terms of language—a notion debunked quite effectively by McCracken (1990, 57–70)—that she never points out that Senegambians themselves seem to have quite a different perspective. And, in an extremely telling lacuna, Heath also neglects to present an etymology for *sañse;* we are simply informed that it equates to fashion. The "language" of Senegambian clothing is thus one that Western representational theory easily supersedes.

6 See Barnes and Eicher 1992 for a similar point. According to them, "The analysis of dress needs to place the complete *objet d'art* into the context of a total cognative structure. A definition must allow room for all types of body supplements and modifications" (3). While "*objet d'art*" suggests a more static display than I am comfortable with, I do like the idea of "body supplements and modifications" and think that an emphasis on clothing practice(s) would necessarily focus on such supplements and modifications.

7 Several chapters in this volume (most notably those of Renne and Hendrickson) interrogate, at least implicitly, the concept of "the traditional" in local African clothing practice.

8 *Agbada* prints are cotton cloth decorated with batik ("wax") designs. These printed cloths are purchased by both men and women and are generally made up into different sorts of clothing designs. Men's ordinary *agbada* clothing style is well represented by Akapa in this drawing; women can have the cloth made either into a blouse and wrapper or into certain styles of Western dress. The key to understanding *agbada* clothing practice, however, resides in whether the print design is new, imported or locally produced, or custom-designed. The cartoon cannot even begin to suggest this information, but my own tendency is to "read" the man's *agbada* as plain.

9 In a further, subtle subversion, these elements work against contemporary northern/Muslim ideas of "modest" dress for women. In this ethos of "modest" dress, women should wear swathed headcoverings; long, loose dresses or robes; and their feet should be covered—wearing flat shoes or sandals, and certainly without high heels.

10 I would argue that the only women who are "all stomach" in southern Nigeria are those most dangerous female eaters, witches. The appropriateness of such an exaggeratedly curved stomach for men, however, is shown in their propensity to "eat" opponents in political and business situations; the now well-known "governmentality of the belly" throughout Africa. (See, for example, Ruth Marshall [forthcoming] on this gustatory representation of governance in contemporary Nigeria.)

11 One of the anonymous readers of this volume informs me, however, that it was not a new fact of Nigerian women's clothing practice: "Yoruba women in Lagos in the early seventies had an 'Alhaji' style of dress that included eyelet (or as they say 'lace') wrapper and an indigo headtie." This is valuable information for a number of reasons. The first is that it shows how the very idea of "*alhaji*" (and possibly the

power attached to it) has transformed over a decade: in the seventies, when the "*alhajis*" ruled the republic openly, women could take on their fabrics and colors, but not their masculine form of attire. Wrappers have been female style since colonial times; the appropriation was incomplete and not nearly as excessive. Later in time and more distant in (political/social/geographical) space, young women could take on "*alhaji*ness" in a more ironic way, playing with a stereotype that was still being constructed in the heyday of their older sisters and mothers. I suggest that what we can see at play here is nothing less than one representation of Nigerian historical consciousness: wearing "*alhaji*" in the late 1980s had different, historical meanings than tying "*alhaji*" in the 1970s. These 1980s meanings, which were commentaries on 1970s realities, will become clearer below.

12   The use of "development" here is in quotation marks because it was the term used by a couple of young women of my acquaintance to describe the prospective impact of their attire on society. The progressivist language of modernization was on every English-speaker's lips in 1987–88; it was one of the most pervasive discourses of Nigerian public life.

13   My anthropological fieldwork took place in fifteen months between January 1987 and March 1988 and was wholly funded by a Fulbright U.S. graduate student grant sponsored by the U.S. Information Agency and administered by the Institute of International Education. Most of the information in this essay comes from the usual anthropological field methodology of participant observation; some from official and unofficial archival sources in southeastern Nigeria. Although not an historian, I am interested in historical issues and present some historical material in the course of the discussion.

14   Cloth traders in Onitsha's Main Market told me that "guinea brocade" actually came into northern Nigeria from northern Africa, specifically from Egypt. These traders, however, admitted that their knowledge of the cloth's provenance was limited to what they heard in the markets of Kano and Kaduna—where they bought their own supply of brocades.

15   The conflation of political interest and politicized (male) attire is made constantly in Nigerian public discourse. For example, Niyi Osundare (1992) recently editorialized in the weekly newsmagazine *Newswatch*: "Civilians tell us they do not need our votes to rump into power (true, since our voters' list is always crammed with ghost entries); their military counterparts will never let you forget that you never voted them into office. And so whether in *agbada* or khaki, political power is a victim of the Nigerian Factor [official corruption]."

16   In the late 1980s, when I did my fieldwork, these younger men had also resuscitated the European suit for formal and important business wear. These suits were a far cry from the grey wool three-pieces favored by their professionalized fathers and grandfathers, however. They were the products of a new western sensibility about color and line in men's fashion, exquisitely tailored or loosely draped and often in colors like taupe or nontraditional blues.

17   I will address the historical reconstruction of the loose, mission "frock" into the tight silhouette of the 1950s elsewhere. In this essay, I consider more recent transformations. Westernized emphases on the legs and an elongated torso were only beginning to make inroads into female dress consciousness during the late 1980s. Although women's legs were on view in frocks, bodily aesthetic appreciation was definitely *centered*. From pictures showing the mini-wrapper fad of the early 1970s, it would seem that even shortening the ankle-length, "traditional" wrapper was meant more to emphasize the waist and hip area than to display thin and shapely legs. (The photographs invariably linger on the bosom/waist/hip region, often cutting off the legs at the knee.) When the legs were shown in 1970s photographs, people would point out their elaborate platform shoes to me and talk about how awkward it was to walk in them.

18   It also tended to display the back of the body more than frocks would; the interplay of women's back muscles in dance, for example, was more evident (and much commented on) when dance performance took place in wrapper.

19   The condition of "wetness" in women is associated, throughout the Igbo-speaking region, with health, fecundity, wealth, and weight. A "wet" woman is a woman whose skin glows moistly, whose body is nicely rounded (in older women with a neck displaying rings of fat), and who exudes an aura of prosperity. Like water—or the gold that should adorn her neck, ears, and fingers—she gleams.

20   Madame I, the mother, did not have an income of her own, and this was one source of tension within the family. This was only one instance in which Madame used her husband's considerable monetary resources to purchase clothing that he knew nothing about, out of her "household" funds. Her husband thought that she was a bad household manager, but he grudgingly continued to give her extra money. Madame's personal store of rich wrappers and Western frocks was extensive. By turning her husband's wealth into clothing and jewelry, she was actually giving herself a wealth base in the oldest Igbo fashion: a woman's clothing and jewelry constitute her private estate, usually inherited at death by her daughters. The aggressive use of clothing in their mother's domestic struggles was obviously not lost on her children.

21   The question was made more poignant for me by the fact that I, in an anthropologically influenced clothing practice, was wearing a wrapper constantly during this period. Young women thought my personal style extremely archaic—although I did convince some of my friends to try their mothers' wrappers on to see how comfortable an outfit it could be. The woman elder, above, had begun our conversation by saying that my wrapper "fit me."

22   I note that a catalog of "African fashion" printed in Chicago in 1992 for a company run by a Nigerian immigrant woman showed an extremely modified design of the "*alhaji*" that included ballooning harem trousers and an embroidered overshirt made of *agbada* cloth. The trousers—if representative of the "latest" in Lagos fashion, as advertised—further subverted the satiric or resistance intent of the original attire, making it more generically "ethnic" while displacing it from specific

commentary on northerners and even on men. This could, of course, be more representative of the immigrant entrepreneur's desire to sell recognizably "ethnic" attire to her targeted local market—both African immigrant and African American consumers. The fine points of sending up Nigerian politics or Nigerian male power structures would be lost on the latter and possibly no longer as important for the former. More research is required into this type of material.

23 Dior's late-1940s New Look tended toward tight bodices, cinched-in waists, and tantalizing glimpses of the female leg. In this way it mediated against the masculinist trend in women's wartime fashion—where women doing "men's jobs" on the homefront often wore menswear-inspired suits; loose, flowing trousers; and other, less body-defining outfits. The New Look was meant, according to the press at the time, to signify the " 'womanly woman' (*femme femme*)" (Charles-Roux 1981, 229). Silverman (1986, 144–45) rightly notes how the New Look and its (male) proponents like photographer Richard Avedon helped to reassert the primacy of the male gaze on Western female bodies. However, as Angela Partington (1992, 145–61) cautions us in her article "Popular Fashion and Working-Class Affluence," the practices of the New Look, once it arrived in working-class homes via 1950s popular media, could actually run counter to this covertly antifeminist agenda. The male gaze can be subverted by female—and even by male—practices. What are missing from theories based on monolithic notions of maleness, like Silverman's above, are the subtle movements and delicate articulations within the monolith, the differences embedded in different male gazes and the differences encoded in female remodelings of male models. Mass theories inevitably generate mass, overdetermined interpretations. The point of essays like Partington's and this one is to look for more historically/culturally specific and hopefully more inclusive models of popular cultural forms.

24 This is beautifully illustrated in Buchi Emecheta's novel *The Slave Girl*, when Okolie—a young man who sold his sister as a slave in the Onitsha market—festooned himself beyond his real means with the proceeds of his sister's servitude. Okolie soon found himself in difficulties: "So before the end of a season Okolie had acquired a title, but one he knew he could not live up to. What was more, he had so impressed the girls, with his dancing and his well-fed body and his expensive outfit, that he was forced to accept the gift of a wife. Although he protested to the girl's parents that he could not pay the bride price, the elders of her people laughed and said, 'Only a foolish man would admit that he is rich. A rich man does not tell people he is rich but his behaviour says as much' " (Emecheta 1977, 84).

25 It seems clear that the father was objecting to more than the cost of his son's footwear. He may also have considered the young man to be representing himself as too politically and socially senior, "too big for his britches," as we say in southern American English.

26 Nnamdi Azikiwe offers us photographic evidence to the contrary in his autobiography, including a picture of himself in American football gear. He did not

reject "traditional" authority only in dress, however, since he espoused "the eman-
cipation of Africans not only from foreign oppression but also from indigenous
tyranny" (Azikiwe 1971, 275). The contradictions between his sense of fashion and
his opposition to colonial rule were evidently not as important at that time as
distancing his bodily representation from that favored by local elders.

27   There were several reasons for this, not the least of which was that a whole generation of southeastern military officers threw their lot in with the Biafran forces
during the civil war. Although some of those rebel officers were readmitted to the
federal military after the war, most Igbo-speaking survivors preferred to go into a
premature retirement and became civilians. The fathers of several of the young
men whose clothing practice I am interested in here fought on the losing side of the
war and did not encourage their sons to take up military service.

28   Nri and its inhabitants hold an unusual position in the imagination of Igbo-
speaking peoples. "Nri men" were, in the past, itinerant ritual specialists whose
presence was required at various important functions—including the holding of
ozo title ceremonies in some towns. (This was not true in Onitsha, where *ndi onicha*
held it to be part of their own special character that they were not under obligation
to Nri.) This young man was related, through his mother, to one of the highest
priestly families. (For more on Nri, see Onwuejeogwu 1981.)

29   This practice continues in contemporary southeastern Nigeria. During my fieldwork, I noted many instances of sisters loaning their brothers spectacular wrappers to enhance the brothers' appearance at important, "traditional" social events.
Young men also depended on their mothers to dress them lavishly for age-grade
outings, etc. Onitsha indigenes usually knew where these men's fashions came from
and would praise women for their generosity in adding to the splendor of male-
dominated occasions.

30   Many Nigerian men already used their *agbada* undershirts to add an African signa-
ture to otherwise unremarkable Western-style trousers and T-shirts. This casual
breaking apart of the *agbada* made for a hybrid look that emphasized the upper
torso at the expense of the legs and feet. Although there was a utilitarian, uniform
quality to this look, it was mitigated by the different prints and bright colors used in
the *agbada* shirt. Men were wearing the same basic silhouette, but they proclaimed
an individuality within the uniform.

31   Homi Bhabha's point about darkness is exceedingly apt here: "Its symbolic meaning . . . is thoroughly ambivalent. Darkness signifies at once birth and death; it is in
all cases a desire to return to the fullness of the mother, a desire for an unbroken
and undifferentiated line of vision and origin" (Bhabha 1990, 85).

32   Elderly Onitsha women still use Yoruba *adire* (indigo printed cloth) as mourning
attire. (Since the Igbo word for blue is also the word for black, Onitsha residents
call this in English "black cloth.") During the first year of mourning, the cloth
is worn with the unprinted indigo side facing outwards. Afterwards, continued
mourning is signified by wearing the faded print side where it can be seen. When I

first debuted an *adire* skirt in the marketplace, I was puzzled at being greeted with "Sorry!" by my trader friends—until I discovered that they thought I was bereaved.

33   Garber (1992, 66) makes a similar point about male-to-female cross-dressing in the West: "Far from undercutting the power of the ruling elite, male cross-dressing rituals here seem often to serve as confirmations and expressions of it. Indeed, what is fascinating about the study of transvestism is precisely that it can occupy such contradictory social sites: stigmatized and outlawed in some circumstances, appropriated as a sign of privilege in others." Matory (1994, 178) makes an interesting intervention about cross-dressing in African ritual contexts that should give us pause, however. He notes that, at least in such cases, cross-dressing may be less about performance and the (momentary) breaking up of classificatory systems than about the "process by which [it] designs new forms of relationship and hierarchy."

34   Dick Hebdige's (1979, 96) description of this process remains apt, if not completely relevant to the present case: "Once removed from their private contexts by the small entrepreneurs and big fashion interests who produce them on a mass scale, [subcultural innovations] become codified, made comprehensible, rendered at once public property and profitable merchandise. . . . Youth cultural styles may begin by issuing symbolic challenges, but they must inevitably end by establishing new sets of conventions."

35   There was some scandal during the 1980s when not only well-to-do young men were taking *ozo* title in Onitsha—but when unmarried and putatively *childless* young men were taking the title. *Ozo* was supposed to be reserved for later middle age, after a man had proved his worth as warrior, farmer, and father/lineage mate. In 1987–88 there was grumbling that *ozo* title was "being ruined" by some of these anomalously youthful titled men.

36   *Ndichie* are those elders who are "living ancestors" for Onitsha people. They have special titles, essentially communally bestowed names, and are only addressed by those names/titles. They make up the *imobi,* or court, of the Obi or King of Onitsha.

37   Women also are not permitted to wear caps or carry these objects of regalia— excepting fans. Women dancers can carry small fans, but usually only fans made from local materials like straw. (The cowhide fan is supposed to be reserved for titled men's use.) Women mourners may also carry horse tails, but they must carry them reversed, holding the tail by the hair and not by its bound handle. I have been told that some women have *ofo* staffs of their own—particularly *umu ada* (first daughters of their lineage)—but I have never knowingly seen one of these staffs.

38   That is, the long flannel or velvet shirts (usually in red or black) decorated with emblems associated with the landed gentry of Europe—hunting dogs, pheasants, coronets, etc.—worn by Igbo and other southeastern coastal elders. See Michelman and Erekosima (1992, 172–73) for photographs of this style of shirt worn by Kalabari male elders.

39   In the film *Paris Is Burning,* the young, mostly gay, New York cross-dressers strive for "realness." Realness, in that context, implies an inner conviction as well as outer performance: you become the military hero or well-to-do society woman you dress as. By practicing the image of model or "superstar" on and through your body, you open yourself up to the experience of *being* the model or "superstar"—and, at least in the recent case of RuPaul, you might even conflate the truth of your imagining with the larger reality recognized by others.

5 DRESSING AT DEATH: CLOTHING, TIME, AND MEMORY IN BUHAYA, TANZANIA

Brad Weiss

Discussions of the relation between memory and objects often focus on the creation of specialized mnemonic forms. This has been true particularly of discussions of clothing (Weiner 1992; Weiner and Schneider 1989), which emphasize the capacity of sacralized heirlooms to preserve continuities across time and space, and thereby provide a means of remembering. While such analyses do draw our attention to the ways in which particular objects become imbued with vital aspects of social identity, they run the risk of overemphasizing the material substance of such objects at the expense of analytic interest in the broader sociocultural problems that create them. At the same time, an exclusive interest in the creation of long-term continuities through the use of mnemonic forms diverts attention away from the crucial role that *forgetting* may play in the sociocultural construction of temporality. In spite of the dichotomy commonly drawn between these processes, forgetting need not be merely an ineffective attempt to retain information or an unintended consequence of the production of new forms of knowledge. Rather, in some instances, forgetting can be seen as an intentional and purposive attempt to create absences that can be crucial to the reconstruction and revaluation of social meanings and relations (Lass 1988, Derrida 1986, Battaglia 1992). I suggest that Haya mortuary practices are one such instance, and that clothing and adornment in particular play a crucial part in the conjoined processes of remembering and forgetting that are occasioned by death.

During my fieldwork with Haya communities in the Kagera region of northwest Tanzania,[1] I was frequently absorbed in the project of trying to understand the wide-reaching implications of death as a sociocultural problem in this area. I was especially interested in the concreteness and specific detail of mortuary and mourning practices that mediate experiences of death for the Haya. Their use of cloth and clothing of different kinds is very important to Haya mortuary practices, as it is to many peoples; moreover, important transformations in the various uses of clothing in this context can be traced over time. The implications of these practices and their transformations, I suggest, raise a series of questions that turn on the relation between persons and objects, continuity and discontinuity, as well as the living and the dead. The analysis I propose here, therefore, is not restricted to a discussion of the uses and meanings of mortuary cloth and clothing, but rather employs such activities as exemplifications of wider cultural themes and processes objectified in the relation between clothing, time, and memory.

Effigies and Heirlooms

Just over one million Haya live in the Kagera region, located in the northwest of Tanzania. The Haya form a part of the Interlacustrine sociocultural area, which includes (among others) the Ganda and Nyoro in Uganda to the north, as well as the indigenes of Rwanda and Burundi to the west and southwest. Haya villages (*ekyaro*, singular) in the rural areas of Kagera, the primary site of the research on which this essay is based, are composed of a number of family farms (*ekibanja*, singular). These farms are also places of residence, and all households occupy farmland. All the farms within a village lie immediately adjacent to one another, so the village as a whole is a contiguous group of households on perennially cultivated land. These residential villages are dispersed across and clearly contrast with open grassland (*orweya*). The primary produce of Haya family farms are perennial tree crops; bananas, which provide the edible staple; and coffee, which provides the principal source of money. Coffee remains the most significant source of a rapidly declining cash income in Kagera today, and this cash is filtered through the Haya community in an informal economy (*biashara ndogo ndogo* in Swahili) of marketing local produce, household commodities, and (most importantly for these analyses) new and used textiles and clothing at local weekly markets.

Let me begin this discussion of Haya dressing practices by addressing certain historical shifts in the use of different kinds of cloth, and explore in particular the temporal forms that clothing realizes and makes tangible over this history. According to ethnographic reports on Buhaya from the earliest decade of this century (Cesard 1937), all of the deceased's clothing was once destroyed as a part of funeral procedures. Indeed, a wide range of objects owned by the deceased, from pots and plates to gourds and even house posts, were destroyed. The central exception to this practice in the case of a male household head was a single animal skin. This skin was used in the installation ceremony that followed the burial, as the heir assumed his senior position by sitting in the chair of the former head and wearing his inherited skin.

In northwest Tanzania in the late 1980s, this array of objects belonging to the deceased, including clothing, is preserved; in fact, my neighbors suggested to me that it would be especially shameful to destroy the possessions of one's dead relatives since these are the principal source of wealth for descendant generations. What is just as important, however, is the fact that the single item of clothing most strongly identified with the household head (my neighbors usually referred to the coat or the *kansu*[2] of a man) is used in the installation process in precisely the same way as the animal skin described earlier. Thus in spite of the shifting relations between persons and objects over the course of Haya history, clothing continues to be a critical medium for articulating descent, and especially for objectifying identifications between the authority of the living and the dead.

There is another intermediate position that clothing occupies, intermediate to both the order of mortuary practices and descent relations, which is worth addressing in order to assess what seems to be the importance of clothing in the construction of symbolic and social authority. Before an heir is installed, the coat or other item of clothing that will mark his ascendance is used by the grandchildren of the deceased for a very different purpose. This generation takes the coat and either creates an effigy of the dead grandfather with it, or dresses up in imitation of him, parading around the village and demanding payment for their performance. In either case, my Haya friends said that this display, which is always received as fairly hilarious, is intended to suggest that the deceased is not actually dead, but is still around and able to make demands of his children.

The Haya call this kind of display "joking" (*okusilibya*) and it is consistent with the character of relations between grandparents and grandchildren during their lives. These alternate generations are, to begin with, *equivalent* in important respects. For example, while marriage with a member of one's mother's and certainly father's clan is strictly prohibited, Haya prefer to marry members of their grandparents' clan.[3] Thus, grandfathers call granddaughters "my wife" and grandmothers call grandsons "my husband." It is appropriate, then, that grandchildren should replicate their grandparents at their death, since, as we shall see in important respects, they *are* their grandparents.

At the same time, it is important to understand why this activity is not just imitation, but joking, and how this joking works. And our understanding turns on the meanings of the clothing through which this activity is achieved. Remember that the same clothing that is used to install an heir in the place of his elder is used to *recreate* that elder through imitation. Here, again, we see that clothing contributes simultaneously to processes of remembering *and* forgetting, for it is only by completely forgetting the "actual" deceased person, as well as the variety of forms that are intended to recreate him, that a memory of the deceased can be reconstructed. The authority vested in the new household head is not an imitation of former authorities, but an instantiation within a continuous as well as individuated set of temporally ordered social relations. Clothing mediates both of these dimensions, reciprocally forgetting and memorializing the dead.

What's more, the imitation of the elder by the youngest generation is actually a means of undermining the authority to which the ascendant generation aspires. For if the deceased is still present, even in this mock form, no heir can assume his place. Grandchildren recognize the irony that is involved in joking as well as the power that is at stake in these actions, for it is they who will be subjected to the final authority of their parents when they assume this position. Thus, as a friend of mine told me, "We joke with our dead grandfathers in order to bother our fathers!"

These activities reveal the ways in which clothing is central to the coordination of intergenerational relations. The basic form of senior-to-junior hierarchy is embedded in the inherited garment, which insures not only the continuity of descent but the *reproduction* of its *authority,* as ascendant generations assume greater power over their own juniors. At the same time, grandchildren are able to appropriate this very same item in order to assert a very different kind of identification with the authority of senior generations. Through their joking and by means of the same clothing that embodies the power of descent, juniors are also suggesting that the nature of authority is grounded, not simply in the relation of seniors to juniors, or parents to children, but in the ongoing reproduction of generations over time. The authority exercised in descent relations does not lie in a dyadic relation but in generative relations. This joking, then, demonstrates that the authority that seniors exercise over juniors ultimately derives from the relation between generations and will inevitably be assumed by these juniors themselves.

These acts, I am suggesting, instantiate different aspects of identity and, consequently, constitute different forms of power. Sons can assert their equivalence to their grandfathers, thereby suggesting that the power of their own fathers is circumscribed by the passage of time. But these fathers assume their positions as household heads by the same actions, and so achieve an authoritative identity. Fathers, in these situations, do not become "the same as" their own fathers. Rather, they become elders in their own right who command a more complete authority over their sons as an aspect of their own, as clearly distinguished from the deceased's, identity.

Clothing, it seems to me, is an especially appropriate vehicle for representing these alternative forms of identity and authority. Put simply, in these contexts a garment can be worn as both an heirloom and a costume. That is, a coat can be worn as an heirloom in order to represent the values that attend to a certain position, or it can be worn as a costume in order to imitate particular figures who occupy these positions. When a father wears a coat imbued with such generational, temporal values, his body is placed in a position identical to others who have worn it. Yet, precisely because wearing clothing both displays and conceals the body, the possibility for imitation and disguise is also introduced. Thus, grandchildren claim not that they occupy the same position as their grandfathers, but that they recreate the same bodies as these elders. In this shifting relation between bodies and clothing, heirlooms and costumes, representation and imitation, shifts made possible in these contexts by the use of clothing itself, we see the construction of alternative models of hierarchy and authority, as well as continuity and discontinuity over time.

The Ironies of Secondhand Style

The former destruction of personal clothing as opposed to its contemporary preservation exemplifies one significant historical change in Haya understandings of the relation of persons to clothing, and especially to the clothing of the dead. And there is another, in some ways more obvious change in Haya "fashion" that requires some explanation. Moreover, it is a change that helps illuminate the place of clothing in the construction of time and memory in these communities. The uses of clothing and other beautification techniques I describe below are clearly historical practices—animal skins have been replaced by coats and *kansu*, bodies once beautified by butter are now adorned with petroleum-based oils. Clearly, these commodities are cultural imports; but clothing in the Haya world has long been a means of relating local communities to other places. In the nineteenth century, Haya merchants traded coffee berries prepared for chewing in order to acquire the finest bark cloth pieces from Buganda. When money was to be made in the 1920s, this time from the *sale* of coffee on the world market, it was reported that the Haya used their profits to procure European finery. As one district commissioner at the time put it: "It is delightful to see well dressed Africans who have given up their skins and rags" (Bakengesa 1974, 20).

In the late 1980s, European clothing of a different sort was available in local markets. Both men's and women's clothing—especially coats, shirts, and dresses—were made available as church and development agencies airlifted containers of used clothing into the region, which local entrepreneurs then sold at weekly markets (cf. Hansen 1994; Comaroff n.d.). Tailors and a very few seamstresses also commonly prepared suits and skirts from bolts of fabric, but this locally made clothing, while cut in a similar "style," was clearly distinguished from used European clothing. This used, imported clothing is called, in the vernacular, *Kafa Ulaya*—literally "Died in Europe." My friends' exegeses indicated that this term meant that "someone has died in Europe, and we get their clothes!" In other parts of Tanzania, I have been told, a common slang insult is *Kafe Ulaya*, "Drop dead in Europe!" In this case, the implication of the insult is not just that the insulted party should die, but that they should die in Europe, where they will surely come back to Tanzania in the form of spare parts. At least then they will be good for something!

These bits of jargon, though they may seem fragmentary, clearly speak to Tanzanians' own sense of themselves as parts of a global order of property relations and values. But it is worth noting, especially with regard to the Haya example, that this form of popular consciousness is expressed in terms of what we have already seen to be a powerful set of relations between clothing and death. In this case, we see again the ways in which clothing concretizes the transformations introduced at times of death; and more importantly, we see the way in which encompassing questions of continuity and discontinuity, of integration into a wider world of circulating commodities, as well as one's marginality to this same world, are engaged through the medium of clothing. And this is a medium which, in the context of temporal transitions like death, is able to objectify the irony of this situation. Indeed, wearing *Kafa Ulaya* has the potential for many of the same deceptions and conceits as making an effigy of the dead. I often heard men who (in the view of their neighbors) thought too highly of themselves lampooned for "wrapping on a tie" or "putting on a coat." Other items associated with European dress, like brimmed hats and eyeglasses, might also be dismissed as simply the trappings of those who aspire to refinement. Of course, the ability to wear such items *and* command the respect of those who see you wear them is a widespread ambition. As in the case of effigies and heirlooms, those who create a "successful" appearance are those who project an identification with the objects they deploy, while the very *same* objects can also be taken as signs of mere pretension. Styles of adornment such as these, therefore, capture the sense of both an appreciation of the values handed down via pieces of used clothing and the prestige that many Tanzanians themselves attribute to possessing such garments, as well as a recognition of the indifference, if not disdain, with which these items are made hand-me-downs by Europeans. Again like the use of heirlooms to create effigies, such items objectify and comment on relations of authority at an extremely wide level. In this context, clothing places those who wear it in a position of both belonging to and being cast off from an encompassing world of property and values.

The Affinities of Bark Cloth

Continuities, as well as discontinuities between the living and the dead are revealed not only by the trajectories of "inherited" garments such as heirlooms or *Kafa Ulaya* but by the clothing in which Haya men and women inter their dead. Funerary shrouds establish important social ties in the context of mortuary relations. The ways in which they are purchased, wrapped, preserved, and ultimately undone concretize and make meaningful a host of relationships. The use of shrouds as memorials demonstrates the ways in which memories are given tangible form, as well as the fact that the necessity of securing memories can be *anticipated* and acted upon. Securing a memorial can, in many instances, provide a basis of *sociality* in Haya men's and women's lives, and the control and disposition of clothing gives evidence of this critical sociocultural process.

The cloth in which corpses are buried is known as an *enzikyo* (from *okuzikya*, "to cause to be buried") or *ekilago* (from *okulaga*, "to sleep"). Until the middle of this century (Sundkler 1974, 70) the material used for these shrouds was bark cloth (*orubugu*, cut from the ficus tree, *omubugu*). Bark cloth was once an important trade good in the Interlacustrine region (Hartwig 1976). This cloth was cut and prepared in the Haya kingdoms and traded north into the kingdoms of Bunyoro and Buganda. During the nineteenth century, control over the bark cloth trade was carefully regulated by Haya monarchs, and in the late 1980s I found many bark cloth trees growing prominently on what were once royal lands.

When bark cloth was used as a shroud, the corpse was first dressed in everyday clothing (Cesard 1937; Sundkler 1974, 70) and then wrapped in bark cloth. Bark cloth was not only used to wrap the corpse but was also worn as signs of mourning by clansmen of the deceased. The sections of bark cloth that provided shrouds were generally quite large (perhaps two by three meters square), and these mourning cloaks were in fact cut from the same cloth that served to wrap the corpse. *Okujwala olubugu*, "to wear bark cloth," is still a term that is synonymous with *okufelwa*, "to be in mourning." This use of bark cloth suggests, therefore, a powerful means of asserting an identification of the living with the dead, as not only the same material but the very same cloth was used both to shroud the dead and to clothe the mourners.

While some bark cloth is still produced in northwest Tanzania, it is no longer as widely available as it once was. Funeral shrouds, with perhaps a few exceptions, are no longer prepared from bark cloth; however, there are some important continuities in Haya mourning styles that give evidence of an ongoing concern with the use of clothing to mediate relations between the living and the dead. In some parts of Kagera, especially in the northern region of Kiziba, men and women in mourning wear printed textiles called *kanga* and *kitenge*,[4] which are everyday women's clothing throughout East Africa, draped around their necks. This practice, which is followed for a few weeks following the burial of a clansman, is still called "to wear bark cloth" in spite of the different materials used today. In other areas, men and women do not wear textiles in this way, but women continue to wear sections of cloth cut from the funeral shroud itself (now made of a white broadcloth known as *Merikani* for its American origins) as a sign of mourning. In spite of a change in textiles, then, shrouds continue to establish links between the living and the dead.

The connections between the living and the dead confirmed through bark cloth and contemporary burial cloth can also be seen to be closely related to material relations between living generations, as well as affinal relatives. According to all of my informants, the *Merikani* now used throughout Kagera to provide funeral shrouds should always be purchased by the spouses of the deceased's children. Those who marry your children, both your daughters' husbands and your sons' wives, can be expected to provide you with funeral shrouds upon your death, and corpses therefore are often wrapped in several layers of burial cloth. Thus, it might be said that such shrouds, which fashion critical links between the living and the dead, also embody an important connection between children and their parents. Parents are dependent on their children to clothe them in the funeral shrouds that will provide the connection between these same generations after death. Moreover, this obligation to clothe the dead is widely recognized as a crucial dimension of intergenerational relationships. Haya men and women often described to me the burden and tragedy of not having children in terms of this obligation and its consequences; as one man put it, "If I don't have children, who will bring funeral shrouds?" Children, then, are not only expected to care for their parents in their old age, but the value of this care takes on its greatest significance at a parent's death. Indeed, a person's relationship with his or her children is often expressly *motivated* by concerns about their own death and funeral, and these concerns are concretized and enacted through the gift of burial cloth.

It is especially important that this relationship between generations becomes fully realized through affinal connections. Children's obligations to their parents at death are actually made possible by their marital relations, since funeral shrouds are purchased by the spouse of one's offspring. This connection between affinity and mortuary, a connection that is instantiated in funeral shrouds, raises a number of points about the ways in which clothing organizes and orients Haya social relations. To begin with, the explicit relationship between one's own death and the having of children—or, to be more specific, the *marriage* of one's children—indicates the close associations between mortality and reproduction, a phenomenon recognized as an aspect of mortuary procedures in an extremely wide range of contexts (Bloch and Parry 1982). In Haya mortuary practices, funeral shrouds do more than simply demonstrate this crucial connection, they establish the relevance of marriage to death by revealing the ways in which the *trajectories* of these productive social relations—that is, the processes of constructing, undoing, and reconstructing these relations as they unfold over time—implicate each other. In effect, death is widely recognized as *the* occasion toward and through which a diverse array of Haya social relations are oriented: parents have children in order to ensure their proper death, parents secure marriages for their children in order to commemorate their own burials, and spouses fulfill their obligations to one another at their in-laws' funerals. These gifts of burial shrouds, then, have to be understood and assessed in terms of the coordination of practices and relations achieved at death.

Death and Bridewealth

If we consider death as a point of orientation in the development of many Haya relationships, we can discern some interesting temporal qualities embedded in the gifts of cloth that instantiate this process. The link of burial cloths to affines, for example, suggests the connection of death to bridewealth. Haya bridewealth, *amakula*, not only allows for the acquisition of important material goods into a bride's family at the time surrounding her marriage, it also ensures the incorporation of extended networks of relations into one's mourning party. The cloth or clothing that is always a central feature of the contributions offered by daughters' husbands, husbands' siblings, as well as their children at the funeral of an ascendant affine might therefore be considered the completion or fulfillment of bridewealth payments. In this respect, Haya marriages and the expectation of ongoing marriage payments anticipate and prepare for the death of one's parent.

These temporal qualities—the ways in which gifts, especially gifts of clothing, can anticipate an event or process—can also be seen in the kinds of objects that are given as bridewealth at the time of marriage. Haya bridewealth payments and prestations have changed considerably in both degree and kind over the last century. New forms of marriage—especially marriages given "official" recognition by both religious and State agencies[5]—have arisen and have greatly expanded the field of possible marital arrangements. They have also extended the strategies for providing bridewealth to recognize and secure such arrangements. However, in spite of this diversity, most Haya men and women with whom I spoke held that certain payments *had* to be made in order for a marriage to be recognized as such; and among the most important gifts that had to accompany any marriage were items of cloth, namely blankets and sheets for the mother (and often the mother's sisters, and their mother, as well) of the bride.

These gifts of cloth at marriage parallel the gifts of shrouds at death, each of which is provided by a daughter's affines. Until factory manufactured textiles became widely available in the region, the blankets (*blanketi*) and sheets (*mashuka*) offered to a bride's matrikin were made from bark cloth, just as funeral shrouds were. But, in addition to these noteworthy similarities in materials, these gifts of cloth constructed, and continue to construct, complementary ways of organizing the temporal patterns of social processes (e.g., their sequencing, duration, repetition, origination, and conclusion) as well as specific experiences of these temporal patterns (e.g., anticipation, recollection, foreshadowing, or forgetting)—that is, the objects exchanged contribute to the generation of complementary *temporal orientations*.[6] For example, Haya men and women told me that blankets and sheets are given to a bride's mother(s) as bridewealth in order to replace the many blankets and sheets that the new wife had undoubtedly soiled as a child herself. These gifts of cloth (which are, in fact, explicitly forms of *clothing*, since they clothe an infant) are, therefore, intended to recognize the (specifically women's) work involved in raising a child. They acknowledge and *recall* the mothers' contributions to the development of the donor's bride. Indeed, according to all of my informants, the "things" (*ebintu*) of bridewealth, from the beer and goats specifically intended for senior male members of the bride's clan to the cash gifts that today accompany any marriage, are given as tokens of thanks and appreciation for having raised a daughter well. These sentiments are significant, for they indicate that rather than serving as compensation for the loss of future services that a daughter might provide or as possible resources that might be drawn on by her brothers for their future marriages (Comaroff 1980, 167), Haya bridewealth prestations are oriented toward the *prior* activities of raising a daughter that make a marriage possible. In fact, the term for bridewealth, *amakula,* derives from the verb *okukula,* "to mature or develop." Such terminology suggests not only that these offerings are able to make a mature woman out of a girl, but that bridewealth recognizes and gives thanks for the process of *maturing* a girl for marriage.

Any offering can be presented or received as a gesture of thanks, a token that acknowledges the efforts made by the bride's natal family, efforts that ultimately will benefit her marital relations. But what is especially significant about the gift of blankets and sheets in this context is that they not only thank the bride's matrikin for their acts of nurturance, they also are intended specifically to replace a set of similar objects that were used up in the course of these activities. Through this replacement, then, these gifts of cloth provide a means of *remembering* the very concrete practices, including the bodily connections of the mother and the bride to the clothing itself, through which the bride was cared for and (ultimately) made ready for marriage. Moreover, by evoking and incorporating the memory of these maternal activities and objects into the marriage process itself, these gifts of cloth might be said to reconfigure their significance in some important respects. Replacing the worn-out blankets and sheets of child-rearing with new ones at the time of marriage connects these life events into a cohesive process. These gifts establish a specific *orientation* to the acts and objects of raising a child, by demonstrating that caring for a daughter *anticipates* her future marriage, itself an event that may explicitly anticipate a future gift of cloth, the funeral shroud.

What is important, then, is that these marital gifts of cloth work to create specific sorts of memories, making material recollections of raising a daughter an aspect of her readiness to be married as a woman. These gifts also give a definitive temporal orientation to the acts of child-rearing and to the qualities characteristic of parents' relations with their children. The blankets and sheets of bridewealth, then, operate in ways that complement the use and provision of funeral shrouds. All these forms of clothing the body (whether of infants, or corpses and mourners) invoke memories, in particular, memories that are features of intergenerational relations. Similarly, the different uses of these kinds of clothing can fulfill expectations or anticipated outcomes—in some cases, even anticipated memorials. Parents may have children in anticipation of the provision of a burial shroud that will ensure their memorialization at death. At marriage, memories of child care invoked by blankets and sheets may cause those actions to be seen as anticipations of that child's maturation and preparation for marriage. Clothing, and the exchange of particular kinds of clothing, it seems, can be seen as crucial media for embedding not just temporal modes of continuities and discontinuities but the experiential qualities of memory, recollection, and anticipation into the very forms of Haya sociality.

Time and Adornment

These gifts and practices demonstrate the capacity of clothing to forge and reconfigure critical temporal features of Haya sociality. I have argued that generational as well as affinal relations are felt to develop over time and are often oriented toward specific events or sequences of events—especially death and marriage, each of which must be addressed as a process in the Haya context. Clothing, perhaps more than any other material medium or item, is the vehicle through which these temporal orientations are concretized. In the passage from generation to generation, from natal kin to marital relations, and from life to death, Haya clothing works to recall certain prior experiences and aspects of identity and to anticipate the fulfillment of others. The question that these capacities provokes is, why clothing? Why is it that clothing seems to be so central to these dynamic dimensions of Haya social process? While it may not be possible to give a definitive answer to this question (that is, one that accounts for the privileged position of clothing *as opposed to* any other available item), it does seem important to address this problem by examining the significance of Haya practices of *wearing* clothing. A Haya aesthetics of adornment (especially mortuary adornment), a consideration of the qualities generated and conveyed both by wearing particular kinds of clothing in particular ways as well as by treating and preparing the body through a variety of techniques so as to produce an appropriate appearance, can tell us a great deal about Haya men's and women's emphasis on clothing in the construction of memory.

Mourners at a Haya funeral, especially those who consider themselves close relatives of the deceased, are generally rather unkempt. As many men and women told me, those in mourning are so preoccupied (*baina ebitekelezo,* literally "they have thoughts/concerns") by their grief that they care little for maintaining a neat appearance. But this apparent lack of careful grooming actually has a persistent aesthetic form. It is women, especially, who take special care to present what we might call a proper mourning appearance. Haya women are generally said to express their feelings more readily than men (as men, I was often told, are "harder," *nibaguma,* than women), and women's physical semblance and comportment is a central means of this expression. When women come to a funeral they almost always present a distinct bearing. As they make their way to the house where the deceased is to be buried, women mourners wail with grief (*obushasi,* literally "pain" or "bitterness"), firmly clasping their hands to the sides of their heads as they cry. Women told me that they hold their heads in this way because they are "so full of thoughts" that it feels as though their heads may split open. After a woman has greeted the mourners at the funeral and cried over the corpse, she will often wear a long, narrow strip of banana bast tied around her head until the deceased has been buried. This strip of bast is not only taken as a sign of mourning but, like a woman's hands clasped to her head, is also intended to restrict the uncontrollable expansion of her "thoughts."

These forms of bodily comportment, holding and even tying the head to control the afflictions of grief, reveal a concern with unbridled dispersal and dissolution. The integrity and closure of the mourner's body are threatened by the death of a relative (however that may be defined), and this threat is manifest most clearly in the physical appearance of mourning women. These aesthetics of mourning are further suggested by the way in which women dress to attend a funeral. In everyday contexts other than funerals, Haya women, especially married women, generally wear two large printed textiles, the previously mentioned *kanga* or *kitenge* (called *ekikongo* in Oluhaya). One piece of cloth is wrapped around a woman's waist, and the second piece is draped over both shoulders; occasionally the second piece is pulled up to cover her head, as well. This style of dress was often explicitly described to me as a way of properly "closing" a woman. Young men and women also suggested that a woman (especially a married woman) who did not drape herself in this way when greeting other men or women[7] would be seen as especially aggressive, perhaps even sexually suggestive, in her attire. Through this style of dress, then, women create an appearance of enclosure that suggests personal restraint. Yet, in clear contrast to this style, Haya women attend funerals wearing only one such cloth, which they wrap tightly across their breasts. Like clasping her hands to the sides of her head as she cries, wearing this single cloth while leaving her shoulders and upper body virtually uncovered, conveys a sense of a women's exposure and dissolution that is characteristic of this aesthetic.

This sense of exposure and dispersal, demonstrated so remarkably by Haya women's style of dress and comportment, is a critical feature of the mortuary process. I also suggest that these adornment practices reveal further aspects of the importance of clothing in generating and configuring Haya memories. It is significant that the appearance of dissolution embodied by women is part of the *initial* response to death. Gradually, these exposed forms are enclosed, and the dissolute is made coherent in the course of the mortuary process. For example, a woman's shift from clasping the sides of her head with her hands, her elbows akimbo, frequently trembling with sorrow, during the procession to the funeral to tying a strip of banana bast around her head prior to the burial of the deceased is an attenuated form of this reintegration and composure that the mortuary process attempts to achieve. It should also be pointed out that banana bast fiber (*ebyhai*) was at one time used to construct what I was told were not very prestigious forms of clothing (Cesard 1937), usually simple short skirts generally worn by those who did not have access to finer skins or bark cloth pieces. In any event, this use of bast strips at funerals might be taken as evidence of the significance of *clothing* (since surely the bast tied around her head is *worn* by a woman in mourning) in reestablishing the bodily integrity and composure threatened by death.

If we consider the significance of clothing in terms of the qualities of enclosure and integrity, qualities that are basic features of a Haya aesthetic, then we can begin to assess the importance of clothing as a medium for constructing temporal continuities and discontinuities, especially in the context of death. Bark cloth pieces, which once provided funeral shrouds and also had strips cut from it that were worn as signs of mourning, display these qualities in many respects. When people talked to me about the virtues of bark cloth (even bark cloth pieces produced in the current day), they emphasized how large these pieces were in contrast to standard cotton sheets that were sold at the market. The methods for producing large pieces of bark cloth, such as those once used for shrouds, bear an interesting relation to these aesthetic criteria. Bark was stripped from the *omubugu* ficus in single sections and then pounded with a grooved mallet over a period of several hours, sometimes even a few days. Cesard reports that from a strip of bark measuring 1 by 0.2 meters, a sheet of bark cloth measuring 3 or 4 meters by 1.2 to 1.5 meters could be produced (Cesard 1937, 107). This vigorous pounding resulted in cloth that could be not only quite large but also extremely supple.[8]

The aesthetic concern with creating a cohesive and integrated appearance, a concern that attempts to refashion the expansive disintegration that begins the mortuary process, can be seen to be embedded in the form of bark cloth. As these production techniques indicate, large sheets of bark cloth, which will eventually clothe both the deceased and those who mourn, present a seamless whole. Rather than composing a cloak from separate elements that can be fastened together (as might be the case for fiber skirts, animal skin belts, or contemporary suit jackets and house dresses) the bark cloth artisan creates an uninterrupted form, a single and singular piece that embodies the kind of coherence that funerary practices and aesthetics seek to establish. This seamless shroud not only draws attention to the identification of mourners with the deceased (as it emphasizes the fact that both are clothed not only with the same type of cloth but with sheets of cloth that are separated from a single, unitary piece); it also creates the aesthetic form of coherence across the surface of the enclosed (enclothsed) corpse. That is, the form of seamless integrity embedded in the bark cloth shrouds becomes iconic of the processes through which it is both manufactured and worn.

Temporal Surfaces

In addition to the surface appearance of these various styles of dress, Haya women and men pay special attention to the surface of their skin, especially in the course of events—like birth, marriage, and death[9]—that constitute the life cycle. Haya men and especially Haya women told me that beautiful skin is soft and shiny, or clear (*okuela*, the descriptive verb used, can mean "to be clear," "to shine," "to be white"). To give their skin this appearance, Haya men and women often apply oils to their skin. In the past, butter (*amajuta g'ente*, literally "cow's oil") was applied to the skin as well as to animal pelts, in order to make both of them more shiny and supple. Using large quantities of butter on an everyday basis, which required both access to cattle as well as the finest animal skins to be effective, was a practice especially associated with Haya nobility (*abalangila*); yet even commoners and low-ranking Haya farmers (*abairu*) and tenants might be expected to provide a daughter or wife with butter for her skin in preparation for her marriage. Indeed, the term for the events that prepare a bride for leaving her natal home on the day of her wedding is *olusigilo*, which derives from *okusiga*, "to smear, or coat" (i.e., with butter). In the present day, butter is no longer smoothed on the skin, but a variety of petroleum-based oils, available in shops and markets, are still widely used in this way.

The smooth, clear, even white appearance created by applying oil to the skin clearly relates to the kind of seamless enclosure created by bark cloth as well as by the two-piece styles of dress worn by most Haya women. Such applications of oil demonstrate the integrity of the body on its very surface by creating a uniform appearance, uninterrupted by blemishes or other marks. I further suggest that this concern with surface appearance and form as a focus of Haya aesthetics has an important temporal dimension, one that may be significant to the ways in which memories are constructed through clothing and adornment more generally, especially in mortuary contexts. The smoothness and whiteness of well-oiled skin, according to the descriptions of Haya men and women, projects a kind of pristine appearance, one that suggests, in temporal terms, a return to an original, unsullied condition. For example, newly married women oil their skin quite often in an attempt, as they say, to become as white/clear as possible. This whiteness, then, is characteristic of the beauty and prestige of the *initial* stages of marriage. Furthermore, this white condition is associated with the pigmentation of a newborn child; in effect, a newly married woman reverts to the pristine condition of infancy. This oiling creates a condition preceding the experiences of socialization (and sexuality) which, at least in Haya men's accounts, makes them more susceptible to the sexual control of their new husbands.

Moreover, a woman who has recently given birth is also described as shining and white, just like her new infant, and this postpartum appearance is relevant to her husband's attempts to reassert his access to her sexuality and reproductive capacity. After a woman has given birth, her husband will attempt to establish the clan membership of the next child to whom his wife gives birth at any point in the future. This right is secured by being the first to have sexual contact with a woman after she has given birth. The initial semen (*ebisisi*, literally "embers") of this sexual act ensures a husband's "paternity" over his wife's next child, regardless of when that child is born (see also Reining 1967, 151; Swantz 1985, 72–73). This understanding of paternity and clan identification connects sexuality to reproduction through a definitive sequence from an *initial* act of intercourse through to any *future* pregnancy and childbirth. The whiteness of a woman who has just given birth embodies this temporal orientation. The original, new, pristine condition of a new wife, new mother, or newborn child is visibly apparent on the gleaming surface of their skin.

These temporal shifts and efforts to project a pristine appearance are not restricted to these processes of matrimonial and reproductive renewal. Haya women, and occasionally men, oil their skin as often as they possibly can. After scrubbing and washing, especially one's hands and feet, a really thorough "cleaning" is best achieved by rubbing oil into your exposed skin. While the brilliant, shiny appearance created by oiling in this way was not unremarked upon by my informants, most Haya women and men explained the merits of oiling their skin in somewhat different terms. As one typical account put it, "If you apply oil you won't show any marks." As the woman offered this explanation she scratched a twig along her (oiled) leg to demonstrate how her skin remained unblemished. "When you go out to the fields, the grasses and twigs will leave marks. But they can't if you apply oil to yourself."

This concern with "leaving marks," which was routinely offered to me as a reason for oiling your skin, confirms the prevalent aesthetics of surface appearance. Oiling the skin in these everyday contexts, contexts that entail work and travel (i.e., settings in which one might walk through grassy or wooded areas), provides a means of preserving an unblemished, uninterrupted, seamless appearance. At the same time, there is a distinctive temporal quality to this appearance. The fact that oiling prevents "marks" from appearing on your skin suggests that you can avoid registering the tangible traces of activity. The seamless surface of oiled skin, therefore, embodies a form of spatial integrity and pristine brilliance that also obscures the inscription of time's passing. Oiling the skin not only suggests a renewal and return to an original condition, it also delays concrete appearances that register the passage of time.

I have argued that there is an important Haya aesthetic of surface appearances, an aesthetic that can be seen to organize mortuary styles of adornment, bodily comportment, and funeral shroud production and clothing. What is especially interesting about this aesthetic is that the concern with seamless surfaces and bodily integrity embedded in Haya practices creates a form of spatial coherence that has important temporal consequences as well. As Haya accounts of the surface of the skin suggest, a smooth, unblemished, and uninterrupted skin presents a particular temporal orientation. A smooth skin tangibly embodies a renewed and untrammeled condition that effaces the passage of time. While oiling the skin is not generally a part of Haya mortuary procedures,[10] the practice of shaving the head (*okutega ishoke*) is an important feature of these processes. Shaving creates a surface appearance similar to oiling, which, given the spatial and temporal orientations discussed above, may have significance for the ways in which memories are constructed at these times.

Shaving was occasionally described to me as an onerous obligation but also as a sure sign of mourning that allowed others to recognize your bereavement. Thus, shaving is clearly intended to create an *appearance*, an additional smooth, seamless form, that embodies the condition of mourning. Much has been made of the symbolic value of hair as a tangible medium of growth and expansion of the body. As a substance that grows beneath the skin, and yet extends beyond its surface, hair readily lends itself to discourses and practices concerned with the manipulation and negotiation of sociocultural boundaries and the distinctive expression of collective forms of identity (Turner n.d.; Vlahos 1979; Comaroff 1985). The identification of those in mourning is an important and frequently cited effect achieved through Haya shaving practices. Moreover, the importance of surfaces and enclosure that I have discussed as characteristic of Haya aesthetics indicates that shaving produces a newly created surface. Just as oiling the skin "clears" a smooth surface that, in Haya perceptions, effaces the passage of time, shaving also removes the concrete evidence of time and growth literally embodied in hair.

However, shaving, I would argue, is a more complex, even ambiguous, form of "adornment" than oiling; this much is at least suggested by the fact that oil-

ing is a practice associated with both everyday appearances as well as a range of
ceremonial occasions, while shaving is strictly reserved for periods of mourning.[11] Shaving draws upon the tensions of the skin as a surface that conjoins
internalized activity, growth, and vitality with external expansion and extension
of the physical body. A shaved head, for example, clearly presents a smooth, uninterrupted surface. And Haya mourners, in fact, make a special effort to prevent blemishes from appearing on a newly shaved scalp (this was always the reason given to me for applying banana leaves to your head after shaving), thereby
accentuating once again the importance of seamless integrity. But shaving not
only presents the appearance of enclosure, it also produces a form of potentially
dangerous exposure. Haya men and women often comment on the fact that a
shaved head is particularly susceptible to the effects of the hot sun, and colloquially refer to a sun "strong enough to shave with." Exposure of this sort can
lead to lethargy and even madness if it is not controlled. Shaving, then, like the
mortuary process to which it is so integral, conjoins elements of enclosure and
restriction with those of exposure and dissolution in an attempt to recreate—in
bodily as well as collective terms—the integrity of those in mourning.

   The timing of this procedure and the sets of social relations engaged in
shaving are especially important to the meanings of adornment that have been
addressed thus far. Two to three days after the deceased has been buried, men
and women in mourning for their clansman will have their heads shaved.
Anyone who considers themselves a "relative" (these days the Swahili term for
"cousin/brother," *ndugu*, is used) of the deceased can elect to have their head
shaved. This may include agnates and affines, or even particularly close friends.
It is interesting to note, however, some important connections between shaving
and funeral shrouds, connections that turn on the relations of affinity so closely
linked to the development of Haya sociality and the temporal structuring of
memory and anticipation. A few days after the burial of the deceased, and
roughly coincidental with the shaving of the mourners, the deceased's daughters return to their marital homes from the site of the funeral. The next day they
bring with them enormous pots of cooked food, which are used to feed and
thereby give thanks and acknowledge the prior contributions of those who have
attended the first several days of a funeral. Like the blankets and sheets of
bridewealth that recall those spoiled during childhood, these pots of food are
intended to recall the troubles that those in attendance at a funeral have en-
dured. The term for these pots of food (at least in the southern regions of
Buhaya) is *engembe*, which, according to several senior informants, is a somewhat antiquated word for razor.[12] These gifts of food, therefore, are closely
related to the shaving that (very roughly) coincides with their presentation.

These gifts of food and the shaving procedure can further be associated with the provision of funeral shrouds. These pots of food are (stereotypically) provided by daughters of the deceased, who prepare the food at their husband's homes (usually aided by members of their matrilocal funeral association, *ekyama*) and transport it back to their natal home for consumption. This pattern of provision and consumption follows that of funeral shrouds, which, as we have seen, are provided by the affines of one's children. The parallels between these offerings also extend to the specific ways in which they establish connections between affines and agnates, as well as the mourning community as a whole. Like the funeral shrouds provided for the deceased, the "razors" will ultimately be used to create an appearance for those in mourning. That is, just as the mourners' gift of funeral shrouds that wrap the deceased provide the cloth to be worn by those in mourning, the foods (or "razors") prepared by returning daughters is associated with the shaving of those in mourning. Mourners, in both instances, fulfill an obligation to *others* (the deceased and those who attend the deceased's funeral) by means of tokens that create *their own* appearance as mourners. These agents simultaneously *perform* and *represent* the meanings of their social positions.

There is, moreover, a similar aesthetic of seamless surfaces created by shaving, which complements the material form of funeral shrouds (especially bark cloth shrouds). I would further argue that the most important feature of these prepared pots of food with respect to the structuring of these various social relations has to do with the significance of food itself and its precise place in the mortuary process. However, the range of culturally configured practices, concepts, and debates that are entailed in food-related activities is far too wide to adequately address here.[13] For present purposes, it is sufficient to point out that food provision and preparation are practices critical to demonstrating household self-sufficiency. Haya domestic arrangements, from the spatial distribution of crops on a family farm to the cooking techniques of boiling and roasting at the hearth, are all oriented toward securing internalized control over food as a means of achieving household independence.

Given these very basic concerns, the gifts of food at this particular point in the mortuary process exemplify a set of spatial and temporal tensions similar to the dynamic orientations of Haya adornment aesthetics. On the one hand, these gifts of cooked food are taken into the house of the deceased and redistributed to those who have attended the funeral. This ability to feed one's friends and neighbors, especially on the usually sumptuous food prepared for such offerings, suggests a degree of control over food. A house in mourning (which eats very poorly for the first few days following death) thereby begins to reestablish its integrity through this use of food. At the same time, this food is clearly provided and, just as importantly, cooked by those from outside the household itself. Accepting food that has been grown on distant lands and cooked at hearths far removed from the hearth that is a focus of domestic productivity also demonstrates that the mourning household depends on others to sustain it at these times. Thus, the pots of food provided by children of the deceased from their marital homes convey a sense of the tensions characteristic of the mourning process. Both the emerging control, enclosure, and integrity of the mourning household, as well as its continued dependence upon and potential susceptibility to outsiders at these times are concretized in the pots of cooked food.

Conclusion

These food presentations establish certain direct connections with Haya adornment practices. Their description as "razors" links them to shaving, and their provision ties them to the central affinal offerings of funeral shrouds. But, more importantly, the orientations instantiated by these gifts of food implicates them in the *aesthetic* common to shaving and wearing funeral shrouds. These pots of food not only share a pattern of distribution with these other items, they tangibly incorporate the values and contradictions posed by presenting an *appearance* in the course of the mortuary process. All of these related activities and offerings draw attention to the specific sociocultural problems of integrity and coherence in the face of death, problems that are made concretely evident in the surface forms of mortuary. The tensions of productive enclosure and the susceptibilities of exposure are combined and revealed in the surface appearance of a mourner's shaved head, the seamless construction of a bark cloth shroud, or the mourning household's distribution of the cooked food it has received. And, as we have seen, these surface appearances also exemplify temporal qualities that complement the spatial ones described. Both continuities and discontinuities are created in the seamless surfaces of Haya mortuary practices. Shaving can suggest a form of renewal in the sense of reinitiating a process of growth; the gift of a funeral shroud can be seen to complete the anticipated outcome of an ongoing relationship. There are spatiotemporal *dis*continuities, as well. The severance of shaving or the separation of shrouding—and thereby the concealing of the deceased—imply a rupture in the temporal forms of the body as it is positioned in the establishment of Haya sociality. These dynamics also recall the qualities of heirlooms played upon by grandchildren's effigies, a practice that disguises and deceives through the appearances it reveals. These, then, are the shifting and ambiguous potentialities of a surface form—possibilities of enclosure and disclosure, integrity and dissipation—that make not just clothing but the broader activities of adornment and creating an appearance such an extremely rich field for constituting the temporal orientations out of which Haya memories are created and recreated.

Haya understandings of clothing, then, suggest that adornment is an important aspect of the construction of identity and sociality over time. In the specific context of Haya mortuary practices, adornment often concerns processes of memorialization, of remembering the dead while participating in, undermining, or transforming aspects of the deceased's identity. From a more general perspective, I have also argued that the significance of clothing to processes such as these has to do with actually *wearing* clothing. Haya activities surrounding death demonstrate that the complex questions entailed in wearing clothing and the variety of ways in which it can be worn make clothing more than just an object that mediates interpersonal relations, but a medium whose objective qualities emerge in the course of social practice itself. In particular, the practices of clothing the body and the array of activities in which clothing figures work to generate appearances, surfaces that are not merely facades but rather tangible embodiments of the dynamic orientations of social process. Such appearances create dynamic surfaces that expose and enclose, reveal exterior and conceal interior dimensions of the body. The Haya adornment practices through which they create appearances give clothing the capacity to articulate alternative constructions of identity—to contrast seniors and juniors, agnates and affines, Europeans and Tanzanians—and to embody, through time, continuities and discontinuities, anticipations and memorials.

Notes

An earlier version of this essay was presented at the annual meeting of the African Studies Association in November 1991. I would like to thank Misty Bastian for developing the conference's panel on clothing and for encouraging me to develop some of the most important aspects of my argument. My research was funded by a Fulbright-Hays doctoral dissertation fellowship. The Tanzanian National Institute for Science and Technology (UTAFITI) enabled me to live and work in Tanzania. I would never have had the opportunity to carry out this research had it not been for the tremendous generosity of Severian and Anatolia Ndyetabula.

1   This essay is based on field research carried out in 1988–1990 in the Muleba District of the Kagera Region in Tanzania. In this essay the words I have cited in translation are from Oluhaya, except in those cases where I have indicated that the word is Kiswahili, or have given both Oluhaya and Kiswahili terms.

2   *Kansu* are long white robes, rather like a cassock, that Haya say they have "borrowed" from Muslim styles of dress.

3   Provided they aren't agnates themselves—i.e., this excludes only one's father's father's clan; all other grandparental clansmen are possible marriage partners.

4   *Kanga* and *kitenge* are commercially produced printed textiles. *Kanga* worn in Tanzania are often produced in Tanzanian or Kenyan factories. The printed design is often a central image (an animal, a kerosene lamp, or a political leader, to cite only some of the most popular images) with a surrounding border. Often, a Swahili proverb is printed as part of the border design. *Kitenge* are also printed textiles, but they have a much broader range of designs and origins. I have seen Indian saris, Indonesian batiks, and Rwandan cloth worn as *kitenge* in Kagera.

5   Such marriages (*okukaitwa* in Haya, *Kufunga ndoa* in Swahili) are not commonplace. In the late 1980s, only a small percentage of rural Haya marriages (perhaps less than a third) had ever been "officially" sanctioned in this way.

6   My ideas about the construction of time and space and of sociocultural practice as producing concrete orientations of time are derived from Merleau-Ponty's phenomenology (1962). I develop my analyses of Haya temporal and spatial orientations more fully in Weiss 1996.

7   I should point out that a woman engaged in manual work in the fields or around the house would not be expected to enclose her upper body in this way. Still, many women would wrap a second cloth across their backs while working, thereby freeing their arms for work, but also maintaining the propriety of a second cloth.

8   While my Haya friends remarked on how large bark cloth could be, they bemoaned the fact that it was no longer as smooth and soft as many of them remembered.

9   Indeed, the term *obugenyi*, which is most frequently used for "wedding," can be used to describe any of the celebrations that accompany either a marriage, birth, or death. As one friend told me, "A person has three celebrations [*obugenyi*], not just a marriage [*obugole*]."

10   While people may well oil themselves in times of mourning, I never heard anyone describe this as a common mortuary practice.

11   Indeed, I was often told that it would be improper to shave your head at other times, because, being so strongly associated with mourning, it would suggest that you wished ill of a clansman.

12   The Swahili word for razor is *wembe*, which is a cognate of the apparently archaic *engembe*. In contemporary Buhaya, the vernacular for razor is *jileta*, derived from the ubiquitous Gillette brand of blades.

13   See Weiss 1996 for a more detailed discussion of the many values of Haya food.

III INTERCULTURAL RELATIONS AND THE CREATION OF VALUE

6 DRESSED TO "SHINE": WORK, LEISURE, AND STYLE IN MALINDI, KENYA

Johanna Schoss

Introduction

It's lunch time. A group of four young men enter the small eating establishment, loudly greeting the men already gathered there at several long tables. The restaurant is filled with men, all of whom seem to know one another. Conversation and good-natured joking flow between the groups of diners. The men entering together are dressed in similar fashion: slacks in solid colors—either blue or red, sharply pressed button-down shirts, expensive watches, leather loafers. A few moments later another group arrives. They are dressed in a more varied fashion; one wearing jeans, a T-shirt emblazoned with the Hugo Boss insignia, and sneakers; another in brightly colored windsurfing shorts, tank top, and plastic flip-flops. They enter with a commotion, calling out loudly: "*Ciao! Ciao belli neri!*" Animated conversation, now in Italian, ensues back and forth across the room.

This could be an unremarkable scene in a trattoria somewhere in Italy, possibly near the ocean. But the scene is Malindi, a mid-sized town on the Kenyan coast. The eating establishment is a small, wooden, thatch-roofed kiosk located along a dusty footpath, in the back regions of the open-air marketplace. And all of the men present are Kenyan, largely Swahili. What, then can explain this behavior—the range of Western clothing, the inclusive conversation in Italian?

To an observer leaving the restaurant, passing through the marketplace crowded with retailers of varied ethnic identity, Malindi would appear a rather typical East African coastal town. In one direction, the dusty roads of the town center are lined with two-story, white-plastered, balconied shops in an architectural style found throughout Kenya and other parts of the former British empire. Behind the market, moving away from the town center, is the densely populated neighborhood of Shela, with its single-story, thatch-roofed houses, built of coral stone blocks. It is only as you walk east from the town center, toward the Indian Ocean, that a second and seemingly discontinuous Malindi appears. Here the road, popularly called "Tourist Road," is lined with luxury hotels whose verandas face the bright sand beaches and glistening Indian Ocean. The picturesque dhows of local fishermen dot the horizon, and tourists, in various European styles of street- and beachwear, can be seen on the beaches and roadways.

Over the past twenty years, tourism has transformed Malindi from a fishing and agricultural village into a multiethnic urban center that annually hosts thousands of tourists, largely Italians and Germans. Malindi has a long history as one of the earliest mercantile towns of the East African coast, towns that have been involved in trade across the Indian Ocean for nearly one thousand years. The Swahili people who historically have populated these coastal cities are the descendants of Arabs who settled in the region and intermarried with Bantu-speaking Africans living along the coast.[1] Traditionally, Swahili people, who were urban-based, distinguished themselves from their non-Muslim, rural-dwelling African neighbors, though the rigidity with which these two populations identify themselves as distinct ethnic groups appears to have increased over time under the influence of the British colonial administration (Willis 1993). Currently, the vast majority of the rural population surrounding Malindi are Giriama, an ethnic group that is among eight closely related groups collectively called the Mijikenda. Malindi today is highly ethnically heterogeneous, with both Swahili and Giriama living in town, along with numerous relatively recent arrivals from other parts of Kenya. Tourism has served as a major impetus for in-migration to the area.

The restaurant of our opening scene, which offers home-style Swahili food, is a favorite lunch spot for men working in the tourist industry. Given their structurally central position, such people act to some degree as mediators, or "culture brokers" (see Cohen & Comaroff 1976). While tourism infiltrates all arenas of the Malindi community—as a force of social, cultural, economic, and political change—the critical encounter between locals and foreigners takes place through the intermediation of specific members of the host community.[2] That is to say, certain individuals, most often through their employment activities, either formally or informally, have intensive and ongoing contact with European tourists. Thus, they serve to mediate between tourists and other members of the local community, many of whom have little regularized contact with the foreign tourists. Evans (1976, 192) captures several key characteristics of the culture broker when she describes such individuals as "often bilingual, innovative, analytical about their culture, and active in introducing change and mediating between the local group and outside agencies."

While there are many kinds of culture brokers in Malindi's tourism economy, in this essay I focus on one category—tour guides. Within this category I
include men who work specifically as tour guides as well as the vehicle drivers
who escort tourists on safaris or daily outings and the people employed in tour
and car rental agencies. Individuals engaged in tour guiding are found in both
the formal and the informal sectors of the tourism economy. Those working in
the formal sector are employed directly by tourism enterprises such as hotels
and tour agencies; others are self-employed, independently offering tourists
their services as guides. The men working in these two domains exhibit significantly different sets of practices, while at the same time they all share one
critical characteristic. Unlike others working in the tourist industry, who earn a
living by providing a particular service—such as waiters who work in hotel
restaurants and who mediate tourists' experience of Kenya in the process—tour
guides earn their income exclusively through their abilities to act as cultural
mediators. In practice, tourists have much more intense and sustained interactions with tour guides than they do with other members of the Malindi (or any
host) community. Several studies (e.g., Smith 1989, Almagor 1985, de Kadt 1976,
Towner 1985) have focused on the role of such mediators in structuring tourists'
experiences of foreign locales. Erik Cohen (1985), lending an historical perspective to the inquiry, notes that the role of tour guide has undergone several
transformations, but ultimately derives from two roles—those of "pathfinder"
and "mentor." The contemporary tour guide incorporates the qualities and
functions of both of these earlier roles. In the pathfinder mode, the tour guide
leads visitors not through uncharted territory, as in times gone by, but through
the tourist landscape, in particular "providing [tourists with] privileged access
to otherwise non-public territory" (Cohen 1985, 10). In the mentor mode, the
tour guide is likened to the tutor who accompanied the pupil/traveler on his
European Grand Tour, providing the pupil/traveler with the insights with
which to interpret his experiences. In this respect, the tour guide serves as a mediator and educator, responsible for translating and interpreting local culture
to the tourists. The tour guide also becomes a mediator between tourists and
local residents; by providing tourists access to the local culture and community,
the guide also becomes responsible for both buffering tourists' experience of
the unknown and protecting the community from the European "Others."

Perhaps the most important role played by these culture brokers is that of
interpreter. Cohen (1985, 14–16) refers to this aspect of the guide's role as the
"communicative function." The tour guide acts as an interpreter in multiple
ways. First, he literally acts as a language translator because he is competent in
the languages of both the tourists and the local community. Further, rather
than simply showing tourists what is there to be seen, the tour guide essentially

creates the landscape (both physical and cultural) that tourists view by his selection of "attractions." With these "attractions" he directs the tourists' gaze (see Urry 1990), both by revealing to them the local life and landscape and by concealing other possible scenes and objects from the tourists' view. This process of structuring the tourist gaze is one way in which tour guides engage in cultural brokerage, but it is also an act of interpretation, in that the guides provide a context for the tourists' reading of and consumption of the local scene. And finally, tour guides are translators in that they provide tourists with a "translation of the strangeness of a foreign culture [that of Malindi, of Kenya, and of Africa more generally] into a cultural idiom familiar to [them]" (Cohen 1985, 15).

The tour guides' ability to translate from one cultural idiom to another stems from their possession of what Hannerz (1990) calls "the cosmopolitan perspective." The "cosmopolitan," as opposed to the "local," is someone who is exposed to a multiplicity of cultures, but more than this, Hannerz (1990, 239) suggests that the cosmopolitan perspective is

> a stance toward diversity itself, toward the co-existence of cultures in the individual experience, . . . a state of readiness, a personal ability to make one's way into other cultures through listening, looking, intuiting, and reflecting.

Malindi's tour guides are characterized both by this intellectual and aesthetic orientation toward "the Other," and by possessing the requisite competence to maneuver their way through alternative cultural systems.

The cosmopolitan identity of Malindi's tour guides is based upon their understanding of, control over, and successful deployment of Western goods, practices, and cultural knowledge. Through their sustained interaction with Europeans, tour guides have become very adept at understanding how tourists of different nationalities behave in terms of dress, speech, and action, as well as learning to anticipate what tourists expect and even—as many tourism entrepreneurs would say—how tourists think. These locals have also learned to embody European styles of dress and behavior. A Malindi formal-sector tour leader, explaining the nature of this knowledge, once pointed out to me that Coastal people really understand Western tourists and "The West" in general far better than do "up-country" businessmen and bureaucrats. He highlighted his point with images of dress and "style," saying:

> One time a group came here from Nairobi [Ministry of Tourism officials] in their suits and ties . . . They have lots of formal education but no hands-

on experience, so they really don't understand these things [i.e., tourism, Europeans] . . . We Coastal people have no education, but we are really more sophisticated. . . . You people have made us this way. You [Europeans] taught us how to talk, how to dress, how to walk . . . They [the bureaucrats] have their white-collar shirts and ties on, but if you look at them from behind, there's nothing there—only a shirtless collar.[3]

What the tour leader implies here is that it is not enough to *know what clothes to wear,* as do the suit-wearing bureaucrats. Rather, one must also *understand how to wear the clothes*—the bodily comportment, the cultural competence that makes the act of wearing believable. These "upcountry" bureaucrats control the overt forms of Western culture, but somehow fail to grasp its substance. For dress, it seems clear, is synecdochic for Western material forms and cultural understanding in general.[4] Thus, it is not surprising that Malindi's tourism professionals present and represent their involvement in the global tourist economy and their relations with European tourists through their selection of particular styles of Western dress and comportment. The choice of styles varies quite markedly between the group of men who work in the formal economic sector—employed by largely foreign-owned tourism enterprises—and those men who are self-employed in the informal economic sector. I will return to these stylistic variations after a discussion of tour guiding in Malindi.

The History of Tour Guiding in Malindi

As I mentioned above, there are different categories of tour guides in Malindi, distinguished most importantly by their operation in either the formal or the informal sector of the tourism economy. In Malindi, with the exception of one or two tour guides of either description, these men are locals—both Swahili and Giriama. Tour guides working in the formal sector are those employed by European tour agencies on a salary plus commission (on sale of safaris, etc.) basis. In keeping with the terminology used in the tourist industry internationally, these people are called tour leaders. They, along with the safari drivers and tour agency personnel, constitute the group of what I call "professionalized" tour guides. This category of employment arose with the development of the tourist industry itself. At least as early as the mid-1970s there were a growing number of Malindi residents employed by tour agencies and car rental firms as drivers, managers, office personnel, and tour leaders. Currently, all local tour agencies, the vast majority of which are foreign-owned, employ local tour leaders who are responsible for the daily overseeing of tourists. These individuals assist tourists from the moment of their arrival at the airport and throughout their stay. They arrange for the tourists' daily entertainment and excursions, assist them with any problems, inquiries, and explanations. Tour leaders have primary responsibility for their agencies' clients and have the most extensive contact with them. At the same time, tour leaders must work in perfect concert with safari drivers and tour office personnel in order to successfully manage their tourist clients. Thus, I include the men working in these positions as part of the larger category of professionalized tour guides. In keeping with the characteristics of the tour guide outlined above, these men are professional culture brokers who act as the interface between tourists and their experience of Malindi generally.

At present the group of men involved in formal-sector tour guiding activities—either as tour leaders, safari drivers, or other tour agency and car rental personnel—includes men ranging in age from their early twenties to late forties. These men have mixed educational backgrounds, some with secondary school education and beyond, others with little or no formal schooling. As with most forms of tourism employment in Malindi, people gain the bulk of their job-specific training through experience and through informal networks. Younger men are taught such skills as languages, knowledge of how the tourist industry works, and information about wildlife, bird species, geography, and so forth, by men with more extensive experience and knowledge. This teaching occurs both on the job and at informal gatherings. There is no tourism training institution in Malindi. The national tourism training institute—Utalii College, located in Nairobi—offers degree-granting programs, but enrollment is quite limited and few Malindi residents have the opportunity to attend. Some employees in formal-sector enterprises are sent to Utalii College by their companies for additional training through short-term, intensive courses.

In addition to this group of men employed by formal-sector agencies, there is another fairly large group of men who work as tour guides, though they do so independently. Operating without the structured relationship between themselves and specified groups of tourists assigned to them by tour agencies, they "freelance," plying the streets and beaches of Malindi to create their own relationships with tourists. They do so by soliciting passing tourists—whom they refer to as guests (*wageni*), rather than tourists (*watalii*)—with offers to arrange safaris, provide tours of Malindi and the surrounding area, or assist them in shopping for curios. In fact, they provide much the same services as those orchestrated by tour leaders, only without the legitimacy of having formal employment positions. Since they are not salaried, they earn their income based either upon commissions paid by safari companies and shopkeepers, voluntary remuneration from the tourists (in the form of both cash and gifts such as clothing), and more rarely, by charging set fees for the tours they provide. There is no explicit Swahili word to describe these men. Rather people describe what they do: *wanatembeza wageni,* "they tour guests around." Colloquially they are commonly referred to as "beachboys" by Malindi residents, including foreigners involved in the tourist industry, although this term carries some ambivalence. While they may use the term among themselves, the men who do such work sometimes reject the label when it is applied to them by others. Like those working in the formal sector, these men range in age. Most are between their early twenties and middle thirties, although there are also some much older men who engage in this work.[5]

The history of the development of this group sheds some light on the ambivalence with which they and their activities have been viewed. Quite early on in the expansion of the tourist industry, by 1968, the term was used to refer to youths of Kamba ethnicity who hawked wood carvings to tourists on the beaches. These men were not involved in the sort of tour-guiding activities described above. By the beginning of the 1970s, however, a new group of young men entered into the tourist economy. These men were Swahili secondary school students who initiated closer interactions with tourists. Their activities met with much resistance on the part of Swahili elders and school officials, and eventually most of these youths were forced out of their beachboy activities. It seems that many of this original group later sought employment in the formal sector of the tourist industry, and eventually they became part of the "professionalized" tour leaders and tourism employees (Peake 1984, 82–124; my interviews confirm this).

Peake (1984, 86–87), who conducted research in Malindi between 1981 and 1982, notes that at that time men working as independent tour guides fell into two groups. The first group consisted of those older men who had begun such activities while still in secondary school and had not been dissuaded by community pressure. The second group were younger boys, ranging in age from sixteen to their early twenties. He does not say how this group originated, but the following story gives some clues. The story, told to me by several different people, seems to be factual in its essential details. I believe it can also be read both as an origin myth of the Malindi beachboys and as a morality play.

Although many Swahili children living on the Coast never attend formal secular school, virtually every one attends Madarasa, afternoon Islamic schooling, for two or more years. There are numerous Madarasa in Malindi; attendance is frequently organized on a neighborhood basis. About seventeen years ago, one of the Madarasa was run by Musa, a local businessman. Musa, it is said, was one of the most learned scholars of Koran in the community. At that time (the early 1970s) tourists—largely from Germany, Austria, and Switzerland—were just beginning to visit Malindi. Musa taught his students to sing songs in German and French and when he heard tourists passing by on the streets outside, he would stop classes and invite the tourists into the classroom. The children would line up along the walls, from the smallest to the tallest, and entertain the tourists with their singing. He told the visitors that the students were orphans and he would appreciate any contributions to assist them and the school which he ran. It is said that he kept the bulk of the money himself and gave the children only a few coins or some candy. As one former student reports, the first generation of contemporary beachboys[6] to work Malindi's streets were the products of this training. He reports that as they became teenagers, the boys from Musa's Madarasa class became beachboys. Many of this original group, now men in their mid-thirties, continue in this work today. In 1986, Musa went blind rather suddenly. One afternoon while I was sitting with some Swahili men—some, beachboys and others, taxi drivers—someone commented about Musa as he passed by on the street. One man who was a member of this original group of beachboys, remarked ironically, "Yes, he was our great teacher. He taught us to follow the Europeans." Pausing, he added, "that is why God has made him blind." I later heard a somewhat different account of Musa's sudden and mysterious blindness, during a conversation with several young men who have formal sector employment in the tourist industry. This group described the events leading to Musa's blindness as follows: He is diabetic and his doctor had given him a bottle of some solution which, when added to a urine sample would indicate his blood-sugar level. Upon leaving the doctor's office, Musa promptly forgot how to use the solution. While having lunch with a business associate he ingested some of the liquid and immediately began to lose his vision. He never saw again, despite several trips to Europe for treatment. Hearing this account, I remarked that I thought God had made him blind for hiding the Koran from the children in his Madarasa. The group collectively responded, "Yes, of course. Why do you think he forgot how to use the solution?" Thus, regardless of the explanatory mechanism, the basic interpretation of this event remains the same. Musa's blindness is interpreted as punishment not because he profited from tourism, but rather because he profited in an inappropriate way. He deceptively used the skills of others, namely the children, to his own advantage. Beachboys and tour leaders, on the other hand, utilize their own *ujuzi* ("wisdom," "practical experience"), which is part of the cultural information encoded in their cosmopolitan styles of dress and comportment (see Schoss 1995).

Peake (1984, 29–44) offers some additional historical information which helps to bring into clearer focus the sociological parameters of these groups of tourism entrepreneurs and their relationship to Malindi's Swahili community at large. In August 1982 there was an election for the seat on the Malindi Municipal Council that would represent Shela, the very old neighborhood that is the heart of the Muslim community. Musa was one of three candidates to run for the position. Despite the fact that Musa can trace his family back to the very earliest arrivals in Shela, he had some difficulty gaining neighborhood support and was ultimately unsuccessful in his bid for election. His difficulties were linked directly to the activities described above. As Peake describes:

> Some years ago [Musa] was a much respected Islamic scholar, and many Shela young men were taught by him in the local Muslim school. However, amid some scandal he was forced to leave his teaching. He had invited some tourists into his school and had shown them various sacred texts. This was considered intolerable disrespect, especially as he had received money from the tourists for the sacrilege. However [Musa's] scholarship is still recognized; for example, he is still regularly invited to lead the prayers at grave sites. (33)

Beyond this, Musa had engaged in even more direct tourism activities. He had "organized several trips for tourists into parts of Shela" (33). In recent years, beachboys offer the very same excursions, bringing tourists directly into the domain of Swahili daily life. Much of Musa's constituency were, in fact, beachboys. His detractors called him "the beachboy elder," and accused him of corrupting the Muslim youth (33).

The "professionalized" men involved in tourism, both at that time and today, attempt to distance themselves from the beachboys and their ambivalently viewed practices. Yet in the early days of tourism development, they too were seeking some way to negotiate between the relative isolation of their Muslim community and their own involvement in tourism. Recalling the early days of tourism involvement, one Malindi tour leader[7] recounted that the confrontation with community elders was often quite heated and frequently voiced in religious terms. Muslim elders expressed their antipathy by condemning the youth who interacted with Europeans, calling them "*watoto wa motoni*" ("children of/in the fire," i.e., "damned") and thieves who would burn for their sins. In response, he and other young men, including both beachboys and the newly emerging group of "professionals" working formally in the tourist industry, took up the banner of Islamic fundamentalism, claiming the elders were misinterpreting Koran and that interacting with Europeans was not in itself evil. In addition to joining Islamic revivalist groups, these young men also engaged in forms of resistance that were in explicit contradiction to Islamic teachings, such as the wearing of numerous gold chains and medallions, including crosses.[8] Peake (1984, 36) gives further evidence of this strategy: In response to the criticism of his involvement in tourism, Musa took the position that he was actually acting in the interest of Islam, arguing that "Islam was an evangelical religion, and therefore Muslims should never be afraid of dealing with out-siders." Further, he suggested that introducing outsiders to the value of Islam and demonstrating Muslim generosity and openness could only serve to prove the religion's superiority and relevance for the modern world. His stance found fertile ground among the "professional" youths, many of whom supported his candidacy.

Clearly Musa was an early tourism entrepreneur and a self-conscious culture broker, and yet it was not his involvement in tourism per se that was prob-lematic. Indeed, at the time of his election bid, and today as well, many Swa-hili residents of Shela earned a living through some involvement in tourism. Rather, the key issues under debate concerned precisely how this involvement should be enacted.[9] And this debate is still underway, as the following incident illustrates. In March of 1990 on the first day of Ramadan,[10] I was with a group of beachboys on the street near the center of town. One of the beachboys had just finished telling me that because it was Ramadan he was fasting, not working, and not planning to work for the entire month of the holiday, when Hamud approached. Hamud is the same age as the other young men, speaks Italian quite well, and works in the formal sector for an Italian company. He imme-diately began to berate the group of beachboys, saying they had disappointed him and marveling that they could claim to be fasting.[11] It seems the beachboys had been at the Baobob Cafe[12] the night before, drinking until the early hours of morning. Afterward, as Hamud described, "they came into the village[13] in the morning, drunk and making a commotion (in Swahili, *fujo,* "disturbance," "uproar") which everyone could hear." Other beachboys passing by or sitting within earshot joined the conversation, many of them supporting Hamud in his criticism of the accused youths. Interestingly, the conflict between Hamud and the other young men is not about the evils of such Western ways as alcohol consumption, but rather how such activities are pursued. Hamud himself fre-quents discos and drinks alcohol, though not during the month of Ramadan. His disapproval stems from the combined fact that the others were *publicly* drunk, particularly during Ramadan, and they brought their activities "*into the village.*"[14] As this incident shows, such actions can potentially meet with disap-proval from both professionalized tour guides and beachboys. Thus, although beachboys in general mark their involvement in tourism activities through a far more gregarious demeanor than their formal-sector counterparts (as I discuss below), the question of just how far one can acceptably go is still very much under debate, even among beachboys themselves.

In part, the conflict turns around a question of domains—that is, what places, activities, and practices should remain distinct from touristic influence. The boundaries of the domains are under constant debate, but Musa's blindness could be attributable in part to his failure to recognize the boundaries at the time. By mixing tourist entrepreneurship with Islamic sacred texts he incurred divine punishment. The ambivalence toward beachboys and their activities has significantly lessened in recent years, to the point where their activities are generally accepted as a legitimate occupational alternative. Beachboys have gained this recognition by developing a code of acceptable and "proper" work practices that is quite palatable to more conservative Muslim sectors of the community (Schoss 1995). Musa, I would argue, did not conform to this code, a factor that may help to explain the contemporary analyses of his sudden affliction. In the end, Musa did not win the election, and he has since given up any attempt at political life. The harshness with which both beachboys and professionals describe his blindness is, I believe, an indication that in the ongoing debate over how to engage in the tourist economy, Musa's personal strategies have been found to be inappropriate.

Cosmopolitan Styles in Malindi's Tourism Economy

As the opening description of tourism employees suggests, both formal- and informal-sector tour guides wear Western clothing. Certainly it is true that many Malindi residents (both men and women), regardless of their occupations, wear Western clothing routinely. In addition, more traditional items of clothing and styles of dress are still very often worn throughout the community.[15] The most commonly worn local items of dress include the *kikoi*, the *sarong*, and the *kanga*. The *kikoi* (Swahili; plural *vikoi*) is a male item of dress, very often worn by fishermen. It consists of a colored length of sturdy cotton fabric (five feet long by three-and-a-half feet wide), fringed at the short ends, with a decorative band running lengthwise at each edge. It is worn tied lengthwise around the waist and held in place by rolling down the top edge, as if to form a waistband. A somewhat different version of the locally produced *kikoi* originates in South India. It is also called *kikoi* or, more commonly, *sarong*, and is constructed of softer, more intricately decorated cotton. This fabric is purchased already sewn into a circular column. It is worn in the same way as the locally produced *vikoi*—wrapped tight at the waist and rolled down at the top to secure it. Such items of clothing are "traditional" in that they have a long history of use on the Kenyan Coast among both Swahili and Giriama men.

Another quite similar item of clothing is the *kanga* (plural *kanga*), also called *leso* in Coastal areas. Like the *kikoi*, it consists of a rectangular length of cotton, with an elaborately decorated border and complementary field design. In most cases, there is a proverb written in Swahili at the bottom of the central field. These items are produced in Kenya, as well as in other countries (China, India, the Arab countries), and are worn throughout Kenya. Among Swahili people, they are considered strictly women's apparel and worn in matched sets of two pieces, one wrapped at the chest, or at the waist if worn with a shirt, and the other wrapped over the shoulders. Among Giriama, however, men will also wear *kanga*, tied at the waist as are *vikoi*.

As detailed below, Malindi's tourism culture brokers wear these traditional items of clothing in some settings, but they more typically wear Western clothing. In wearing this garb, they stand out from the local community, even those dressed in Western-style clothing, in quite overt ways. Both beachboys and tour leaders dress so as, it is said in a local idiom, "to shine." Their appearance draws attention to itself, marking their access to expensive goods and a comfortable lifestyle. Minou Fuglesang (1994) has discussed this notion in Swahili society, looking at the *kupamba*—the ritual during which a bride is publicly presented to the women of the community for the first time. For this ceremony the bride's hair, skin, and body are carefully prepared through beautifying treatments. If the preparation is successful, the bride will "shine," meaning that her inner beauty has been brought out, but also that she has properly chosen and worn fine clothing, makeup, jewelry, and other accessories. Thus, Fuglesang further notes that "to 'shine' is associated with new commodities and the 'trendy'" (128). And indeed tour guides "shine" because their garments stand out for their notable newness, quality of manufacture, and European origin (as opposed to Western-style clothing produced in Kenya or elsewhere in Africa). Beyond the particularities of the items worn, tour guides' dress is marked by a high degree of self-consciousness about the act of wearing these garments. Unlike the often haphazard ways in which other locals may mix and match Western clothing, tourism employees conscientiously combine items of clothing into a consistent and identifiable style; a style that is intentionally cosmopolitan. But, formal-sector tour leaders and beachboys assemble Western clothing into two different, very distinctive cosmopolitan styles.

These styles encompass not only dress, but also bodily comportment and consumption practices. Thus *style*, as I use it here, refers not merely to a way of dressing, but more importantly to the way in which people present and represent themselves to others in a manner that implies an underlying ideological vision (see Hebdige 1979). Style, in effect, is a way of being in the world; one that demonstrates conscious choices and speaks to differentiated sociocultural systems of value and meaning. Indeed, these two cosmopolitan styles are readily distinguishable through distinctions that, to the outside observer—be it the anthropologist or the tourist, seemingly lie "on the surface," in the visual forms and appearances of the garb and in the observable behavior patterns. And yet, the crucial distinction between the two styles lies beyond the realm of the visible, embedded in differing ideological orientations. These styles become the tangible markers of two very different strategies through which formal-sector and informal-sector tourism employees engage with the tourist economy. I will return to this point after a detailed discussion of each style.

The formal sector: tour leaders, safari drivers,
car rental and tour agency personnel
Tour leaders (including the range of men working in formal-sector tour enterprises) deploy a constellation of Western goods and practices in what I have called the *professionalized* style. Typically, these men wear slacks, button-down dress shirts or polo-type sport shirts—always clean and carefully pressed—and shoes imported from Europe. They may also wear jeans or logo-embossed T-shirts, but these items are always very crisply pressed and new-looking. They may also wear khaki safari suits; this is particularly common among safari drivers. On occasion, they opt for traditional clothing in the form of a *kanzu*, a long gown often worn for prayer at the Mosque and ritual events.[16] Most often, however, these men wear slacks in solid and somewhat subdued colors. In fact, most tour agencies have some kind of uniform, which consists of solid color pants of one or two designated colors (such as red or blue) and white shirts— short-sleeved and buttoned-down, with buttoned front pockets and epaulets. Nevertheless, employees have a good deal of liberty in adopting such uniforms, liberty that they fully exercise in their daily choice of clothing—for example, by pairing the appropriate solid-colored slacks with a striped or patterned shirt. Overall, their style is what would be described locally as "smart" (in Swahili, *smarti*)—that is, polished, sharp-looking, and well put together.[17]

It is this very practice of maintaining a look that is perfectly "put together" that so clearly and immediately marks the professional tour guides. They dress very much like their European clients and employers, and yet somehow more so than the Europeans themselves. Dick Hebdige describes a similar phenomenon with British youths who adopted the "Mod" style in the early 1960s:

Unlike the defiantly obtrusive teddy boys, the mods were more subtle and subdued in their appearance: they wore apparently conservative suits in respectable colors, they were fastidiously neat and tidy. . . . The mods invented a style which enabled them to negotiate smoothly between school, work and leisure, and which concealed as much as it stated. . . . the mods undermined the conventional meaning of 'collar, suit and tie,' pushing neatness to the point of absurdity. . . . They were a little *too* smart, somewhat *too* alert. . . ." (1979, 52, emphasis in original)

Malindi's professionalized tour guides similarly endeavor to effect a Europeanized look that even the Europeans cannot quite match. What one notices about their dress, without being able to immediately point to it, is their uncanny ability to look at the end of a ten-hour work day in the equatorial sun, precisely as they looked when they first got dressed—gleaming shirts, still pressed razor-sharp and unsoiled by the day's heat; never appearing less than absolutely neat, contained, and "smart."

These formal-sector employees maintain this professional appearance most of the time, both at work and in their free time—at discos in the evening with friends, for example. In a few limited contexts tour leaders allow themselves to "dress down," wearing shorts or *vikoi*, casual T-shirts, sneakers, sandals, or even bare feet. Such contexts include occasions when they escort clients on beach outings, in their own homes, or on Friday afternoons or Sundays when relaxing with friends at their *maskani* (meeting place).[18] Only the first of these contexts is work-related, and in this case casual attire is appropriate. Tour leaders would consider dressing in slacks and shoes for a beach or fishing outing to be as ludicrous as bureaucrats who arrive for a tour of the Marine Park wearing suits and ties. The other two settings that are exceptions to this strict code of "professional" appearance are settings completely outside of tourist domains. Private homes and local *maskani* are places where tourism professionals can truly relax, because these places are, for the most part, inaccessible to tourists. While beachboys may bring tourists into their neighborhoods, and even to their own homes, they would rarely bring them to a neighborhood *maskani*. Friday afternoons or Sundays are significant because, during the peak tourist seasons, these are virtually the only times tourism professionals can escape the demands of their jobs. Even when not officially working, tour leaders consider themselves to be in the public eye in professional terms whenever they are in public spaces that are accessible to tourists. Thus, they maintain their professional appearance and demeanor when relaxing in the evening with friends at restaurants or night clubs, even if they are not accompanying clients.

For the most part, these men purchase much of their clothing directly from Europe. Other items they have custom-made for themselves by local tailors. Apart from items like *vikoi,* they rarely buy clothing produced and mass-marketed in Kenya. Professionalized tour guides explained this antipathy for locally produced clothing in two ways. First, they complained that Kenyan-made clothing intended for local consumption was poor in quality and shabbily constructed. Second, other items intended for the tourist trade were considered to be rather absurd. One tour leader, wryly commented on such mementos by saying, "What kind of clothes would I buy here in Kenya? A 'JAMBO KENYA' T-Shirt with elephants on it?" Such attitudes toward clothing highlight the activities of guides as culture brokers. They are able to convincingly direct the tourist gaze toward the stereotypical commodity representations of "Africa," at the same time rejecting those images as characterizing or encompassing themselves.

Independent tour guides: the beachboys
The beachboys have a much more flamboyant and unpredictable style, which consists of often outlandish and wild combinations of colors and patterns of European clothing and accessories. They commonly wear shorts; bright colored windsurfing pants are among the more popular, but long and baggy, or shorter running-style shorts are also common. Jeans are another common clothing item; in 1989–1991 many beachboys were wearing the stylishly torn variety. These items are paired with brightly colored and variously patterned shirts or T-shirts, sneakers or bare feet. In terms of "traditional" dress, beachboys will wear *vikoi,* though only one beachboy in Malindi routinely wears *kanzu* and most of the others rarely do. Another typical feature of beachboys' attire is the fanny pack—called *kipauchi* in Swahili, an item that is apparently very popular in Europe. Such packs are ubiquitous in Malindi now and are used by formal-sector tourism employees as well, though among beachboys they are practically de rigueur. Locals get these packs either by trading with tourists, or by gaining access to those given to tourists by local tour agencies. As with other clothing items, beachboys prefer the brightly colored fanny packs. Among the goods that make up the beachboy style are items of clothing that I call "indigenous chic." These are clothing items made from some transformation of a local item—one example is *kikoi* or, more typically, *sarong* material tailored into a pair of loose-fitting, drawstring trousers. These pants, and other similar items, have an interesting history in that they were initially transformed into pants by local tailors on demand from tourists. Tailors and shopkeepers began stocking them as a part of their regular stock; beachboys eventually took up wearing

them, and now tourists buy them, thinking that they are adopting something of the local style (though within the local community, *only* beachboys wear such items). Another "indigenous chic" style is clothing made from three-inch squares of many different fabrics. Local tailoring shops use their scrap materials to make pants, vests, and hats that have a dazzling, multi-colored, quilted appearance. In general, beachboy style draws upon both the more avant-garde and funky elements, and more casual trends in popular Euro-American fashion.

The "indigenous chic" items of the beachboy style are purchased locally in tailoring shops that also make clothing for tourists. Most other items are European in origin, but unlike their formal-sector counterparts, beachboys are less likely to purchase these items directly. Rather, they get a lot of their clothing by trading with tourists—as, for example, in exchange for wood carvings. They receive other items as gifts or as payment for tour guiding services they have provided. And in some cases, they may purchase items directly from Europe, or receive them through the mail as gifts from clients. Unlike the dressing style of formal-sector tour guides, that of beachboys is highly marked within the Malindi community. In local slang it is sometimes referred to as "*kichizi*," a word that has the sense of funny, comical, or unconventional. One adolescent boy described beachboy dressing habits to me in the following way:

> They wear very short shorts. They wear the same clothes for months at a time, without washing them, until you can not even tell what color they are supposed to be—they are the color of mud.

While the description is not empirically accurate, it does reflect the ambivalence with which beachboys' dress and overall comportment is sometimes viewed by the community at large. Of course, there is a good deal of variation among beachboys with regard to both clothing and comportment, and some beachboys dress in a more conventional style, similar to their formal-sector counterparts. For the most part, however, their self-presentation is unconventional, as indeed is their insistence on creating their own niche in the tourist economy rather than simply choosing among the opportunities offered by the formally structured industry. By dressing in the "beachboy style," these men both practically and symbolically preclude their formal-sector employability (see Ewen 1988, 64–77ff).

Other Clothing Styles

Many local Swahili and Giriama men continue to wear the *vikoi* or *sarong* described above. For example, fishermen, particularly older men, typically wear *vikoi*, often belted at the waist with wide belts made of tightly webbed canvas and equipped with built-in, leather-covered, waterproof pockets. Over their *vikoi* they wear cotton, long-sleeved, button-down shirts. If they are actually going out to fish, they may trade their button-down shirts for T-shirts, saving the former for wear during less arduous activities. When walking out to their boats, they roll up the bottom of the *kikoi,* pulling the back panel up and tucking it into the waistband at the front, creating a billowed, shorts-like effect. Similarly, Giriama men often wear *vikoi* of the locally produced sort, topped by some kind of shirt. Men working at such enterprises as fish markets, selling produce in the central market, or as proprietors or employees of local shops, lodges, and restaurants may dress in this manner.

People who work in tourist hotels or other European businesses are expected to wear standard Western dress. In everyday situations the majority of Muslim women continue to wear the traditional *buibui*—a black, loose-fitting, ankle-length garment over their dresses, together with a scarf-like headcovering. In recent years, an increasing number of young Swahili women are finding employment in tourist shops or hotels, but the management of these enterprises does not allow the women to wear *buibui* on the premises. Many women, in such cases, continue to cover their heads while at work and simply carry their *buibui* with them, taking it off as they approach the hotel or shop entrance, and putting it on again as they leave work. Men working in tourist hotels and restaurants as waiters, barmen, and so forth are generally required to wear uniforms provided by their place of employment. Those working at management levels can choose their own work clothing, and like the formal-sector tour leaders, they dress in a "smart," "professional" style. Young men who are members of the local elite—such as the sons of the wealthy, business-owning Arab families of Malindi—also have access to the expensive, European clothing worn by formal-sector tour leaders. Unlike the tour leaders, however, they tend to dress more casually on a daily basis, wearing their more expensive-looking European clothing for evening outings. Another group of people working in Malindi's tourism economy are those who own small curio retail kiosks.[19] Like the beachboys, they are also informal-sector tourism entrepreneurs. They dress in Western style and, like the beachboys, sometimes receive clothing from tourists in exchange for items from their shops. Yet, while they may keep some of these items for their own wardrobe, for the most part they prefer to resell these clothes to other locals in exchange for cash. In contrast to beachboys and formal-sector tour leaders, they will wear clothing purchased locally and of Kenyan manufacture.

Women working as prostitutes have a dress style that is highly marked and in some ways similar to that of the beachboys. They also have access to expensive European clothes and accessories, which they receive from clients or purchase from Europe. Many of these women have been to Europe and brought clothing back. These women are very style conscious and spend a good portion of their earnings on fashionable European clothing. In addition, they often wear "indigenous chic" fashions, such as *vikoi* pants or items made locally from African fabrics, which are sold for the tourist market in expensive Malindi boutiques. Thus, like the beachboys, they are often the innovators of local fashion trends which are then adopted by tourists.

Though many Malindi residents wear Western-style clothing, most residents do not routinely wear clothing marked by its quality, newness, and obvious foreign manufacture, as do the tour guides. In addition, tour guides (both formal and informal sector) and prostitutes prominently wear accessories such as expensive watches, Ray-Ban sunglasses, gold jewelry, Italian leather shoes and belts—items that are often not available locally.[20] Thus in some cases, the distinctions between these cosmopolitan styles and other local dress styles that I am describing are readily discernable. For example, as noted above, many of the items worn by Malindi cosmopolitans are readily noticeable because they are either not available locally, they are markedly superior in quality, or they look expensive and beyond the means of most locals.

In other respects, however, the distinctions between cosmopolitan styles and the average dress of most Malindi locals are more subtle. In part, this is due to the nature of the Western fashion industry itself. Styles change very rapidly and often in almost imperceptible ways. As consumers and residents living in the West, we are bombarded with these changes on a daily basis to the point where our ability to discern what is "fashionable" or "stylish" is often intuitive. For example, a person may be wearing what seems to be a perfectly straightforward cotton, button-down shirt, but yet the person somehow does not seem quite "fashionably dressed." This stylistic misfire may be due to an alteration of cut, such as the shirt lapels being a fraction too wide to accord with current fashion. This is often the case with Western clothing available in Kenya and elsewhere in Africa, with regard both to clothing produced by the local clothing industry and that available through the secondhand market. The items are Western in pattern and style, but the cuts and the detail of design are such that they do not quite meet the demands of the most contemporary fashion trends. Though Kenyans are exposed to changes in Western styles (and consumer goods more generally), they have differential access to the "volatility and ephemerality of fashions" (Harvey 1990). Malindi's cosmopolitans are marked by their ability to discern subtle changes in fashions in Euro-American terms—that is, they take pains to stay apace of the rapid changes in Western consumption practices.

An additional factor that plays into the styles of the beachboys, professionalized tour leaders, and prostitutes is the self-consciousness with which items of clothing are put together to create a particular "look." This "look" becomes embodied not merely through wearing the clothes but also through mastering the sensibility, the attitude appropriate to the style. Part of this is the ability to put together items in a way that accords with conventional norms and "genres" of dress—rather than, for example, pairing a red plaid work shirt with a wide blue-striped tie. This ability to "coordinate" an entire "look" is something Malindi's cosmopolitan tourism employees acquire through self-conscious effort and an intensive knowledge of the fashion code. The ability of tour guides (and prostitutes) to "pull off" these styles also depends upon their control over many other items of European cultural capital as well, such as language, cultural norms, and a detailed empirical knowledge of European society.

Other Elements of Style

Items of dress are not the only Western goods consumed by local tour guides in Malindi's tourism economy. Commodities that are less tangible, those that may be best thought of as commoditized practices, also enter into the equation of cosmopolitan styles. Among these practices, perhaps the most apparent one is leisure. Both beachboys and professionalized tour guides, particularly the younger men, participate fully in the cycle of leisure activities that are intended for the consumption of tourists. For example, the discos held nightly in various hotels are, without fail, packed with these men, whose presence in number sometimes overshadows the tourists themselves. This is so despite, and in conscious opposition to, various past and present efforts to limit locals' presence in such places. Peake (1984) details how in the early 1980s hotel managers and local police authorities made efforts to restrict local access to tourist areas; efforts that angered many locals, particularly beachboys. While most of the hotels sponsor a disco featuring a popular deejay one night of the week, in 1984 there was only one enterprise that operated strictly as a disco every night. The management of this disco, Club 28, held a dance contest every Saturday night, with prizes for the winners. Although this marketing ploy was geared toward tourists, beachboys and prostitutes, with the tacit assistance of the disc jockeys, soon began to dominate, consistently winning nearly every contest. The management responded by opening a new and more impressive disco, the Stardust, with entrance fees double those of Club 28. Peake (1984, 120) notes that "the 'capture' of Club 28 was hailed as a great victory by the beachboys." Between 1989 and 1991, Club 28 continued to be a favorite nightspot for beachboys and other local cosmopolitans, as did the Stardust, despite its high entrance fee.

Local cosmopolitans consume tourist-designated leisure activities throughout the year,[21] but do so particularly during the days between Christmas and New Year's Eve (the peak of tourist high season). At this time of year, even locals who never routinely attend the discos will go as part of the holiday festivities, and tour guides will be present every night. During this time, the hotel managements raise the disco entrance prices to often astronomical levels (sometimes equivalent to the price of nightclubs in Manhattan), but nevertheless the dance floor is always dominated by an overwhelming proportion of locals. By New Year's Eve, the disco is so crowded and the beachboys so rambunctious in their dancing that tourists rarely brave the dance floor.

Indeed it is an essential aspect of the cosmopolitan style of tour guides that they dine in tourist hotels and restaurants, frequent discos, drink expensive liquor, travel by taxi or private car, and so forth. Unlike many other members of the local community, they have incomes that allow such expenditures, but more importantly, their legitimacy as cosmopolitans depends upon it. As with their choice of clothing, beachboys and professionalized tour guides consume leisure in markedly different ways. They make use of similar leisure settings and practices, but in doing so they comport themselves in strikingly distinct ways. Similarly, they represent their participation in and consumption of such activities in significantly different ways.

Tour leaders, in such settings, (and this is true of their practice overall) present themselves with an extraordinary degree of reserve; they must, as they say, remain "cool."[22] They drink alcohol, but not to excess. They avoid loud, obtrusive, or unruly behavior. In part, tour leaders' decorous behavior is linked to their rationale for being in tourist settings at all. They often justify spending time in nightclubs because it is part of their work. Indeed, they often serve as host to their agency's clients, escorting them to Malindi's various leisure settings. Even when they are not with a group of clients, however, they maintain this demeanor, because they are always, in effect, "on the job." They see themselves as always in view of tourists, tourism investors, and managers. Thus they carefully guard their "professional" appearance both within the tourist economy and in front of the local community. At the same time, tour guides behave with this remarkable reserve because it is this quality that they hope to put forward, both to the local community and to the participants of the tourist economy, as their defining personal and professional characteristic. In short, their "reputation" (in the sense of the Swahili notion of *heshima*) rests upon representing themselves as confident, dependable, highly qualified, and always in control.

Beachboys, on the other hand, engage in such leisure activities with an abandon that is often not matched even by the tourists themselves. They have a fairly earned reputation for making a public display of drinking heavily, fighting in public places, and generally causing scenes. On occasion, some beach-boys' behavior results in their being thrown out of these leisure settings. At such times they can begin to frequent the disco or bar again only after long negotiation with the establishment's management. Their behavior during these evening outings frequently becomes a topic of disapproving conversation in the local community the following day. In their tendency toward excess, they seem to consume leisure in its most marked, most "tourist-like" form.

There is one important issue that needs to be clarified at this point. The practice that the culture-brokers consume, the "leisure" in which they engage, is explicitly leisure as conceived and constituted by Western cultural understanding. It is leisure as Urry describes it: "leisure activity which presupposes its opposite, namely regulated and organized work" (1990, 2). Leisure, in this sense is very much an historical development, linked closely to the emerging industrial economies of nineteenth-century Europe. Detailing the legislative and organizational changes surrounding nineteenth-century industrial work forces in Britain, Urry points out that along with increased routinization and control over industrial labor forces, formalized recreational events and structured holidays increasingly came into effect. Such policies followed on the theory that structured breaks from work helped to increase labor-force efficiency and workplace discipline (Urry 1990, 17ff; also see Cummingham 1980). These institutionalized holidays, in turn, were directly linked to the rise of the British seaside resorts, one of the early sites of contemporary mass tourism.

This form of leisure, as structured nonwork, stands in marked opposition to local practices in Malindi, where social interaction, "relaxing," and labor are continuous and undistinguished activities. Thus, for example, beachboys spend much of their time while on the streets looking for clients, sitting casually and talking with groups of friends. To a foreign eye this looks like a form of leisure, but by local consideration it is merely an unmarked aspect of daily life and an aspect that is integrally interwoven with labor activities (cf. E. P. Thompson 1967). In fact, it is an essential part of their daily work, in that beachboys exchange important information and keep each other updated as to the current tourism situation in Malindi through such informal conversational settings. While tour guides are often furthering their business interests while "at leisure" in such tourist facilities as hotels and nightclubs (seeking clients, etc.), they are also *explicitly* consuming structured leisure for its own sake, as do the tourists. Urry, in his discussion of the rise of tourism and its linkages to the rise of structured participation in "leisure," suggests that "acting as a tourist is one of the defining characteristics of being 'modern' " (1990, 2). Indeed beachboys are explicitly trying to appropriate the practices of tourists—including leisure styles and practices, in effect making themselves members of an international tourist class. And yet they consume leisure practices in a manner that sets them outside of this international tourist class, because—unlike the tourists who return to the routine of work when the vacation ends—beachboys act like tourists throughout the year. Just as the formal-sector tour leaders surpass Western tourists in the manner of wearing of Western fashions, beachboys exceed the tourists in their continual and conspicuous pursuit of fun-seeking.

Indeed overt displays of conspicuous consumption are the most striking feature of beachboys' participation in tourism-linked leisure activities. For example, beachboys often will celebrate a successful day of work by spending all their earnings in a lavish public display, buying all their friends drinks and demonstrating their control over large amounts of cash. Some beachboys even express the philosophy that if they do not spend their often substantial income readily, they will not earn more money the next day, but if they do spend their earnings freely, they can feel confident that they will earn more the next day. From many beachboys' point of view, it would appear that the whole point of earning good incomes working as tour guides is to enable themselves to spend that income publicly. At the same time, many beachboys use their earnings on private forms of consumption, such as household expenses or remittances to their extended families.[23] When among their fellow beachboys, however, they generally downplay or in some cases completely hide these private expenditures. Other beachboys, however, redistribute very little of their often substantial earnings to their immediate or extended families and/or to other members of the community.

The professionalized tour guides also earn relatively large incomes, and their professionalized style and identity indeed depends upon having this financial security. They also spend money on leisure activities, but they do not make their spending publicly known through conspicuous displays in leisure settings, as do many of the beachboys. On the contrary, they spend a good portion of their incomes on the support of their own families as well as assisting extensive networks of kith and kin, a practice that is widely recognized within the local community. In doing this, the professionalized guides reinvest their earnings in traditional Swahili values of social reproduction as economic providers, and in doing so they index their own status as social adults (cf. Fuglesang 1994, 193). In fact, such men are quite willing to severely limit their consumption of leisure activities during the low season,[24] but even at this time of year they would find it difficult to refuse a request for assistance. In part this is because the obligation toward family and community assistance is so integral to their "professional" reputation and style, and in part because they are loath to admit publicly to financial hardship themselves. One tour leader described this dilemma as follows:

> During the low season, some days when I'm really broke I'd rather carry no money at all. That way if someone asks me to give them something [i.e., money], I can say: "Sorry I don't have any money with me today. Ask me tomorrow and I'll give you something." You see, if someone asks me for help, I can't say no if I have money in my pocket. I have to give them something . . . and these days I just can't afford to, so it's better if I go out with my pockets empty.

These distinct consumption and expenditure patterns—which I argue are crucial features of the beachboy and professionalized styles, respectively—yield a relationship of unequal interdependence between the two categories of tour guides. The professionalized tour guides' obligation to assist others extends to the beachboys as well. Beachboys, who do not have the same reserve toward admitting financial hardship, call upon tour leaders' largess for both direct financial assistance and aid in work-related matters. For example, formal-sector tour guides assist beachboys through such practices as arranging for the particular beachboys to accompany them and their clients on shopping outings and allowing the beachboys to collect a commission payment instead of keeping it themselves. While beachboys make such demands upon formal-sector tour guides with whom they have such a relationship, tour leaders would not call upon beachboys for such assistance.

This relationship of interdependence manifests itself in other domains as well as through these economic exchanges. As noted above, some beachboys periodically find themselves in trouble because of their leisure activities. In such cases, it is often professionalized tour guides who intercede on their behalf in negotiations with hotel management, local authorities, and so forth. In these situations, the professionalized tour guides are able to call upon their considerable networks of contacts, built up largely through their employment position. Their negotiating ability is reinforced, however, by their public reputation (both within the local community and the tourism economy), which gives them a mien of legitimacy and respectability. On the other hand, beachboys quite readily endeavor to build up this reputation (i.e., *heshima*) for the tour leaders with whom they closely interact. This respect is apparent in the way beachboys speak of and interact with their formal-sector counterparts. And at times beachboys will actually take action to maintain a tour leader's reputation and "cool" demeanor. On one occasion at a disco, a tour leader was being harassed by a local youth. The tour leader was surrounded by other formal-sector tourism employees, but when it appeared that he and the young man might come to blows, he was suddenly surrounded by a dozen beachboys who appeared seemingly from nowhere. The beachboys ushered the tour leader away, insisting that they would do any necessary fighting. Thus, in many respects their contrasting behaviors work in concert, with beachboys protecting professionalized tour guides from scandal and professionalized tour guides assisting beachboys who find themselves in trouble.

What these interactions suggest is that beachboys are in certain respects subordinate to the professionalized tour guides. This relationship is sustained by the Malindi community at large, which views beachboys with some ambivalence while according professionalized tour guides a good deal of respect. The ambivalence commonly felt toward beachboys is grounded in generalized community disapproval of the extreme examples of outlandish beachboy style (both in terms of dress and behavior) in which some individuals engage. It is further linked, I would argue, to the fact that some beachboys wield their identity explicitly to avoid family and community financial obligations. And yet, ironically enough, parents and other elders often excuse beachboys from such obligations on the basis of their "subordinate" position, with the effect of inadvertently encouraging the relationship of unequal interdependency between the two groups. That is to say, in many cases beachboys choose to pursue work as independent tour guides rather than becoming professionalized tour leaders or seeking other more formalized employment, precisely because as beachboys they can avoid the often burdensome obligations of family and community financial assistance. Despite the facts that, on the one hand, beachboys often earn quite good incomes through their activities, and on the other hand, many still resist pressures to redistribute this income, parents and other elders will sometimes excuse these young men from their obligations with justifications that they, as it is said, are "jobless," or at least do not "have good work."[25] Men working in formal-sector employment as professionalized tour guides, safari drivers, or other tour agency employees could not similarly use this logic to avoid community and family obligations.

Conclusion

These two categories of tour guides clearly exist in an interdependent but unequal relationship to one another. While this relationship entails a hierarchical status distinction between the two groups, such status distinctions do not yield an arena of serious competition or struggle for social and economic power between the two groups. Rather, the arena of struggle in which both categories of tour guides are involved is that over social and economic power between locals and the Europeans who dominate the tourism economy, both as investors and as tourists. In this context, beachboys and tour leaders are engaged in a debate over how to insert themselves into the changing economy. It is only in light of this debate that the distinctions in style between these two groups become intelligible. Indeed, these two distinct styles embody alternative strategies by which locals position themselves within the political economy of international tourism.

Both beachboys and professionalized tour guides not only seek to gain access to the tourism revenues that figure as a relatively new but increasingly important feature of the local economy, they are also endeavoring to assert some measure of control over the economic and social changes that tourism is bringing to Malindi. It remains an undeniable fact that the tourist economy is dominated by European investors who have the capital necessary to establish large tourist facilities and who largely control the flow of tourists into Malindi. Beachboys and professionalized tour guides have chosen to locate themselves quite differently within the overall structure of the local tourist industry. Professionalized tour guides, in choosing formal-sector employment, place themselves in the very center of the European-controlled tourist industry. Indeed their dress style materially indexes this socioeconomic position. From this position they utilize their cosmopolitan knowledge and competence in order to make themselves indispensable producers of the tourist experience. Specifically, they employ their multicultural capital, which on one hand includes intimate knowledge of the local situation—such as the ability to recognize and package tourist attractions, or an ability to coordinate all facets of the local tourist industry and Kenyan services—and on the other, a detailed understanding of European practices, languages, and tourist expectations. In this way, tour leaders make their European employers dependent upon them for the smooth operation of the tourist industry. Their professionalized style, with its emphasis on a "smart" appearance and a "cool" demeanor, embodies this effort to place themselves within the tourist economy according to the terms dictated by the European-dominated structure of the industry and yet maintain a position of considerable personal and professional control.

The beachboys, by contrast, have a rather different agenda. They too seek financial reward from, and some measure of control over, the changing tourist economy. Like professionalized tour leaders, they use their cosmopolitan knowledge and identity to this end. At the same time, however, beachboys also venture to place themselves within the tourist economy by appropriating touristic spaces and experiences altogether. Thus they insert themselves into the political economy of Malindi's tourist industry, not only as producers of the tourist experience but principally as consumers of that experience.

A major feature of this strategy, and indeed a hallmark of the beachboy style, is the beachboys' refusal to participate in wage labor. Although these young men have the necessary qualifications to work as tour leaders for European agencies, they refuse to do so. Their casual and avant-garde dress style further marks this refusal because it is inappropriate to an office setting (and equally so to the mosque). Those beachboys who have worked for a time in a formal-sector agency, or in another form of wage-labor employment, quickly give up their jobs and return to working as a self-employed tour guide. The beachboys' extreme distaste for formal wage-labor is directed toward its regimented structure and its discipline-like features and rationale. In particular, beachboys note that they "could not take a job in a hotel or company because you are always being sent here and there," or "your boss can even tell you what to wear and how to use your time." In general, what these men seem to contest in such work settings is the lack of control over their person and the required conformity to institutionalized patterns of behavior, the very features that historically came to typify European notions of "work" and the industrial workplace (see Foucault 1979, 170–76; I discuss this issue along with a detailed analysis of Swahili cultural conceptions of work in my dissertation: Schoss 1995).[26]

It is precisely these features of the emerging European industrial workplace that structured leisure practices were designed to complement. Thus, the beachboys' refusal to engage in "rationalized wage-labor" stands in marked contrast to their ardent consumption of "rationalized leisure," since the two come as a pair in a Western work/leisure paradigm. And yet beachboys' leisure practices are in keeping with the internal logic of the beachboy style—that is, they are part of a strategy aimed at inverting the objective structure of the tourist industry as it exists in Malindi, and of the tourist encounter itself. A further indication of this strategy takes the form, among many beachboys, of a complete refusal to save money, or if they do so, to completely conceal this fact. They choose instead to engage in conspicuous expenditure, because they seek to present their consumption of those leisure activities geared toward tourists as utterly unproblematic. Through their distinctive style they suggest that whereas tourists spend money freely while vacationing, they themselves do so on a daily basis as a matter of course. The leisure beachboys engage in is not merely the rationalized opposite of work, but an extreme form that parodies the work/leisure contrast.

In effect, both beachboys and professionalized tour guides, through their cosmopolitan styles, assert and represent themselves as being sociological and economic equals of the tourists. Hebdige describes style as "intentional communication" that "gives itself to be read." Thus, subcultural styles

> are *obviously* fabricated. . . . They *display* their own codes. . . . In this they go against the grain of a mainstream culture whose principal defining characteristic . . . is to masquerade as nature. (1979, 101–2)

And, he further argues, they do so in order to highlight sociological difference and group identity. In the case of British subcultures this may well be "the point" behind distinctive styles. However, there are other contexts in which, though style is a motivated form of intentional communication, the point of this communication is to reject sociological difference and indeed to present the "obviously fabricated" style as fully natural. This is the case with cosmopolitan styles of Malindi's tour guides.

Beyond a rejection of difference, the styles inhabited[27] by Malindi tour guides make claims for the guides' membership in a supralocal cultural identity, that of cosmopolitan participants in "world culture." Numerous authors have noted the role of tourism, global mass media, and increasing mobility of and dislocation among the world's population in creating new arenas of cross-cultural visibility and dialogue. Many suggest that such forces are contributing to the development of a "global ecumene" (Hannerz 1989, 1992) or a transnational "public culture" (Appadurai and Breckenridge 1988), arenas of economic exchange in which new cultural forms and identities are being formulated and debated. Deena Weinstein (1989) suggests that it is "cosmopolitanism" or "transnationalism" itself that is the major commodity being exchanged in this arena. As an exchangeable commodity, "cosmopolitanism" (or "transnationalism") takes various forms, such as highly celebrated world events, style, consumerism, and perhaps most importantly, the knowledge of these forms and events. Further, the transnational event or form becomes a sort of symbol that both stands for itself and offers a coherent meaning—it offers its audience, the consumers, "membership in a world community transcending national, ethnic, or class communities; a community in which only the human as consumer and the consumer as human are relevant" (Weinstein 1989, 65). Although this process has accelerated during the last half of this century, Stuart Ewen notes that global consumer culture has its origins beginning with nineteenth-century factory production. He suggests that a "new *consumer democracy,* which was propelled by the mass production and marketing of stylish goods, was founded on the idea that symbols and prerogatives of elites could now be made available on a mass scale" (1988, 32). Membership in this global community of consumers, then, implies a state of cross-cultural equality. It is this theoretical equality to which one young Malindi man was referring to when he answered my queries about his newly adopted beachboy style of dress. "What do you mean?" he responded. "They're only clothes, aren't they? Anyone can wear them."[28] I would suggest that the styles of Malindi tour guides are indeed cosmopolitan, or transnational, forms of this sort. And as such, tour guides (and other local culture brokers) consciously draw upon this symbolic value of "equal membership in world culture" in their ongoing effort to reconfigure the terms of tourist interactions.

Yet, the emerging "global cultural economy" (Appadurai, 1990), to which mass tourism acts as a major contributor, is not giving rise to *one* newly forming modernity, *one* homogenized cosmopolitan identity. Rather, transnational contact lays the ground for the emergence of a *multiplicity of cosmopolitanisms*. Equally, "Westernization" is not a process that presents itself whole cloth—or perhaps I should say, fully clothed. The distinct styles through which local cosmopolitans incorporate and deploy Western goods and practices encode conscious attitudes and coherent strategies for addressing the globalizing tourism economy, and the encounter with the West in general. Style, consequently, articulates both alternative cosmopolitanisms and alternative means of managing social, cultural, and economic transformation.

Notes

This essay is part of my dissertation, *Beach Tours and Safari Visions: Relations of Production and the Production of "Culture" in Malindi, Kenya*. The dissertation is based upon twenty-two months of ethnographic fieldwork, conducted between May 1989 and February 1991. The observations presented here come not only from direct interviews and discussions with the tour guides described in this essay but also from my observations of and participation in the daily life of Malindi, as well as discussion with its diverse residents. I gratefully acknowledge the assistance of the Government of the Republic of Kenya and of the Institute for Development Studies at the University of Nairobi, with which I was affiliated. I also thank the Department of Education (Fulbright-Hays Program) and the Wenner-Gren Foundation for Anthropological Research, Inc. for their financial support of the research. In addition to the countless people of Malindi who took me in, aided me in so many ways, and taught me about tourism and much more, I must particularly thank my research assistant, Peter K. Ndaa. Though I have tried to bring the voices of many Malindi residents into this essay, all the names used are pseudonyms.

1   For a recent account of Swahili history and a discussion of the often debated nature of Swahili ethnicity, see Middleton 1992. Numerous other valuable sources exist,

including: Eastman 1971; Salim 1973; Allen 1974, 1981, 1993; Chittick and Rotberg 1975; Arens 1975; Nurse and Spear 1985; Sheriff 1987; and Freeman-Grenville 1988.

2 Indeed I would argue that Malindi is not unique in this respect, but rather that such loci of mediation (both human and geographical) are structurally inherent in virtually all tourist economies. Moreover, the notion of specialized social roles through which (inter-)cultural contact occurs is not particular to the study of tourism. Neither, indeed, is the process that it implies (on the notion of inter-cultural role networks (see Social Science Research Council 1954).

3 The broader context for this comment and the entire exchange is the Kenyan stereotype that Coastal people are backward and not fully engaged in the develop-ment progress (progress that is implicitly framed as "Westernizing" development) being made in other parts of Kenya. Fuglesang (1992) presents an interesting anal-ysis of how Coastal people view government officials as misinterpreting Islamic belief and practices (in this case, the practice of veiling by Swahili women) as backward and antidevelopment.

4 This same tour leader went on to elaborate that in contrast to such Kenyans (i.e., "Westernized" bureaucrats) who "think an *mzungu* (Swahili for "a European") is an *mzungu*, we [i.e., Coastal people) know how to deal with . . . how to actually live with an Italian, or a German, or a British person." A critical component of tour guides' cultural understanding is competence in European languages, especially Italian and German. Tour guides repeatedly express the notion that by engaging tourists in even the briefest exchange of greetings, they can immediately determine their nationality and even region of origin. Having ascertained that much, the tour guides maintain that the encounter to follow holds no surprises, because they know just what to expect of different categories of tourists. Through the control of this multicultural capital (see Bourdieu 1984), the tour guides are able to set certain of the key parameters of their encounters with tourists.

5 There are younger men taking up this work all the time, particularly those who have just finished secondary school and have not found other employment. Many of these new arrivals do not pursue such work for long, either because they find other work or because they find that they cannot successfully compete with the more experienced and skilled independent guides. Generally, the ones who do succeed in making tour guiding a viable career are those who have been taken on by older men and trained through a form of apprenticeship. This phenomenon of training and assistance made available through personal networks also occurs in the formal sector, as well as between the formal and informal sectors. That is, professionalized men will at times recruit beachboys into the formal sector, helping them to secure employment and training them in the necessary skills. There are very few women who work as tour guides in Malindi. It is usually the case that the women who work as tour leaders have formal training, often in the form of a degree from Utalii College, the national hotel and restaurant school. The men who hold such positions in Malindi, however, almost never have any formal training

and many have very little formal education of any kind. Most of them learned the business, including language skills, through experience, much of it gained by working in the informal sector for some time (as beachboys). As more young local women (particularly Swahili women) begin working in the tourist industry in clerical or concierge positions, this distribution may change somewhat. These young women have at least completed secondary school. The tour guides working in the informal sector, the "beachboys," are all men. There are apparently women who do such work in Mombasa (the larger Swahili port town one hundred and twenty kilometers to the south), but not in Malindi. Some government officials in Kenya have suggested to me that women who appear to work as prostitutes are actually informal-sector tour guides as well. It is simply not the case that any women in Malindi do the sort of work in which beachboys are engaged.

6   That is, the first group of beachboys as described in this essay, as opposed to the secondary school youths who briefly toyed with the practice.

7   This tour leader had briefly worked as a beachboy early on and was a student of Musa's Madarasa class. He is now employed by an Italian tour agency and is one of the professionalized, formal-sector tourism employees.

8   Although Muslim women wear gold and are expected to receive gold jewelry from their father upon their marriage, men are prohibited by Islamic law from wearing gold and silk. Fuglesang (1994, 135) notes that these items are discouraged for men because their beauty and shininess "distracts the worshipper during prayer." When worn by women, however, gold (or silk) is thought to "reflect the light (*nuru*) which is considered a divine quality, a visible manifestation of God's will working in the world."

9   In Musa's case, Shela residents argued that "it was one thing to work in the tourist industry outside of the Old Town, but quite another to invite tourists into the Old Town" (Peake 1984, 36). Peake refers to the neighborhood of Shela as the "Old Town." This is in keeping with the way locals refer to the early-settled Muslim/Swahili neighborhoods of Mombasa as Mombasa Old Town. In Malindi, however, I never heard Swahili refer to Shela this way. Rather, they call Shela "the village," as opposed to the rest of Malindi, which is referred to simply as Malindi or "town."

10   The ninth month of the Islamic year observed through fasting.

11   He said: "*Wanafunga vipi?*" literally "In what manner are they fasting?"

12   A small cafe and bar located near Shela and frequented by Malindi residents of various description, as well as foreign "travelers" (i.e., younger, low-budget tourists and backpackers).

13   I.e., Shela (see note 10).

14   Though this conflict was not generational—as the men involved are contemporaries as well as neighbors and, in some cases, relatives—Hamud expressed the problem in generational terms. Reminiscent of the early days of tourism, Hamud noted that the *wazee* (elders) reacted to the incident by pronouncing a *laana* (a curse) to the effect that the youths' entire lives would be of this sort. Hamud stressed, "And they're young. How does it look? Their parents will say something to

someone, but everyone will know that their son is like this . . . Their parents will have no face (*uso*) in public." The difference in positions of the men involved also manifests itself in the clothing each side wore. Hamud was wearing clean, pressed jeans and a pressed, button-down shirt; the others were wearing shorts or *kikoi* pants (a native style) and T-shirts in bright colors.

15   I do not intend to give a thorough discussion of traditional dress in this essay. I also am not discussing women's styles (either within the tourist industry or in nontourism contexts) in any detail so as to focus only upon those individuals involved in these two forms of tour guiding activities—who, as noted previously, are predominantly men.

16   When tour guides wear such traditional garb as the *kanzu,* they do it with a conscious intent of asserting Swahili ethnic identity—as they say, to "let these tourists know that I am a Muslim." In effect, at these moments, the guides deploy traditional Islamic dress in much the same way that the first generation of African nationalist leaders employed "traditional" garb—as a way of stressing that, yes, they are *fully knowledgeable about* and *competent in* the ways of Westerners, but that does not mean they wish to *be* Westerners.

17   Fuglesang (1994, 300) notes that young professional men (i.e., those working in "white-collar" office positions) similarly wear "well-pressed long trousers and spotless shirts."

18   Most adult Swahili men have some location where they gather in the evenings with a fairly regular group of friends to relax and converse. These meeting places can range from small coffee kiosks to a street corner or a shady tree.

19   This group includes both men and women, though the vast majority are men. Ethnically they are Kikuyu, Kamba, Kisii, and some Giriama, and most have come to Malindi over the past twenty years from other areas in central and western Kenya.

20   Leather shoes are certainly produced in Kenya and available in Malindi, but the quality does not compare to Italian shoes. Also, many locals wear less expensive, locally made canvas sneakers, plastic sandals, or flip-flops on a daily basis.

21   There is a noticeable drop-off in disco attendance during the tourist low seasons, in part because people simply have less ready income. During the bulk of the year, however, young men routinely attend the discos several nights a week, to the point where days of the week can be referred to by naming the location of the deejayed disco.

22   "Cool" as used by Swahili speakers in this sense stands in opposition to *moto* ("hot"), which carries the sense not only of hot with respect to temperature, but hot as with fever, bad or uncontrolled temper, or a lack of personal stability and centeredness. A useful comparison may be drawn between Swahili tour leaders' notion of "cool" in this sense, and R. F. Thompson's notion of "cool" as the guiding aesthetic principle in much of African dance. He notes that "cool" implies a sense of balance and order that combines vigorous bodily energy with controlled decorum. For example, he points out the Yoruba dancer who "maintains the whole

time she dances a 'bound motion' in her head, thus balancing a delicate terra-cotta sculpture on her head without danger, while simultaneously subjecting her torso and arms to the most confounding expressions of raw energy and force" (1966, 97). He further observers that the aesthetics of "cool" implies a moral imperative to proper conduct, a point I think equally applicable to Malindi tour leaders' "cool" comportment as well. The Swahili word that encompasses this principle is *utaratibu*—"orderliness" or "quietness" (see Schoss 1993 and 1995).

23 Some beachboys are married, though the majority express a desire to avoid mar-riage specifically because of the costs involved in first arranging a wedding and later providing a wife with clothing and other commodities.

24 That is, the off-peak season (May through July), during which the volume of tourists, and consequently tourist revenues, drops tremendously.

25 Fuglesang (1994, 196), looking at the new trend for young Swahili women in Lamu to finish secondary school and seek formal-sector employment, notes that it is far more difficult for young men to find employment upon completing their school-ing. The same is true in Malindi and this is one of the reasons that, unlike Swahili girls, boys often show little interest in formal schooling (see Schoss 1995). The real difficulties young men experience in finding formal-sector employment on the Coast contributes to the sympathetic attitude that elders take toward beachboys.

26 The men working as professionalized tour guides and employees are generally critical of the beachboys' style, attitudes, and practices. At the same time, however, they occasionally express a sort of admiration for the beachboys' ardent rejection of wage-labor and its implications of dependency upon European employers and lack of personal autonomy.

27 I use the term "inhabited" here because these styles are not merely superficially affected, that is, styles of dress that are copied from European images. Rather, these styles imply a radically reconfigured social identity, marked by the control over consciously acquired multicultural capital.

28 At the time of this exchange, this young man was in the process of undergoing an apprenticeship to a somewhat older and well-respected beachboy who tended toward a more professionalized appearance. During the course of his training, his appearance was completely transformed, presumably under the instruction of his mentor. Where the young man had formerly worn unremarkable, locally produced clothes in drab colors, he began to wear the new and brightly colored, European-produced garments typical of the "beachboy style." The more striking change, however, was in his choice of decorative items. He had always worn as a necklace a leather thong with three colored plastic beads on it and similar beads braided into one piece of his hair. This kind of necklace is commonly worn by young, somewhat urbanized Giriama men, and while it may be considered stylish locally (i.e., in and around Malindi), it is not appropriate to the internationally focused cosmopolitan style of tour guides. Soon after he was taken into training by the older beachboy he stopped wearing the necklace and cut off the long beaded lock.

7 "SUNLIGHT SOAP HAS CHANGED MY LIFE": HYGIENE, COMMODIFICATION, AND THE BODY IN COLONIAL ZIMBABWE

Timothy Burke

Before European influence . . . natives lived more or less like wild animals and in a general state of filth.—Native Commissioner, Gutu District, 1909

There is a custom which the old mothers do of bathing the babies' faces . . . When I came to stop them from doing that, some of them said, "our fathers and mothers were doing this, and we are well and strong" . . . How shall I answer them when they say this? —Elizabeth Mhombochota, teacher, 1935

This essay examines some of the intersections between race, bodies, and cleanliness in colonial Zimbabwe, with reference to recent scholarly models for recounting the social and historical role played by the human body. Such "body history" and related Foucauldian notions of "bio-power" and the "body surface" have attracted increasing amounts of interest over the last decade. This scholarship offers some powerful tools for interrogating colonial visions of the body, but it requires a considerable degree of historical precision in its application to African experiences. As it stands, body history is already acknowledged by many to be a loosely connected group of writings; this point was dramatized by the title of the three-volume anthology *Fragments for a History of the Human Body* (Feher 1989; Culianu 1991). At the most general and long-term level, such studies have pursued two intertwined concerns: the history of figurations, ideologies, and descriptions of the human body; and the related history of practices and uses of the body. One especially dominant strain in contemporary writings about the body follows on the work of Michel Foucault, especially his *History of Sexuality* (1980a). In his later works Foucault identifies a distinctive mode of modern power that produces its effects from within the sphere of the self—through regulation, inhibition, and introspection—a mode that he calls bio-power. Foucault's choice of defining prefix in this instance is not incidental;

his most memorable accounts of the functioning of bio-power have all involved institutions and practices concerned with the regulation and "inscription" of bodies—such as medicine, punishment, and sexuality. Some Foucauldian scholars have argued that his later texts offer the body as an anchor for a new political and ethical dispensation: Judith Butler, for example, identifies the body surface as a uniquely important locus for the configuration and reconfiguration of identity, sexuality, and gender (Foucault 1980a; Butler 1990).

Many Africanists have also taken an interest in body history in recent years. Rene Devisch, for example, has written recently of the use of body imagery in discourses among emotion among the Yaka of Zaire, in an article that clearly descends from a longer and more complex ethnographic lineage of writing about the African body (Devish 1990; Blacking 1977). Other recent Africanist studies dramatize both the advantages and dangers of using the body as a unit of social analysis. Jean Comaroff's rich and provocative study, *Body of Power, Spirit of Resistance,* sets forth a complex schema for understanding the symbolic and material culture adhering to bodies in Zionist religious practice in South Africa. Comaroff argues, with evident caution, that "the relationship between the human body and the social collectivity is a critical dimension of consciousness in all societies," while arguing that the histories of distinct Tshidi "ritual complexes" have generated distinct and particular uses of the body as metaphor and trope in culture (Comaroff 1985, 6–9). Gillian Feeley-Harnik's complex study *A Green Estate: Restoring Independence in Madagascar* (1991) details the full range of a cultural vocabulary of bodily experience—of death, life, hygiene, sexuality, beauty, and far more besides. Paul Stoller's *The Taste of Ethnographic Things: The Senses in Anthropology* (1986), insists that anthropological writings that included the sensuality of bodily experience would help to radically reconstruct ethnography away from scientific pretensions and toward a new "empiricism" based on rich narratives of personal experience.

Problems arise, however, when a particular local African vocabulary for describing bodies is translated indistinguishably into scholarly language about "the" body. Regarding the body as an invariably significant or coherent subject in any culture must be regarded as a suspect notion; the body as a subject is specifically a product of the peculiar and convoluted history of Western and Christian insistence on mind/body duality. The latest wave of body histories has mostly done a good job of historically contextualizing the particularity of various bodily discourses and practices in European history, although much of this scholarship also flirts dangerously with mistakenly reifying bodies—speaking, for example, about womens' bodies and women themselves as if the two entities were separate. It is far from clear that "the" body is an intelligible unit of analysis across time and space.

Many of these recent Africanist writings about the body, of which the texts cited above are only a few prominent examples, edge uncomfortably toward this mistaken assumption and assume the salience of the body as a subject in all societies.[1] In reality, there is no *inevitable* presence of the body in various discrete moments in diverse African cultures. In particular, bio-power and Butler's Foucauldian use of the body surface makes sense only in reference to historically specific and modern figurations of the body in Western history, and thus have dubious relevance to the pre-colonial and perhaps even contemporary cultural experiences of many Africans (Vaughan 1991).

Hygiene and the Colonial Encounter in Zimbabwe

The African body was an imagined subject that generated pervasive concern in official, settler and missionary discourse. Hygiene, domesticity, and manners were only components in a larger network concerned with the bodies of colonial subjects in southern Africa, a network that also included the discipline of laboring bodies in local versions of metropolitan discourses about bodies at work (Rabinbach 1990) and biomedical practices and discourses, including mine medicine, physical anthropology, and obstetrics and gynecology (Vaughan 1991; Burns 1994). It makes a great deal of sense to speak about the body within the bounds of this intensive and complex production of the physiognomic qualities of racial difference, hygienic and otherwise.

However, it is problematic to lump together various diverse and fluid notions and practices concerned with bodies that existed in pre-colonial and early colonial Shona, Ndebele, and Tonga cultures around the Zimbabwean plateau as functions of "the" body. The repertoires of hygienic, decorative, and mannerly treatments and uses of bodies in nineteenth-century pre-colonial cultures were important parts of everyday life, but they were not necessarily continuous across a single conceived realm of cultural practice or otherwise conceptually linked by their common involvement with bodies.

The most basic and regionally universal of these bodily regimens was "smearing," the regular use of a mixture of soil and some kind of oil or fat to coat most or all of the body. The specific soils used tended to vary depending upon availability and preference; most typically, thick red or yellow clay was used. The oil used was different from place to place—castor bean oil, miscellaneous other plant oils, and animal fat were all common. Some kind of paste from fats and soil, however, was a basic feature of a regular toilette, along with regular washing with water. There seem to have been several basic underlying justifications for smearing. First, the fundamental hygienic concept underlying smearing for most peoples seems to have been a belief that the best way to make bodies safe from dirt and other menaces in the environment was to coat them with a protective layer. Second, smearing was held to keep the skin from cracking or drying. Third, the glossy sheen of bodies and the sensuous feeling of smearing were widely regarded as fundamental components of an aesthetically pleasing appearance.

Beyond that, however, this basic routine alone was fluidly used to define a wide variety of effects throughout the region: marking ethnicity, defining elite status, or achieving gendered idioms of beauty and appearance. Smearing was only one component of larger, heterogeneous vocabularies of difference, not always or even usually narrowly functional, vocabularies that used bodies as canvases in various regional pre-colonial cultures. These included cicatrices (*nyora* in Shona), hairdressing, clothing, jewelry, scents, and plant-derived dyes and cosmetics. In another vein, notions about cleanliness were also a vital part of the rhetoric of ethnic differentiation and contest around the Zimbabwean plateau. The Ndebele and their allies used the Shona word *tsvina* (dirt) to describe their antagonists as *chiTsvina*, "dirty people."[2]

Daily washing was also part of other arenas of everyday life, especially the life of families and the arrangement of labor within the household. Among Shona speakers, men and women bathed in separate groups; children also bathed separately from the adults. Not all peoples around the plateau were able to wash in a river every day, and even those close to water usually refrained during the winter. However, even where river water was some distance away or when the weather was too cold, women usually would fetch water in the early morning. This water would be used for the washing of the face, hands, and other body parts. Again, washing was made into a ritual affirmation of relationships between men and women: in some places, wives were expected to attend to the washing of a husband's face and hands in the morning. Some households also had a *chibekeswa*, a small hut or enclosure for washing, with partitioned sections used by adult men and women in the household. In general, washing and the providing of water was governed by the same rules of deference and service that wives were supposed to observe in serving food to their husbands (Gelfand 1971).

Hygienic practice and bodily manners had many other varied dimensions in Shona, Ndebele, and other cultures and were tied to particular visions of sexuality, childhood, initiation, social malevolence, death, and other aspects of daily life. In any case, it is not clear that any feature of these figurations linked them within the symbolic worlds of the people who actually practiced them. Beyond the tendency of some ethnographic analyses to presume that all cultural practices have meaning and that all symbolic systems are seamless and universally understood by all members of a given community, there may be an even more specific problem with talking about "the" body in pre-colonial Zimbabwe. If we can describe today the pre-colonial body in southern Africa as a subject, or a realm of "alternative" hygiene distinct from the vision of European settlers, this is largely a *consequence* of the definition of linkages between all practices concerning the body under colonial rule.

Envisioning the African Body: Early Colonial Perspectives

Many Europeans arriving in the colonial worlds of the nineteenth century were interested in the sensual, physical, and bodily nature of indigenous cultures, and the early ethnographic texts that often framed their interest in these subjects shared this preoccupation (Pratt 1992; Stepan 1982; Stocking 1987; Gilman 1985). Philip Setel has argued convincingly that nineteenth-century travel narratives about Africa define "a conceptual domain in which health, illness and techniques of bodily display linked Africans to preconceived notions of race, moral status, and savagery . . . [a] hidden template against which the African body/person was measured." Setel also notes that among the vital components of this "template" were cleanliness, manners, appearance, decoration, and odor (Setel 1991, 13).

Early European visitors to south-central Africa, like Robert Moffat and Thomas Morgan Thomas, only fitfully regarded African bodies as filthy and degraded (Wallis 1945, 193; Thomas 1872, 171). Perhaps the only consistent object of commentary was the "greasiness" of local African peoples, a reference to the regional practice of smearing bodies with a mud/fat mixture. Francis Coillard, for example, complained that his shirts had been "borrowed" by an unknown African and thus were left smeared with "ochre and grease" (Boggie 1966, 243).

By contrast, later settler writings usually characterized African bodies as a coherent subject, one that was filthy, depraved, and ugly. European hygienic practices were defined as the essence of "civilization," coinciding with the cementing of intensive personal and social cleanliness as normative in English social life. Most Rhodesians settlers agreed with the author Jeannie Boggie: "The native generally by nature is a filthy animal. What is filth and dirt to a European is not so to a native" (Zimbabwe National Archives [hereafter ZNA] 1944 ZBJ 1/2/2). The African world was seen as a world of universal dirt and filth, and indigenous practices of bodily preparation and sanitation were always regarded as the inverse of "civilized" hygiene. There were occasional exceptions, of course, that inverted this perspective in favor of the stereotype of the "noble savage," praising the African body as natural, unspoiled, and Edenic.

Social segregation, especially the segregation of urban space, was frequently justified in colonial society by an appeal to images of disease, dirt, and pollution, making particular use of the evolving professional doctrines of tropical medicine (Curtin 1989; Vaughan 1991). Donald Denoon has described this process as the forging of "an important link between tropical *disease* and tropical *people*" (Denoon 1988, 125; Andersson and Marks 1988). This overall tendency of southern African colonizers to regard the proximity of Africans as a primary source of contagion has been referred to by Maynard Swanson as the "sanitation syndrome":

> Overcrowding, slums, public health and safety . . . were in the colonial context perceived largely in terms of colour differences. Conversely, urban race relations came to be widely conceived and dealt with in the imagery of infection and epidemic disease. This "sanitation syndrome" can be traced as a major strand in the creation of urban apartheid. (1977: 387).

This syndrome played a powerful role in Zimbabwe's urban history. The Sanitary Boards of colonial Bulawayo and Harare were important arenas for the design of segregated African "locations" removed from the city center and northern suburbs, especially from 1898 to 1911 (Gelfand 1953, 56–60; Gelfand 1964, 74; Yoshikuni 1989).

Educators and missionaries also drew heavily on portrayals of Africans as unwashed and pre-hygienic and subsequently had a major impact on the bodily practices of Africans themselves. The strong promotion by both local and imperial authorities of hygienic training for colonial subjects led missionaries in Zimbabwe to quickly emphasize it in the making of Christian, "civilized" African communities. Changes in the appearance and habits of converts— especially the wearing of clothing and the daily washing of the body—became important outward symbols of what the missionaries hoped would be a complete social transformation of African life. By the 1930s, the Southern Rhodesian Missionary Conference had wholeheartedly and aggressively embraced "the need of instructing Natives in Hygiene," arguing that

> the physique and bodily habits of the Natives were bad . . . The general alertness of natives was increased by cleanliness of person and home . . . Simple handbooks on hygiene should be supplied in the Native tongue. Hygiene should be a matter of first importance in schools. Dirt should be prohibited by superintendents and teachers, either on the person or around the

school . . . That cleanliness is next to Godliness should be taught. (Report of the Southern Rhodesian Missionary Conference, 1932, 15)

Textbooks and other pedagogical documents from this era give some sense of the slant and tone of appeals made to African pupils by teachers (Brackett and Wrong 1930). First of all, pupils were exhorted to rigorously pursue habits of personal cleanliness and to wear and wash clothing suited to their social status. In many cases, teachers enforced this dictum by inspecting students closely and turning away those who failed to keep to class standards. Missionaries assumed that the teaching of hygiene had to proceed from a solid grounding in Christian principles. Therefore, most of textbooks and course outlines began with an explicit linkage between personal cleanliness and Godliness. Missionaries and their allies often preferred to define dirt as an elemental component of immorality, a distilled, vague, and generalized essence of profane living. A "Catechism of Health" circulating in mission schools in the 1920s warned students against both "dirt of the mind" and "dirt of the body," giving the following definitions of each: dirt of the mind was "thinking bad thoughts or not thinking at all," dirt of the body was "to live in a dirty way and to have dirty habits" (Catechism of Health 1926, 6). Additionally, lessons on hygiene were often part of general attempts to promote "civilized" manners and discipline in the comportment of the self and the practice of everyday life (Elias 1978; Hunt 1992).

African women were the most exaggerated subjects of such campaigns. Images of hygienic practice and mannerly, "civilized" bodily habits were aimed at women largely through the intensive promotion of domesticity. In many ways, the imagined body of the colonial subject in Zimbabwe was first black but also crucially female, especially with regard to hygiene. The making of domesticity in Zimbabwe was pushed along by a number of complex factors, including recurrent "black peril" panics, concerns about the supply of male laborers, displaced arguments about the reproduction of black families, and evolving notions derived from metropolitan culture about the proper constitution of private space (Pape 1990; Schmidt 1992). Initially through "Jeanes" teachers— female home demonstrators who were trained and supervised by missionaries and funded by the state and international philanthropists during the 1930s— and later, from the 1940s to the 1970s, through a growing network of womens' clubs, Zimbabwean women in both rural and urban communities were increasingly exposed to settler notions about domesticity and bodily propriety (Ranchod-Nilsson 1992).

Such intensive efforts by the state and by settler society to define and change the African body often produced an equal and opposite effort among Africans to define "true" African bodies that stood in opposition to *chirungu*, the "ways of the Europeans." Native Commissioners' reports and missionary documents make it clear that for the first three decades of colonial rule, many elders forbade their children and grandchildren to attend mission schools; when possible, they sought to prevent such schools from operating (ZNA 1920 N 3/9/1–2). Similarly, home demonstrators in the 1930s frequently met with vigorous opposition, which often centered primarily upon the demonstrators' attempts to teach new practices of personal hygiene and to enforce the use of trench latrines.

Still, as time wore on, many other families and individuals strategically sought to satisfy the cultural requirements of the colonial order—in mission schools, in places of employment, in the public spaces of urban society, in their relations with state administrators. Colonial disciplines of hygiene and bodily manners reproduced themselves within the daily lives of many Africans, especially those with mission schooling. Such reproduction was never robotic or wholesale, but instead was marked by the same kinds of processes of fragmentary inventions and appropriations that characterized the culture of colonialism as a whole.

For example, the Zimbabwean politician and activist Maurice Nyagumbo recalled in his memoirs that when he arrived at St. Faith's Mission for Standard I lessons, he and the other new pupils were marched to the stream while singing

> *Tiri, manyukama,*
> *Tiri, manyukama,*
> *Tine tsvina*
> *Tine tsvina*
> *Hatigoni, kuyeza,*
> *Hatigoni, kudzidza.*

> We are the newcomers,
> We are the newcomers,
> We are dirty,
> We are dirty,
> We do not know how to wash ourselves.
> We have not acquired education. (Nyagumbo 1980, 24)

Some Africans who entered colonial professions, worked closely with the bureaucracy, or saw themselves as strongly religious Christians particularly identified with the ideal of redeeming the imagined and unified "dirty" African body described by colonial rulers.

Because of the power invested in them by the colonial system, figurations of hygiene and domesticity increasingly began to articulate with other sentiments, desires, and strategies within African communities, both among those most directly socialized by colonial institutions and among others more tangentially connected to colonial rule. For example, students, teachers, and other aspirant elites sometimes turned the language of cleanliness against settlers. J. H. Sobantu wrote to the *Native Mirror* in 1933 to complain:

> Why is it that a civilised, clean and well-dressed native is chased away from the sidewalk? Education to that native means nothing because he sees no difference. Missionaries have worked so hard to educate me . . . Is it fair for a civilised man to be dressed in short trousers and walk bare-footed in the street and yet call himself a policeman? I would rather call myself donkey leader or rickshaw boy. (Sobantu 1933, 11)

Nyagumbo's accounts of his travels in South Africa during this era were particularly striking for turning the hygienic tables on white culture. Nyagumbo recounted his youthful obsession with "smart" clothing and style while working in South Africa and described with horror the habits of Afrikaners in the Orange Free State in the 1930s:

> As far as cleanliness was concerned, the Boers of this area were completely oblivious to it and did not understand why a "kaffir" was so sensitive to anything that was dirty. The whole building was infested with swarms of flies. Women came into the dining-room with hair falling everywhere. People blew their noses and spat everywhere in the dining-room. (Nyagumbo 1980, 56)

In the public discourse of the 1930s and 1940s, settler ideals of cleanliness were appropriated in fragmented ways to apply to diverse cultural questions and controversies. One letter writer used cleanliness to explain the desire for "fat girls": "We want to marry fat girls because hygiene tells us that they are healthier than thin ones; few fat people get consumption" (Moyo 1934, 10). Another claimed: "Native women and girls should not follow some white women in the fashion of wearing long hair, which . . . is unhygienic" (Ndzou 1935, 4). The prohibitions against bodily contact with strangers, so important to protecting oneself from *uroyi* (witchcraft), resurfaced with new hygienic language in the following missive:

> Africans are far behind in observing the hygienic rules in their daily lives. Why are Africans now very fond of shaking hands with unknown people?

Is this habit according to the rules of hygiene? It is a way of inviting infectious diseases to your bodies such as syphilis, gonorrhea and yaws. (Siguake 1939, 8)

The power of hygienic and bodily language in daily life continued to grow far beyond the boundaries of settler pedagogy and propaganda. In the late 1960s, Kenneth Green Ntopa, head of the True African N'angas Association, disparaged his competitors by declaring:

Cleanliness is one of the most important things we thoroughly stress on in our work as ngangas [healers] . . . dirty ngangas [are] a "Big Danger" to public health . . . They touch a snake's skin or fats and then they proceed to give a sick person some edible muti without washing their hands with soap . . . A good nganga should wash his hands with strong soap. (True African Ngangas, 1969, 13)

The colonial projection of a racialized body and its racialized hygiene thus partially defined a new domain of interlinked practices among Africans. Some of these practices were oppositional to the colonial vision of African bodies, some of them were responsive to it, and others were wholly tangential to this vision but nevertheless operated with new reference to the body as a unified subject. In Zimbabwe, by the 1940s, the articulation of colonial and hegemonic visions about hygiene and appearance with diverse and unconnected uses of bodies in pre-colonial societies had created a complex, multilayered world in which a domain of the body was interculturally but inconsistently salient. A further understanding of how the meanings and practices attached to the body were interpreted and changed can be found by examining the accelerating process of commodification in colonial Zimbabwe.

Commodification, Advertising, and Colonial Hygiene

In Zimbabwe, the process of commodification has a complex history of its own. This process, by which locally produced objects were displaced by manufactured goods produced by local and transnational capitalist firms, and the meanings of goods were reinvented and reimagined, were shaped by the evolution of the colonial political economy, by the initiatives of prewar merchants, by situational appropriations of newly introduced objects in African communities, by the simultaneous and contradictory construction of consumption as the essence of the "civilizing mission" and as a realm of protected white privilege (Burke, forthcoming).

After the end of World War II, manufacturing in South Africa and colonial Zimbabwe enjoyed several decades of sustained expansion. Many of the settler elites of both countries were ruefully forced to acknowledge that this expansion had been made possible by the growth of a mass market for manufactured goods among the African population and that continued growth would require sustaining this development.

One of the most prominent areas of activity in this industrial boom was the manufacture of soap and other toiletries. Soap manufacture was already well-established in Zimbabwe before the 1940s, and in 1947 the transnational giant Unilever pruned managerial staff and resources from its South African plants to establish subsidiaries in British Central Africa. Lever Brothers was only the first of a number of transnationals to take an interest in British Central Africa during this time; in particular, the implicit promise of a unified and economically vigorous market in the short-lived Central African Foundation spurred interest among American and British investors.

Lever Brothers and other local and transnational firms involved in toiletry manufacture brought a complex apparatus for marketing and advertising to bear on what they identified as the problem of the "African market." In Zimbabwean rural and urban communities, African consumers had been purchasing manufactured items for decades, but postwar capitalists in southern Africa nevertheless continued to imagine African consumption as a mysterious, untouched Dark Continent, shaped by unknown tastes and preferences. To reach these consuming Others, toiletry manufacturers appropriated institutional forms of communication founded by the state and settler voluntary organizations that had previously been used to spread the gospel of cleanliness and other colonial forms of propaganda—demonstration and cinema vans, radio, "African" newspapers, women's clubs, health lectures, mission schools, beauty contests, and fashion shows. Equally, advertisements were carefully crafted to take advantage of prior colonial productions of the proper and mannerly African body.

Additionally, many analyses of advertising have pointed out that as a cultural institution, it tends to have a particular—some would say unique—interest in bodies and sensuality. As one author writes,

> Since capital producing underpants is aiming for a niche in a profitable market, underpants are necessarily in the spotlight. Since they must be saleable at monopoly prices, they must be shown in the right light, and thus, once again, the body is emphasized . . . The advertised underpants are made into a "hit" by underlining the fact that they make the body a

"hit." They become the body's snug marketing package, and thus the concerns of capital appear, as it were, in underwear and, by seeming to take an interest in the body, promote commodities by suggesting that they advertise the body itself. The body, on whose behalf all this advertising is happening, adopts the compulsory traits of a brand-named product; in the same way, it is not the body itself but the effective advertising image which is being promoted. Capital's interest in the body even contains certain aspects which are rather more detrimental to it than the Christian aversion to the flesh, which capital propagates as its missionary in a different constellation. (Haug 1986, 83)

The beginnings of the visual culture of modern consumption in the West were certainly replete with bodily images. In nineteenth-century Britain, for example, a hugely disproportionate share of advertising was aimed at the promotion of patent medicines and toiletries. Critical readings of twentieth-century advertising have pointed out that this trend has accelerated. The pleasures of consumption as represented by manufacturers have been increasingly and explicitly tied to the satisfaction of the body and its hungers during the twentieth century. Given that commodification and advertising in Zimbabwe were very strongly shaped by transnational practices, it is unsurprising to discover that this thematic stress on the consuming body reproduced itself there.

Print advertisements for Lever Brothers soaps like Lifebuoy, Sunlight, and Lux from the 1950s and 1960s provide some good examples of southern African advertising's appropriation of colonial hygienic training. Lifebuoy was presented by the company in southern African markets primarily as a "strong" soap suited for washing particularly dirty bodies. As a consequence, the advertised image of Lifebuoy ultimately drifted inexorably toward both masculinity and blackness. With the disinfectant carbolic added to it, Lifebuoy has a distinctive, unforgettable odor. Given the weight of the settler vision of "dirty" Africans, it is unsurprising that a soap with extra disinfectant, a soap that gives users a distinctive odor connoting cleanliness, was thought by white manufacturers to be particularly appropriate for use by Africans. The speed with which a soap with properties of "strength" was firmly attached to black male bodies suggests how much power the depiction of Africans as "dirty" continued to have in the postwar era.

The basic Lifebuoy slogan in the 1950s and 1960s was "The Successful Man Uses Lifebuoy." Its first incarnation, in the 1950s, featured the aforementioned slogan accompanied by drawings of an African man dressed smartly in a suit and tie, sometimes holding a pen, beaming from ear to ear. At the end of the decade, these pictures were replaced by an alternating series of photographs featuring African men in various "typical" work clothes. One of the photographs still featured a well-dressed clerk, but others showed a miner, a bricklayer, and a teacher. The slogan remained the same, simultaneously recalling established associations between African masculinity and dirt, between labor and pollution, between professional success within the colonial system and rigorous hygienic purification. The other Lifebuoy campaign used in the 1960s and 1970s in African media played in a different way on the same ideas, with the message "Keep Healthy . . . Keep Clean . . . Use Lifebuoy, the *Health* Soap." Again, the ads almost always featured men, this time often already lathered up and in the shower, clutching a bar of Lifebuoy. In the first campaign, the soap was offered as the force that kept the body successful under the social rules of the white-controlled workplace; the second campaign stressed Lifebuoy's power to guarantee the ability of men's bodies to work by securing continuous good health.

Sunlight Soap was Lever Brothers' oldest and best-known soap product, a higher-quality, brand-name version of cheap "bar soaps." Sunlight Soap advertisements in England, written by Lever himself, promised to relieve the burden of domestic work, improve the durability of clothing, make the lives of housewives healthier and easier, and make their relationships with their husbands better. Sunlight was one of the most ubiquitously advertised commodities all over Africa well before the postwar boom, and its familiarity and seeming prestige also had made it popular among southern Africans, despite its higher price. Sunlight, like other bar soaps, was used by many of them as an all-purpose cleanser for the body, clothes, and the home. Unlike poorly made cheap bar soaps, which were known to shrivel as they dried, losing most of their substance, Sunlight was reliable. Its usage could be paced slowly, by chipping small pieces off the bar. Early ad campaigns in African media took advantage of Sunlight as a known quantity and showed scenes of young children and adults washing in tubs with Sunlight, accompanied by the slogan "Use it for Face, Hands, Bathing and All Home Cleaning . . . Best for All Washing."

However, by the late 1950s, the company was hoping to teach African consumers to use Sunlight strictly for laundry purposes and to purchase other tablet soaps for toiletries. Older African consumers were said to resist by continuing to use Sunlight as an all-purpose soap (Mkele 1959, 130). The new ad campaigns for Sunlight seized hold of domesticity and the concerns of urban African women in a series of narrative comic strips. These ads aimed in particular at the increasingly powerful local image of the "good, Christian, club-going wife," the proper and mannerly woman. Just as many advertisements for products played on men's concerns about remaining healthy and energetic enough to work, the capacity of women to satisfy male demands and organize their households was represented by advertisements as being under siege in a hostile world.

For example, advertisements for Feluna Pills (iron supplements) ran regularly in African media from the early 1940s to the 1970s and were typical examples of these themes. In one Feluna ad, a mother wishes her daughter good-bye when she goes to her new husband, telling her to "be a good wife and bear strong healthy children." The young woman replies, "I love babies and hope to have some." Her mother then tells her all her own children have been strong because Feluna Pills have "kept my blood strong and pure." Feluna advertisements, and a number of other similar product promotions, usually boiled down to the fundamental message: "A Woman Can't Work If She Is Sick." Work in this instance was often portrayed in terms of reproduction, in terms of bodily functions—maintaining households, satisfying husbands, and raising children.

The Sunlight ads of the 1960s played on related themes. In one, a wife is excoriated by a husband who cannot get a good job because his shirts look "so old and dirty." His wife admits to a friend, "Ben is right . . . I am a bad wife." Her friend tells her, "You must change to Sunlight Soap." The change is made, and the wife exults, "Now everything is going right . . . because I wash my husband's shirts in Sunlight!" Not only is the woman's success as a wife threatened, but her failure is also represented as threatening her husband's success. In another storyline, a woman worries, "I'll never find a husband. My clothes look so old and dirty." Again, a good Samaritan intervenes, sharing the secret that Sunlight makes clothes look like new again. Redeemed, the young woman confides, "Sunlight Soap has changed my life . . . and soon I'll be a happy wife!"

If Sunlight advertisements were striving to make connections with African women trying to live up to the ideals of club-going domesticity, then Lux was pitched to African consumers as the way to achieve a "smart" body, a modern body. Lifebuoy and Sunlight worked off hygienic imagery linked to working-class bodies, bodies within the sphere of Christian morality, labor and domesticity, while Lux mined another vein of ideology about manners and bodies, the thread that dealt with "modern living" and "civilized fashion." One advertisement featured the heads of a young couple above the slogan: "Be like smart people, insist on . . . LUX Toilet Soap." The ad went on:

Today, in the homes of the *smartest people,* you'll find Lux Toilet Soap in colour as well as white. You'll see pink, green, yellow and blue tables . . . so pretty to look at . . . so pleasant to use. And the people who use Lux Toilet Soap *are* smart. Their skin is clean and smooth and sweet smelling.

In later ads, an African model held the soap next to her cheek, accompanied by the slogan "a rich, creamy lather to keep your skin soft and smooth . . . expensive beauty oils . . . a lovely new perfume. Three good reasons why Africa's loveliest women use Lux beauty soap." The sensuality of Lux was stressed, its feel on the skin was described insistently. Lux advertisements also implied that urban living was perpetually strained by sexual anxiety, by the burden of ugly bodies. Women were advised that they could use Lux to achieve glamor, to enhance their sexual control over men, while appeals to male audiences for other toiletries often depicted a forlorn man who has been persistently rejected by women because he is too ugly, not yet hygienic or "smart" in his use of commodities.

In like fashion with a range of other toiletries and cleansers—body lotions, skin lighteners, cosmetics, perfumes, toothpaste, detergents—Zimbabwean manufacturers took control of colonial codes of hygiene, bodily appearance, and domesticity and attempted to install them within the essence of various products. The definition and subsequent regulation of "the" African body's hygiene and appearance by the colonial order was reconfigured in the postwar era as a set of commercial propositions about the unmet needs of the people who comprised the mythologized "African market."

The Production of the Body: Toiletries in African Lives

However, there was a disjunction between the imagination of needs, the manufacturers' projection of "official" meanings and uses of goods through advertising, and the heterogenous practices that have actually made use of toiletries and other goods in various Zimbabwean communities over the last five decades. A few particular selections from the "biographies" of soap, Vaseline, and toothpaste—recalling Igor Kopytoff's phrase in his essay on commoditization (Kopytoff 1986)—should suffice to demonstrate the gap between the intentions of white marketers and the actions of African consumers. The making of the meanings of commodities was a process that involved a plurality of different interests within African communities, it was a process that activated complicated struggles and negotiations between classes, genders, and ethnicities and mediated relationships between urban, peri-urban, and rural lifeworlds. Keeping this in mind, the ways in which toiletries have come to define social bodies among Zimbabweans clearly bears the historical imprints of both the colonial production of the hygienic body and the diverse range of unconnected forms of material culture around pre-colonial bodies.

The hygienic needs that have become fundamental to African communities in Zimbabwe, and yet lie most invisibly within the realm of "common sense," involve on one hand soaps and on the other, Vaseline, Pond's Lotion, and similar lotions. It may seem peculiar at first to consider soap and Vaseline together, but in fact, the two types of commodities have existed in close dialectical relationship with each other, constituting separate but closely linked hygienic ideals.

In the postwar era, soap—from Sunlight to Lifebuoy to "blue mottled"— became a nearly universal presence in the everyday life of Africans, rich and poor, men and women, old and young. Soap by that time had been heavily promoted by colonial institutions connected with domesticity and hygiene as the material embodiment of their campaigns to produce "modern" bodies and manners. Soap marketing from the 1940s onward reinforced the image of soaps as the essence of hygiene and began to segment this essence into more specialized "needs." The public promotion of cleanliness, its concerns with manners and practices of the body, by the 1950s had empowered soap to wholly embody the "hygienic ideal."

As a consequence of these accumulated connections, soap has come to be seen as a fundamental part of daily life. In Zimbabwean author Shimmer Chinodya's novel *Harvest of Thorns,* blue mottled soap is depicted as one of the characteristic intimate smells of the human body (Chinodya 1989, 243). During the *chimurenga,* [war for independence], soldiers of both ZANLA and ZIPRA (the armed forces of the two main factions of the independence movement, Zimbabwe African National Liberation Army and Zimbabwe People's Revolutionary Army respectively) had local villagers procure supplies that they regarded as absolute necessities. The delivery of such supplies was one of the most perilous aspects of the conduct of the war for soldiers and peasants alike. Requests had to be kept to a minimum, and it is therefore notable that after food, the item many soldiers regarded as essential was soap (Staunton 1990). Former school pupils, especially those educated by missionaries, as well as women who were active in women's clubs or remain active in church congregations today, noted during interviews that they had been taught that soap was a basic part of good hygiene.

Many of the informants questioned during this research strongly advocated the usage of specific soaps to address particular needs. Lifebuoy, for example, was praised by most people, many of whom said they had used it regularly for decades. Informants were able to trace some of the attributes of Lifebuoy to definable sources. For example, most argued that the soap was generally healthy and specifically good for children, especially for "measles" or other skin ailments. This, they said, was taught by clinics, teachers, and parents alike. However, other common opinions of Lifebuoy were taken almost directly from advertising copy, without any awareness on the part of speakers that this was so. The masculinity of Lifebuoy or its ability to cleanse a laboring body have become part of "common sense," generally known but without specific provenance.

Equally, the historical effectiveness of other campaigns for toilet soaps became clear in interviews. Lux and Palmolive were occasionally said to be good beauty soaps, though once again, few were certain where they had learned this. Both soaps were also said to be recommended specifically for washing infants under six months old, which people said had been taught by clinics and womens' clubs for many years. The separation between household soaps and toilet soaps, which soap manufacturers stressed increasingly from the 1950s onward, has also been effective; the few who said that they have used household soaps for washing their bodies confessed that they no longer do so or only rarely continue this practice, because it is more economical.

Thus, soap, while having been seen as a fundamental need by most Africans since at least the 1950s, has been closely tied to the visions of clean bodies promoted first by missions and the state and later powerfully and massively reproduced in postwar advertising. Vaseline and other face and body creams, by contrast, were purchased and used in large amounts in the postwar era without any significant initiatives by manufacturers, who realized only slowly and with surprise that they had a ready-made market requiring no commercial sermons. Companies manufacturing Vaseline and body lotions found themselves producing for hygienic needs conceived independently among Africans. Indeed, other companies, like Lever Brothers, even felt it necessary to take steps to protect products like margarine from being misinterpreted as hygienic substances that could meet these demands.

These products were used to reinvent the practice of "smearing" so common in nineteenth-century southern African cultures. It is difficult to say when exactly the mixing of red or yellow soil and some sort of oil as part of a daily hygienic regimen began to disappear in south-central Africa. It has never disappeared completely in the region as a whole, but *none* of the Shona individuals with whom this study was discussed had ever heard of the practice, including individuals in their fifties and sixties who had lived much of their lives in rural districts. However, the basic concept behind pre-colonial practices—that a clean, mannerly, and aesthetically pleasing body should be coated after washing with a paste to protect it from dirt, keep it from cracking or chafing, and give it a rich, shiny appearance—has remained strongly rooted in all walks of life in Zimbabwe.

In the wake of the intensive colonial interest in imagining the proper African body, many people searched during the 1940s and 1950s for a commercially available commodity that could be used for the purpose of smearing. Cooking oil, margarine, and the oil from the top of peanut butter jars were among the substances turned to this purpose. Soap was also used—one washed with soap, rinsed, and then worked the soap into a lather; this lather was then applied to the skin and allowed to dry. In particular, soaps advertised as having "glycerine" and being good for the skin were turned to this purpose.[3] Today, the use of margarine or food oils on the body still occurs, but virtually everyone, from Mbare squatters to middle-class homeowners, regards these substances as undesirable substitutes for skin cream or Vaseline, and as a last refuge for the impoverished. In any case, experimentation with new substances ultimately uncovered wholly satisfactory commodities for use in smearing—both petroleum jelly and body lotions like Pond's and Camphor's.

My own interviews, as well as surveys and various texts, suggest that by the 1960s, most, if not all, Africans in urban areas used these products as often as they could afford, and that many rural people did so as well. Virtually all of my informants agreed that they simply did not feel clean without using some sort of cream or lotion after washing. Everyone had practiced or tried to practice smearing throughout their entire lives. Many also alluded to the cracking of the skin that follows when smearing cannot be performed and the pleasing feel and smell of skin when it is covered by lotion.

In the Tashinga squatter camp near Mbare Musika bus terminal in Harare, many have been unable to afford substances for regular smearing for much of their lives and displayed worn or cracked skin to demonstrate what they clearly regarded as an extremely serious form of deprivation. In a recent anthology of testimonies by Zimbabwean women, one woman describes the desperate poverty that overtook her family after her husband abandoned them: "I wrote many letters to my husband but he never responded. He no longer sent money: he did not care about us any more. . . . My feet began to crack because I had no lotion or Vaseline to put on them and I had no shoes" (Staunton 1990, 217). In interviews, the preferences expressed for different brands or types of lotions mostly seemed to be idiosyncratic and personal, though many people noted that Vaseline has long been regarded as superior for winter use because it provides a thicker coating. Equally, a number of people noted that in summer, dust sticks to Vaseline. Some also noted that Vaseline has long been preferred for use on children. Few of these suggestions were ever voiced in advertisements prior to independence. Unlike Lifebuoy, Lux, Palmolive, or other toilet soaps, whose suggested meanings were carefully controlled by manufacturers, Vaseline and similar products were advertised inconsistently and spottily.

The relationship between the two different hygienic and bodily ideals embodied in the fetishisms of these two commodities has been neither a case of irreconcilable contradiction nor of blissful coexistence. Rather, the needs that each kind of product have satisfied have been in uneasy and subterranean dialogue with each other. One kind of "common sense," a product of decades of colonial teachings and propaganda, has come to rest in a variety of soaps, while another kind, rooted in disconnected indigenous aesthetic notions about proper bodies, is still invested in the practice of smearing—for the last five decades a practice largely defined around commodities manufactured by capitalist factories. At various moments in Zimbabwean culture during the postwar era, the subtle articulation of these two practices has flashed into visibility, idiomatically attached to social class, gender, generation, or migrancy. A persistent thread running throughout such moments, however, has been shifting and contingent notions about "tradition" and "modernity," shadowed by a complex and fractitious relationship between several generations of Zimbabweans. In the postwar era, cleanliness (and the commodity fetishisms that defined cleanliness in Zimbabwe after World War II) thus often concerned the ambiguous ways in which history—and the authority of history—was constituted. It is here that we most clearly see both the utility and the peril of body history. Part of the reason that smeared bodies and Vaseline have never become fully realized oppositional bodies—distinctive uses of the body surface that refer to an active, alternative subjectivity—is that the persistence of smearing comes out of cultural practices that were either not at all referenced to a notion of "the" body or, at the very most, only partially connected to such notions.

As noted previously, colonial ideals about clean and mannerly bodies had already infiltrated much of daily life by the 1950s, while explicit resistance to this infiltration was becoming more diffuse. For many, especially for people born and grown to adulthood since that time, cleanliness, hygienic needs, and daily bodily practices have been shot full of unvoiced misgivings and uncertainties. This has been reminiscent of the ways in which the Mayers's "School Xhosa" reproved their "Red" cousins for supposedly being filthy and backward:

Xhosa, themselves, when asked to explain the Red-School opposition, do so in terms of cultural differentia: Red people do things this way while School people do them that way. "The difference between a Red man and myself," said a young School countryman, "is that I wear clothes like white people's, as expensive as I can afford, while he is satisfied with old clothes and lets his wife go about in a Red dress. After washing, I smear vaseline on my face: he uses red ochre to look nice." (Mayer and Mayer 1971, 21)

Similarly, postwar Zimbabwean associations between dirtiness and "traditional" or rural life have not focused on smearing with Vaseline or other manufactured goods, but on a more elemental stereotype—one that envisions a complete lack of any hygiene.

For example, one of the standard genres of modern Shona literature is the "urbanization" novel, in which "modern" and "traditional" lifestyles come into conflict (Kahari 1990). Frequently, the ambitious urban character in such works, who may have left his family or his background behind in his search for success, regards his parents or other rural relatives and friends with disgust—a disgust that frequently is conceived in primarily hygienic terms, often with powerful overtones of class consciousness as well. In Ben Sibenke's play *My Uncle Grey Bhonzo*, the title character is a rich man who maintains a studied distance from his poorer relatives. Sibenke saddles Grey with a severe hygienic obsession. Grey walks about his house pursuing minute qualities of dirt and calling servants to completely cleanse even the slightest imperfection. When his brother and young nephews come calling, Grey is horrified by their appearance, telling the servants to bring Vaseline for them, telling them, "You must learn to bathe. To play with water. Learn smartness and neatness, you see?" Grey's ill-mannered children mock their cousins, waving handkerchiefs in front of their noses and complaining, "There is a bad smell in here" (Sibenke 1982, 23–24). For Sibenke, Grey symbolizes the urban elite's odious assumption of the cultural habits and bigotries of the settlers. Sibenke depicts a fixation on "modern," commodified hygiene as one of the most emblematic of these habits. Once Grey receives his inevitable comeuppance, his fellow businessman, Hey Zuwa, reminds him and the gathered cast of characters that the wealthy must not behave arrogantly, and that relatives—even poor relatives—are the keepers of tradition. After all, notes Hey, "Is it not our relatives who will bathe our dead?" (Sibenke 1982, 41).

Thus, the contemporary person obsessed with "modern" living has been depicted by authors as negatively judgmental of the hygiene of others, as judgmental of the bodies of people who one way or another fall under the sign of "tradition." However, this picture is further complicated in such discourses by the envisioning of what constitutes "traditional" hygiene. Though the fetishisms associated with Vaseline and lotions may be invested with a good deal of "traditional" significance, the use of these products also has been viewed as acceptably "modern" by urban and rural people alike. For example, Grey offers his nephews Vaseline to correct their "dirtiness," and despite his condescension, they eagerly smear themselves when he gives it to them. Many of my informants similarly stressed the "modern" acceptability of smearing with commercial products. Similarly, soap can lie within the field of "tradition." Many medicines prepared by a *n'anga* (healer) need to be applied in concert with washing, and many informants agreed that there are precise rules involved about whether and when one should use soap in these procedures. Soap has itself become a "traditional" medicine in a few cases—for example, it is sometimes used in witch-finding procedures (*muteyo*), smeared onto the anus of a person undergoing the trial (untitled article, *Parade* 1991, 29).

The complications of these relations between one kind of "modern" commodity, involved in a "traditional" practice of smearing, and another kind of "modern" commoditized cleanliness, rooted in the use of soaps and "beautifying" toiletries, have emerged in a number of Zimbabwean texts. The cleanliness embodied in soap, especially scented or fancy toilet soap, as well as related toiletries, has suggested complicated transformations of the self, simultaneously desired, criticized, and feared. In Chinjerai Hove's novel *Bones*, one of the peasant narrators of the novel, Janifa, muses about "good things" and how "those who have them always want to make rules so that others cannot get to the good things." She continues,

> "Good things are not for everybody," Manyepo says. Even when he smears good smells on his body, he says not everybody must have those good things because good things are not for everybody. But why does he not allow even the baas boy to smear those good scents on his own body? Or give the baas boy the way to make the rules? (Hove 1988, 97)

In Tsitsi Dangarembga's *Nervous Conditions*, this kind of desire spills forth even more intensely. The narrator's brother, who dies early in the novel, is sullen upon his return home from school, disdaining his surroundings and his family. Among the impositions he objects to is "travelling by bus . . . the women smelt of unhealthy reproductive odours, the children were inclined to relieve their upset bowels on the floor, and the men gave off strong aromas of productive labour" (Dangarembga 1988, 2). At school, he has clearly discovered a new commodified body, and he cherishes it, for it confirms his new status and power. When the brother dies, the narrator, Tambudzai, is sent to school in his place. She foresees a similar bodily transformation as emblematic of the larger freedoms she can now grasp:

> When I stepped into Babamukuru's car I was a peasant . . . It was evident from the corrugated black callouses on my knees, the scales on my skin that were due to lack of oil, the short, dull tufts of malnourished hair. This

is the person I was leaving behind. At Babamukuru's, I expected to find another self, a clean, well-groomed genteel self who could not have been bred, could not have survived on the homestead . . . This new me would not be frustrated by wood fires. (Dangarembga 1988, 58–59)

At her wealthy uncle's house, she finds cleanliness and soap: "The joy of that bath! Steaming hot water filled the tub to the brim . . . I washed and scrubbed and rubbed, soaping myself three times over" (Dangarembga 1988, 90).

At the same time, such desires have been tempered by a knowledge of their sources. Another of Hove's narrators, torn by unrequited sexual need, ambiguously implores the woman he desires but cannot have: "Look how I have washed and cleaned myself so that I smell the smells of the white man" (Hove 1988, 84). In his distinctive manner, author Dambudzo Marechera also addressed the ambiguous racial and cultural history of hygienic products and practices:

> I had such a friend once. He is now in a lunatic asylum. I have since asked myself why he did what he did, but I still cannot come to a conclusive answer. He was always washing himself—at least three baths a day. And he had all sorts of lotions and deodorants to appease the thing that had taken hold of him. He did not so much wash as scrub himself until he bled. He tried to purge his tongue, too, by improving his English and getting rid of any accent from the speaking of it. (Marechera 1978, 93)

Tambudzai, the narrator of *Nervous Conditions,* also discovers that "modern" commoditized cleanliness is more complicated than it first appears:

> I was in danger of becoming an angel, or at the very least a saint, and forgetting how ordinary humans existed . . . The absence of dirt was proof of the other-worldly nature of my new home. I knew, had known all my life, that living was dirty and I had been disappointed by the fact. I had often helped my mother to resurface the kitchen floor with dung. I knew, for instance, that rooms where people slept exuded particularly human smells just as the goat pen smelt goaty and the cattle kraal bovine. . . . Yet at a glance it was difficult to perceive dirt in Maiguru's house. After a while, as the novelty wore off, you began to see that the antiseptic sterility that my aunt and uncle strove for could not be attained beyond an illusory level. (Dangarembga 1988, 70–71)

Tambudzai wistfully reflects that the price of living within this hygienic ideal, of bathing in tubs with soap, is losing the joys of washing in the river near her rural home: "Nor would there be trips to Nyamarira, Nyamarira which I loved to bathe in and watch cascade through the narrow outlet of the fall where we drew our water. Leaving this Nyamarira, my flowing, tumbling, musical playground, was difficult" (Dangarembga 1988, 59).

This subtle and contingent awareness of the hidden costs and subtle attractions of each hygienic ideal, "traditional" and "modern," has originated out of a diffuse consciousness of the history of bodily practice and the meanings invested in soaps and body creams. The costs of the type of hygiene invested in soap have been constituted by its associations with the bodily disciplines of colonialism, of decades of mission teachings and domestic training—but the desirability of soap also comes from the same sources. The clean and mannerly body of "tradition" has been celebrated by some cultural authorities in African communities—but the "traditional" body has mostly been maintained for the last five decades through the use of manufactured lotions and creams.

The balance sheet of hygiene, with its accounting of bodies old and new, has been a small part of a much larger tally of the losses and gains, oppressions and opportunities, under colonial rule. Soap and lotions, and the intertwining of their meanings and uses, have played a key role in generating both "the" contemporary Zimbabwean body and the much more elusive undefined "bodies" embedded within contemporary practice. These bodies and the products that have helped to make them have been neither clearly "modern" nor "traditional" but instead have been uncomfortably and indeterminately both and neither.

Body history as it is presently practiced can uncover the hidden face of domination, and it can equally well reveal the complex mutuality and plurality of colonial culture. But body history can also warehouse discrete practices, ideas, and discourses as unwilling tenants under a single roof. The making of hygiene and domesticity by the colonial Zimbabwean state and by missions was certainly a project that injected colonial power into an organized and connected domain of "the" body, but the diverse practices that existed prior to and at the margins of this study have involved multiple and unconnected "bodies." It makes sense to speak of the postwar commodification of toiletries as being about a unified subject, the body, but only if we keep in mind that some toiletries were also used in reference to invisible, plural, and fluid bodies.

Notes

1   Feeley-Harnik is very careful to avoid this, while Comaroff faces the issues involved squarely, though perhaps not entirely satisfactorily. Stoller, as a counterexample, takes it for granted that inserting sensuality—the anthropologist's bodily experi-

ence of another culture—will inevitably produce a new intimacy in the relationship between the subjects and practitioners of ethnography. Yet it seems to me that the senses are a very unsatisfactory and essentialist shorthand for a much more complicated project of reconstructing ethnography.

2   This was picked up as "*chiSwina*" by nineteenth-century missionaries working at the Ndebele capital and remained a common colonial name for Shona speakers until the 1940s. Not all colonial ethnographies concerning Zimbabwe agree on this derivation, but I think it is basically sound, especially in light of the regionally pervasive, long-term tendency to use vocabularies of "dirtiness" and "cleanliness" to describe antagonists. Nathan Shamuyarira described *chiSwina* as meaning more specifically "those people who are supposed to have remained cleaning and eating the intestines of an animal when other tribes were moving on" (Shamuyarira 1965, 118).

3   These practices were discussed in numerous interviews conducted in Zimbabwe in 1990–91 with consumers and executives. The particular appeal of "glycerine" was mentioned in an interview with executives. Interviews with Cornell Butcher, Francis Makosa, Wellington Chikombero in Harare, Zimbabwe, 26 November 1990.

8 BODIES AND FLAGS:
THE REPRESENTATION OF HERERO
IDENTITY IN COLONIAL NAMIBIA

Hildi Hendrickson

Introduction

Some Herero people in Namibia recently have joked that if you squint at the multicolored national flag adopted after independence in 1990, you will see only the DTA or NUDO colors—that is, the red, blue, and white associated with these two Herero-based political groups. As the Namibian flag's actual dominant colors are red, blue, and green—colors associated with the mainly Ovambo-speaking, SWAPO-aligned (South West Africa People's Organization) majority—these pundits are asserting that if they try, they can find themselves in this image of the new nation. The joke implies that Herero identity is not plainly represented in the flag, but that it is submerged there, that it must be sought after, and that it can be found.

The imagination of Namibian identity, the struggle both to choose representations of the polity and to assign lasting meaning to them, has been developing since the Germans claimed colonial control over the territory of South West Africa in 1884. The public use of political acronyms and specific color associations, which blossomed in Namibia just before independence,[1] was not a trivial undertaking, nor was it simply characteristic of the southern African idiom of nationalist political expression. Rather, I argue that the material expression of political affiliation is historically contingent, emergent within a plural cultural milieu, and essential to the developing imagination of the polity.

While the design of the new flag awaits analysis, I here examine the nineteenth- and twentieth-century Herero use of colored cloth on the body as a central symbol through which a Herero polity has come to be imagined. The hand-knitted scarves and hats bearing the red, white, and blue of the DTA[2] party, or the yellow, green, and black of the NPF,[3] which were ubiquitous in 1989 (see fig. 8.1), are only one example of how color and clothing have been used to lend authority to Herero notions of polity. In this essay, I examine the process by which the idea of the Herero polity has been expressed in bodily symbolism and has emerged out of relations with other cultural groups in the region since the mid-nineteenth century.

There have been many of these other groups (see Drechsler [1966] 1980; Esterhuyse 1968; Katjavivi 1988; Pennington and Harpending 1991; Stoecker 1986). Before the Germans asserted themselves in the region, groups of Ovaherero alternately raided and joined forces with groups of other Africans in central Namibia. After a failed attempt to defeat the Germans in 1904, the Herero population was divided between those remaining in Namibia and those who moved east into Botswana. In Namibia, Ovaherero continued to face subjugation by English and then Afrikaner colonialists, who governed from South Africa. Colonial domination of Herero people ended in Namibia only in 1990. In Botswana, independence from British colonial control was achieved in 1966.

By examining the life history of a class of objects (see Appadurai 1986; Kopytoff 1986), I here identify an idiom within which Herero ideas of the polity have been expressed during the last century, and I uncover changes in Herero images of the polity since that time. I discuss the use of colored cloth on the body in the context of Herero "troop" or "flag" ceremonies of remembrance for nineteenth- and twentieth-century heroes. I trace the roots of this style of representation to nineteenth-century practice and discuss how oral histories of the troops reconstruct the meaning of this practice. I then explore the fact that Europeans in Namibia at the time attempted to inculcate Herero people with the idea of a colored flag as a representation of themselves as a unified polity.

True to their own interests, idioms, and agendas, Herero people turned colored cloth into an individual statement of personal loyalty to charismatic leaders. Over time, these collective representations have had the largely unintended consequence of being associated with a hierarchy of Herero leadership and a unified, "traditional" Herero social identity. Wearing colored cloth on the body expresses a peculiarly Herero understanding of the relation between the individual and the polity, which European flags do not articulate.

In this analysis, I seek to better understand the long-term, unforeseen consequences of different social groups using material symbols in culturally specific ways in the struggle for particular kinds of legitimacy and power. As Weiner (1992) has shown, such symbolic media may be critical to social systems in which there is little tolerance for the assertion of lasting claims to ranked leadership status. Further, the Herero case suggests that material media play a pivotal symbolic role in the development of relations between cultural groups before languages are known in common. I argue that the concreteness of material forms may make them lastingly effective upon social structure, though unintentionally so. I thus follow Peirce (see Buchler 1940) in identifying linkages between the form and meaning of symbolic vehicles.

The Herero search for meaning in the new flag and their long-standing interest in colored cloth does not appear to have been created only through contexts of commodity exchange. Rather, in the display and wearing of colored cloth there appears to have been a circulation of *images* and potent, multilayered, historically accumulated referents in which value has also been created. I thus investigate what Appadurai (1986, 32) has called the "visible act of consumption." The creation of value, and perhaps more importantly the reproduction of value, in this class of objects, appears to have emerged out of small-scale episodes of intercultural contact in which new forms of representation and notions of social identity arose together.

Wearing Flags on the Body

The most elaborate public use of color and body symbolism in the articulation of Herero social groups has occurred in the context of a ceremony formalized in 1923 (fig. 8.2) and performed annually thereafter.[4] This ceremony is that of the Herero "troops" and the larger organizations, the "flags," of which they are a part.[5] For many,[6] the use of colored cloth to express national political affiliations is the direct extension of its use in this context to express local, gendered, and historical identities.

The common Otjiherero word for both cloth and flag is *erapi*. Both the national flag, *erapi raNamibia*, and the Herero "flags" discussed here can be denoted by the use of this term. Members of a Herero flag meet once or twice yearly to visit the burial places of its nineteenth- and twentieth-century heroes. There are three flag organizations, known in Otjiherero as *Otjiserandu* (literally the Red or the Red thing), *Otjingirine* (the Green), and *Otjizemba/otjiapa* (the Banded or White flag). As the structure of these words suggests, the flag organizations are intimately associated with particular, contrasting colors.[7]

The flags are alike in the ways they organize people and events, but they are also defined in contrast to one another. In their differing emphases in constructing and memorializing the actions of nineteenth-century heroes, they assert common moral values while attempting to distinguish themselves from one another. The flags express but do not ultimately resolve a basic tension in Herero society created by valuing individualism while striving to create unity and by idealizing heroic leadership while expecting such leaders to be subject to the approval of followers and kin.

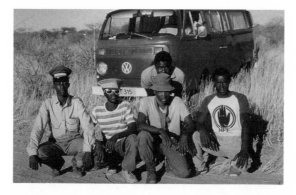

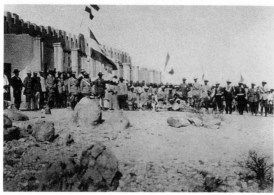

8.1   Young men at a troop ceremony show off their political and Green flag associations. Photo by D. Jacobson.

8.2   The funeral of Samuel Maharero, 1923. National Archives-Windhoek (NAW) photo no. 6956; used by permission.

Herero flag ceremonies unfold in chosen places over a three-day period at specific times of the year in both Namibia and Botswana. Today, celebrations are held in Ndauha, Botswana, in April; Okeseta and/or Otjunda, Namibia, in June; Okahandja, Namibia, in August; and Omaruru, Namibia, in October;[8] and they appear likely to continue to proliferate. For ordinary participants, the troop ceremonies take place over two days[9] in sites defined by the presence of heroes' graves (fig. 8.3). The particular heroes vary between the three flags, though loyalty is implied to the families of the chiefs Maharero among wearers of the Red, Zeraua for the White, and Nguvauva for the Green.

As the central figures vary, so do the images of history that each flag asserts through its ceremonial activity. The flags reflect and perpetuate an internal division in the Herero-speaking community. The Red and White flags are associated with Herero speakers who call themselves Ovaherero, while the Green flag members call themselves Ovambanderu to emphasize their different historical experience since the nineteenth century. Thus, flag membership implies a commitment to a particular reading of Herero history.

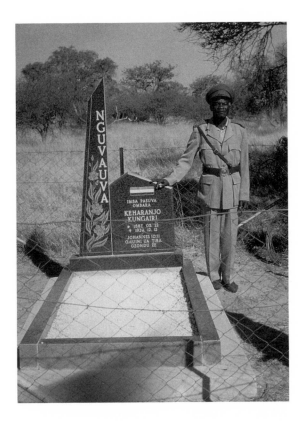

8.3   A Green flag celebration site outside Maun, Botswana. Photo by H. Hendrickson.

Green flag performances vary more from those of the other two flags than the latter do from each other. Green flag participants visit a sacred hearth before going to the graves (fig. 8.4) and can ask for healing to be performed there (fig. 8.5). Still, the flags are alike in their aim to embody a model of moral society and moral leadership, the creation of which is a critical dilemma in Herero social organization. It is through the remembering of events and people in the past that claims about the present and the future are made.

The ceremonies combine practices associated with the veneration of the ancestors at the sacred hearth and observances at the graves of the important patriarchs with military-style drilling, paraphernalia, and uniforms. The elements common to all the ceremonies are encampment near an important grave, sharing of food, singing praise songs, dancing, troop marching, horse-back riding, prayers and introductions to the ancestors, and speeches (figs. 8.6 and 8.7). The climax toward which the action moves is the moment when the participants ask for blessings from the ancestors at their graves (fig. 8.8). The participants and ritual specialists labor to ensure that the ancestors will be attentive as the faithful pass by to touch the graves, make contact with dead male relatives, and ask for blessings.

Before going to the graves, which can be several kilometers from the places where participants camp, participants organize themselves into previously de-fined marching troops associated with a town, village, or school (fig. 8.9). The place associated with a troop is the key factor in determining who marches in it. To be the most legitimate kind of participant in these ceremonies, one should march with a troop. And wearing a uniform is the prerequisite to marching in the troops at the ceremonies. I follow Herero practice in calling the dress worn at these ceremonies "uniforms" when using English; there is no equivalent word in Otjiherero. This type of dress has all the characteristics associated with "uniforms" in Barnes and Eicher's (1992, 20–21) recent classification, except that it does not demand "instant recognition of the right of the wearer not only to make decisions but to use force to maintain social order or wage war."[10]

The uniforms mark both the varying rank and the congruence between indi-vidual troop members, and they do this in slightly different ways for women and for men. Overall, the uniforms subsume any individual into a representa-tion of the whole, while allowing for the recognition of individual achieve-ments within the flags' standards of behavior and morality. Variation between

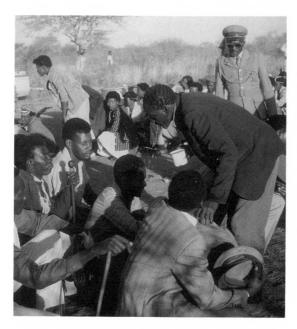

8.4   An *ondangere* pre-pares troop ceremony par-ticipants before they visit the graves. Photo by H. Hendrickson.

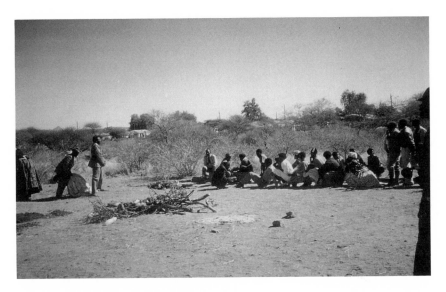

8.5   Green flag members receive healing at the
troop celebration. Photo by H. Hendrickson.

uniforms from individual to individual is seen only in specific aspects of the
design. Differences in men's and women's uniforms reflect differences in their
everyday dress.

For men, the cut of garments is not standardized, nor are there requirements
as to the kind of accessories one may wear. It is necessary to wear a stiff shirt or
jacket (*ombaikiha*) and trousers (*omburukweva*). These may be ordinary store-
bought, European-style work clothes, but jackets and hats of the type worn by
the military and police are more highly valued. Most men in uniform also wear
a hat (*ekori*) and a belt (*ekwamo*), and either may be military in style. Teenaged
boys wear the kind of short-sleeved shirts and shorts that they wear to school.

What is essential to the men's and boys' uniforms is that one's affiliation to a
flag be represented somewhere on the body by the use of color. Most men wear
khaki-colored clothes with small pieces of fabric in the color of their flag
attached to their hatbands, upper sleeves, cuffs, or epaulettes. These markers
may be red or red/black for the Red flag;[11] green or green/white/black for the
Green flag; and black, white/grey/blue, or blue/black with white polka dots for
the White flag. Ovaherero call these colored badges *ovihako* (plural), or ear-
marks, as in those given to cattle.

These cloth bands may also bear a set of initials associated with a specific flag,

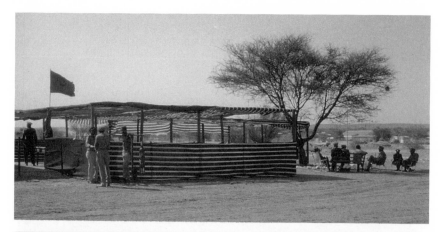

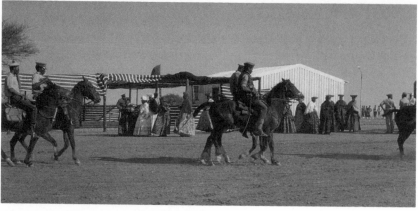

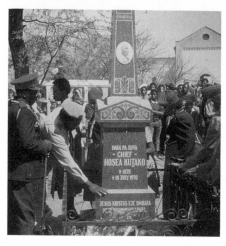

8.6   The Red flag's central plaza area in Okahandja before the ceremonies begin. Photo by H. Hendrickson.

8.7   Troop participants ride in formation around the White flag plaza in Omaruru. Photo by H. Hendrickson.

8.8   Uniformed participants touch the graves of their ancestors. Photo by D. Jacobson.

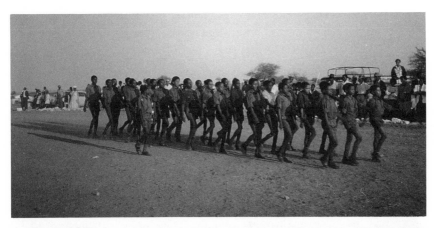

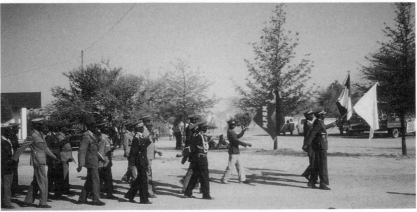

8.9   A troop of young men marches in unison. Photo by D. Jacobson.
8.10   High-ranking troop participants at a White flag ceremony
lead the procession to the graves. Photo by H. Hendrickson.

making reference to the particular heroes that flag remembers in celebration. For the Red flag, the initials read M.P.S.M. or M.P.E.S.M., for *Mukuru puna ete* Samuel Maharero or "God be with us, Samuel Maharero." For the White flag, the initials M.P.E.W.Z. stand for "God be with us, Wilhelm Zeraua"; and for the Green flag, N.K.M.G.M.P. refers to members of the Mbanderu house of Nguvauva. These letters are also inscribed or sewn onto the flags that are now carried during the troop ceremonies. All such marking is done informally by individuals without a great degree of standardization as to design or technique of application.

In recognition of their sustained participation in activities associated with the flag, uniformed members of the troops may be awarded military-style ranks by the highest-ranking flag leaders (fig. 8.10). Stylized crowns, crossed swords, stars, and stripes associated with particular ranks will then be worn on members' colored badges. For example, a major general (*Ogeneralmajora*) may be represented by two crowns and one set of crossed swords and a major (*Omajora*) by one crown. The titles and symbols for various ranks vary somewhat from place to place, but some system of symbolizing rank is used within all the flag organizations.

The emblems of rank are sewn or inscribed in ink on shoulder epaulettes, hatbands, and other cloth markers. At any one celebration, I estimate that one third of the participants have some mark of rank, and more men than women on average wear these. There are roughly ten to twenty members with the highest ranks at any one flag ceremony, and those with the highest ranks are all elderly men. The highest ranking woman I have yet encountered is a major, a rank also held by a number of men at the celebrations. Rank is also recorded in the personal membership book, in which participation in a ceremony is recorded with a stamp.

Ranking male members of the troops may wear a whole suit of clothes in the color associated with their flag. In addition, men with rank and some of the ordinary marchers may carry walking sticks or riding whips and wear medals, leather leggings, and/or military belts made with a strap crossing the body.[12] Some wear pistols in holsters and carry rifles. Some men wear skins or pieces of fur on their hats or hanging down their back (fig. 8.11). It is older men who wear more leather military items and fur, while younger men may wear berets and buttons or scarves with political acronyms on them. Knitted garments such as vests or sweaters in flag colors are also worn.

The clothing worn by the specialists and chiefs involved in the ceremonies differs from flag to flag. Chief Munjuku of the Green flag wears a specially made costume known as royal wear (*ombanda youhona;* fig. 8.12). It consists of a green robe and a three-cornered hat with black-and-white trim. I am told that the chief used to wear everyday clothes to the ceremonies, but that the members of his flag made him this uniform to make him stand out. Chief Zeraua of the White flag has an elaborate blue-and-white uniform with ornamental braid and buttons and a military-style hat with a stiff brim. Chief Riruako of the Red flag wears a similar uniform in red and black.

As is true in daily life, women's participation in the troop ceremonies is somewhat circumscribed in scope and differentiated from that of men, even while it gives women a special role in representing Herero identities. Women

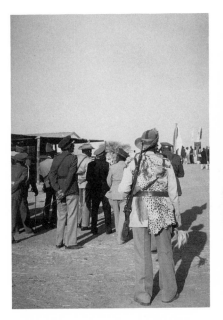

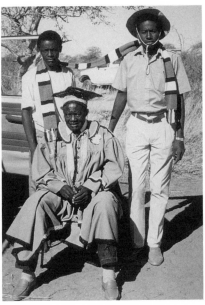

8.11   A high-ranking Red flag member adds an animal skin to his uniform. Photo by D. Jacobson.

8.12   Chief Munjuku II displays the clothing made for him by members of the Green flag. Photo by H. Hendrickson.

march in any troop but are positioned behind the men in line; women can achieve rank but not at the highest levels. Women do not heal or lead the troops to the graves; they may urge on the horseback riders but do not speak to the ancestors at the graves. Nonetheless, it is in women's uniforms that the most impressive expression of flag unity is found.

The basic parts of the woman's uniform include a "long" dress (*ohorokweva onde*), constructed on the same plan as those Herero women are known for wearing every day (see Hendrickson 1994; fig. 8.13). As is true for the everyday dress, the component parts of the woman's uniform are the bodice (*otjari*), the sleeves (*omaoko*), the skirt midsection (*oina*), and the skirt length (*orema*). Women also wear petticoats (*ozondoroko*) and the *otjikaiva* headscarf (*ovikaiva*, plural). For troop celebrations, women wear in addition a special jacket (*eyaki*), which may be worn over the bodice or a shirtwaist blouse worn over the skirt and petticoats. They may also wear badges of rank on their sleeves.

Individual variation in women's dresses is seen in the detailed cut of the sleeves and/or neckline or in the types of topstitching on the skirt length and trim on the jacket. Jewelry worn with the uniform can include necklaces,

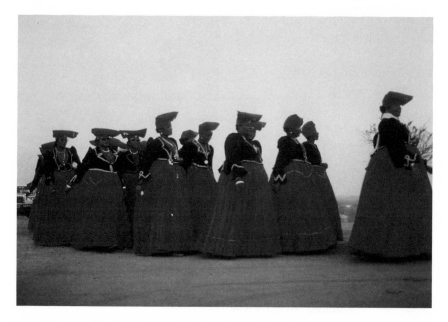

8.13 Women of the Red flag marching in unison. Photo by D. Jacobson.

earrings, pins, rings, and bracelets. Some women may also wear bits of fur in their *otjikaiva*, knitted scarves around their necks, or shawls when it is cold. Some carry handbags and umbrellas.

The use of color is especially pronounced in the women's uniforms, since it is expressed over all the ten or more meters of fabric used to make the long dress. The color properly extends to the *otjikaiva*, for the ideal uniform is one in which all the parts and accessories are coordinated to match or complement the colors of the three flags. Thus, the basic uniform for the Red flag is a red long dress and *otjikaiva*, worn with a black jacket, most often with gold trim and jewelry. As members of the White flag, women wear white dresses and *ovikaiva* with black jackets detailed in gold.[13] Many female marchers for the Green flag wear dark green dresses and *ovikaiva* with black jackets.

Khaki long dresses are sometimes worn by female Red and Green flag members. I am told this color is used to distinguish troop members from Windhoek, who are often of the highest ranks. However, it is also popular with younger Green flag members, who wear khaki jackets, dresses, and *ovikaiva* with a white (*eyapa*) or black (*ezorondu*) shirtwaist with green contrasting stitching and trim. Female Red flag members occasionally wear khaki with a red shirtwaist.

The uniforms ensure that individuals are subsumed into a representation of the group as a collection of standardized units, with some allowance for individual variation at the level of fine details and the marking of individual achievement in leadership. Thus, each ranking troop member is both a leader and a group member, both a recognized loyalist and an ordinary troop member. What we see in Herero troop uniforms is a representation of unity in which the individual units should be exemplary themselves. The same relation of high achievement being subsumed into a unified body is repeated at small and large orders of scale in the action performed by the troops (see Hendrickson 1992).

It is particularly through color that a visual, symbolic statement about troop and flag unity is made. The parade of tens or hundreds of uniformed marchers making their way through the streets or across fields to the graves of their ancestors is powerful on a visual level. The uniforms of women, with their voluminous fabric of matched color, are especially impressive. They are meant to be. Chief Munjuku of the Green flag has likened the troops themselves metaphorically and with pride to cattle whose common color implies shared ancestry (Hendrickson 1992). The marchers in a troop should look the same— like the offspring of a particular pair of cattle.

To the degree that military regimentation confers the same effect, it has been adopted with alacrity. When uniformed troops marching in unison are combined to create a huge procession that proceeds en masse to the graves (fig. 8.14),

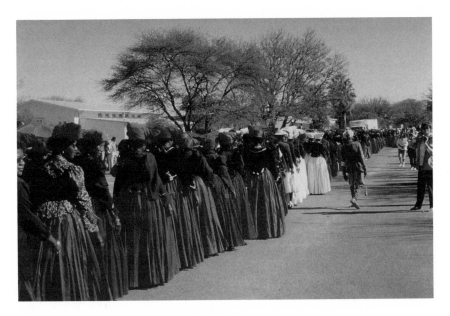

8.14   Onlookers observe part of the procession
to the graves. Photo by D. Jacobson.

both the unity and the internal organization of the whole group is conveyed in the closely defined and detailed use of a few, brilliantly contrasting colors worn on the body. In this unified, moderately hierarchical moral community, a multifaceted model of Herero society is made temporarily concrete.

Hatbands in Nineteenth-Century Herero History

As was the case in other southern African societies (e.g., Comaroff 1985), cloth dress rather than leather came to be worn by Ovaherero in the mid-nineteenth century. At that time (cf. Drechsler [1966] 1980; Goldblatt 1971; Kienitz 1977; Vedder [1928] 1966a, [1938] 1966b; Werner 1989; Wilmsen 1989), Herero speakers, including the Herero proper and Ovambanderu, appear to have been organized into kin-based collectivities around charismatic leaders. Relations between such groups consisted of opportunistic alliance and enmity. This was a time of increasing differentiation between previously intermingled groups of Ovaherero and Orlam, the latter being groups of mixed African and European descent who followed specific leaders north into central Namibia from the 1830s on. In the prime grazing grounds of central Namibia, the Herero leaders Tjamuaha and Zeraua, among others, vied with Orlam leaders such as Jonker Afrikaner[14] for the cattle wealth and renown that would win them followers.

I suggest elsewhere (Hendrickson 1994) that the adoption of the celebrated Herero woman's Victorian-style dress must be seen as resulting from this culture contact and that the Herero use of cloth and clothing occurred within an expanding, indigenous idiom of personal power and bodily treatment. I here draw attention to another aspect of the symbolic use to which men, in particular, put cloth and color.

Ovaherero thought by their peers to be knowledgeable about such esoterica assert that the current symbolic use of cloth and color had its roots in the nineteenth-century Herero use of colored cloth hatbands on men's European-style hats. Hatbands are said to have been used to make visual distinctions between increasingly competitive Herero and Orlam men. As I was told by a Red flag member and respected local leader in Botswana:[15]

First, people wore leather hats . . . When the Herero wore leather hats, there were no Nama [Orlams], so there was no need for a uniform. When the Herero were fighting the Germans, they already had the red cloth. Fighters were supposed to wear the red band so that they could be seen as Herero. The rest of the hat was leather or it was a European hat. We are still wearing the red color now.

This marking of Herero identity is said to be related to the earlier practice of marking of male heroic prowess on the body. As discussed above, pieces of skin and fur are still seen on both men's and women's troop uniforms, and current wisdom links this to the earlier treatment of heroes' bodies and links the use of cloth hat bands to both:[16]

> The new flag was red. This was like when men used to wear a [leopard] skin on their hat for bravery. When the Germans came, the Herero adopted the uniforms because they had no military of their own.

> Men of war wore leopard skin hats in time of Nama war. *Outoņi*[17] was to promote a brave man. You make a mark, scar four marks on a man's chest for one lion—put two marks on either side of the chest. This is for a person who doesn't run and kills the lion.

Among the motivations for this use of markers on the body were ideas about the power and efficacy of European military men.[18]

> After the war [with the Germans], the Herero wore the clothes of their bosses. The bosses, even nonmilitary, were wearing uniforms. Samuel Maharero's generals wore this after the war . . . [As ranks,] General was higher than Hauptmann, which was higher than Kaptain. . . . [The ranks are for] anyone doing a brave deed, not just for elders. It is the same thing as wearing the lion skin, *outoņi*.

> If you wear the clothes of your enemy, the spirit of the enemy is weakened. You are then wearing the spirit of his brothers and then they are weakened. Hereros did do this; there is the sense of this in wearing the German uniform.

Other sources corroborate that the use of cloth hatbands was underway by the last quarter of the century. Photographs taken in 1876[19] show both Herero and Orlam leaders in central Namibia wearing clothes, hats, and hatbands that fit well and look well-worn (figs. 8.15 and 8.16). However, it is not possible to distinguish the use of specific colors from these black and white images. If light and dark color in the photos is taken as an indication, there does not appear to have been a strict association of specific colors with the Orlams or Ovaherero at this early date.[20] Secondary sources also suggest that neither the association of red with Herero groups[21] nor the white with the Orlams was consistent at this time.[22] It is clear, however, that cloth and color were being used to signify identities and the rights that may have flowed from them, and this emerges in other evidence as well (Vedder [1938] 1966b, 208):

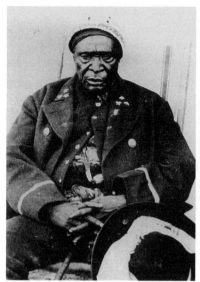

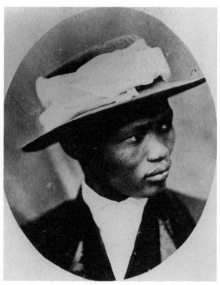

8.15   Maharero with hatband, c. 1885.
National Archives-Windhoek photo
no. 6859; used by permission.

8.16   A Nama school master, 1876. National
Archives-Windhoek photo no. 2829; used by
permission.

Then Jonker had pieces of rag tied to all the raisin bushes, so as to mark them with the tokens of ownership according to ancient custom, but that did not help in the least. When Jonker wanted raisins, he found that other people had been to the bushes previously and had stripped them of fruit. Jonker had the spoors traced up and he had the suspected thieves severely punished.

Sometime between the 1880s and 1923, when the troop ceremonies were initiated in full regalia at the funeral of Maharero's son Samuel, the use of white and red became more standardized. In 1884, Maharero's chief rival Hendrik Witbooi entered the region from the south (Gugelberger 1984), and he became associated with the use of a white hatband. Since Witbooi, Maharero, and their followers engaged in repeated clashes throughout the last decades of the century, it is reasonable to assert that Maharero's association with red took on meaning in distinction to Witbooi's use of white.

The History of a Flag

I turn now to oral histories of the Red flag, to accounts of how Maharero imagined and acted to construct a newly unified Herero polity, and to the ways that commitment to a new ideal of moral leadership was and still is expressed in the wearing of colored cloth on the body. In both the uniformed participation of people in the flag ceremonies and the nineteenth-century coalition of Herero groups around the wearing of red bands of cloth, a degree of social unity has been created through the willing commitment of ordinary people to literally embody certain social principles.

In the 1850s and 1860s, the Orlams were able to use the guns and horses they had obtained before Ovaherero to dominate central Namibia. After the death of his father, however, Maharero moved to organize the first united battles of Ovaherero against the Orlams (Goldblatt 1971; Vedder [1938] 1966b; Lau 1989). In 1863, a force of Orlams was badly beaten at Otjimbingwe by Maharero and others. With their allies Charles John Andersson and his sometime partner Frederick Thomas Green, Maharero's and Zeraua's men waged another successful battle against the Afrikaner Orlams in 1864 at Rehoboth. These battles were fought with guns, by a unified Herero force, and against a common Orlam enemy. As such, they constituted a departure from earlier skirmishes and raids. In victory, Ovaherero were never again to be subject to the Orlams.

Origin narratives for the flag organizations (see Hendrickson 1992) link the emergence of new types of leadership and unified conceptions of the Herero polity to the bodily use of cloth and color at this time. In these narratives, the struggle between the desires of individuals and the value placed on a unified, moral society is writ large in the lives of the ancestors recognized by each flag. Moral leadership is read into the heroic past, male leadership in particular is modeled, and flag membership comes to involve at its widest, a commitment to a view of history itself.

I here consider oral histories of the biggest and best-known flag, the Red;[23] equally important histories of the Green and White flags will be considered elsewhere. The following versions of the story about the death of a Herero hero, Mainuwa, emerged in separate histories of the Red flag given to me, though these were obtained in widely separate circumstances. An account given to Gibson in the 1950's was strikingly similar.[24] These facts suggest that this part of the history of the Red flag is a durable one.[25]

> In 1866, the Herero were fighting the Nama. While they were still fighting, there was a son of Maharero. His European name was Martin, and his Herero name was Mainuwa. This man had a red color on his skin. When the Herero and the Nama were fighting, one Herero shot Martin, thinking he was a Nama. The Herero and the Nama were still fighting. Both had white cloth on their heads. It was just a uniform.
>
> After Martin's death, the Herero returned home thinking about this

death. [They thought] now we are supposed to have a different uniform from the Nama. After the white hats, the Herero decided to find another cloth for the top of the head. Red was chosen because white made us kill the son of Maharero.

Another man gave this version of the story:[26]

The Herero took the red color after Mainuwa was shot by his own people during fighting between the Ovaherero and the Nama in Rehoboth [southern, central Namibia]. Before this, everyone wore a white hatband. This was not a flag.

People wanted to destroy the kraal of the man who had killed Mainuwa, but Maharero said no—that it had happened in battle so it was not the same thing as just killing him. So they chose another color.

Otjiserandu began in Rehoboth when Mainuwa was shot. He had a red skin like the Hottentots. Riarua was the leader of the war after Mainuwa. His skin was red also. Kanaimba, son of Katjimuine, shot Mainuwa. People said that Kanaimba's kraal should be destroyed by Mainuwa's family, the same family as Maharero. Maharero said no. They chose a red cloth (erapi) to wear on the hat. The Nama wore white. Kanaimba sent another man, Kangava, in Mainuwa's place to Okahandja.

A third account went as follows:[27]

The people had decided to use the white flag until 1865. Mainuwa was the son of Tjamuaha, brother of Maharero. He was very handsome; the ombimbi praise song for him says that he was beautiful like a woman. No woman would say no to him. He was a hero of the war.

In 1865, two kilometers east of what is now called Aris [near Windhoek], at a place called Okaokovijaja, there was a battle between the Nama and the Hereros. The Nama were led by Jan Jonker Afrikaner, Christian's brother. The battle began about 8:00 am and went until 4:00 or 4:30. The Nama were defeated and they began to ride away on horseback. The Hereros were under some trees, waiting to get these men as they went by.

Mainuwa was leading the Hereros after them and was killed. He had light skin and white on his hat, on his arm, and also on a stick on his saddle. He was shot by another Herero. Old men recognized him and knew he had been shot by a Herero. They saw that the king's son had been killed. It was the son of Tjitjai who had killed Mainuwa. So after they sang praise songs for Mainuwa, they went back to Okahandja to Maharero. The people wanted [the son of Tjitjai] to be killed. Maharero said no—the problem was that the same color was being worn. He said we need to choose another style of fighting.

These Herero narratives construct a kind of "Great Man" reading of history in which watershed events can be traced to the intelligence and foresight of male leaders who act on behalf of those who follow them. They tell of men who learn to control new resources and allies and whose vision of the future becomes binding upon others. The authority of these heroes is seen as contingent upon proper moral action, however. Further, succession, which Weber (1947) has pointed out is perhaps the most volatile issue of all for such charismatic leaders, emerges as a key issue in these narratives as well.

At stake in these flag charters are new definitions of maleness, leadership, and heroism, which have new nuances of meaning in the present context of Namibian national politics. For each flag, narratives focus on one hero and the innovative acts he performed in order to give his people the advantage in the changing world of the nineteenth-century. For the Red flag, it is confirmed elsewhere that Maharero and Mainuwa are brothers—in this polygynous society, they are in the often contentious relationship of having the same father and different mothers. Maharero was the son of Tjamuaha's first wife and Mainuwa was the son of his third (Schapera 1979, 24). Mainuwa is said to have been a military leader for Maharero; this arrangement may have ameliorated the tensions felt between men of the same generation competing for status within the family.

All these accounts have basic elements in common. The scene is that of ongoing fighting with the Nama over undisclosed issues. In the course of the battles with the Nama, the leader Mainuwa, a relative of the chief Maharero, is killed by another Omuherero who mistakes him for one of the enemy. The people go to Maharero seeking permission to kill the perpetrator in retribution. Maharero refuses to let them do so. Instead, the people begin to wear the red color on their hats, so that they will then be distinguishable from the Nama, who wear white.

The key issue here analytically is that the narratives link Mainuwa's death to his wearing of the wrong color—that is, to the problem of distinguishing Orlam from Herero. There is evidence to suggest that getting caught in friendly fire was one of the hazards of the increasingly more organized fighting that went on in the later part of the nineteenth century. Green, one of the Europeans involved in the unified battles against the Nama, described the battle scene and how easily one could come to be fired upon by one's allies (Lau 1989, 244):

At this time the Damaras [Ovaherero] were becoming fairly dispersed over the mountain and, as we now made our appearance in a position previously occupied by the Hottentots [Nama], we were mistaken for the latter by some of the Damaras. The consequence was we found ourselves exposed to the cross-fire from friend and foe . . . I became so utterly confused that I was at a loss.

What matters more than substantiating whether Mainuwa died in a particular time, place, and manner is the fact that his accidental demise is constructed as the heart of the story. Accidental death is still not a concept that has full acceptance among Ovaherero; rumors of poisoning circulated rapidly in 1989, for instance, when a Herero politician was suddenly taken ill at a political dinner and was hospitalized and underwent surgery shortly thereafter. Retribution by the family of a man killed by other Ovaherero would have been standard in the nineteenth century and still takes place today (Vedder [1928] 1966a, 198–99):

> Vendetta takes a very important place beside private revenge. The relations of the slain person have the right of instituting proceedings against the murderer or manslaughterer, but the chief does not interfere on his own accord, as the avenging of the blood of a relative is legally recognised. . . . But blood-vengence [sic] may not be wreaked within the own oruzo [patrician] circle. It may only be applied to members of foreign tribes or members of the own eanda [matriclan] . . . When a man has been killed, his brothers and his mother's brothers are entitled to avenge his blood. Instead of taking blood-vengence, they may choose to plunder the town of the perpetrator.

In Mainuwa's case, the people may have had especially good reason to want to gain retribution, since it was the chief's family that had been threatened by the death. He may have been a likely target for jealousy and treachery given that he was a military leader and a man known for his beauty and attractiveness to women. One account says Kanaimba sent a man to Okahandja, Maharero's base, to replace Mainuwa. This implies that some kind of retribution was in fact gained by Maharero's people for the death.

Red flag histories characterize Maharero as proposing a novel solution to the problem posed by this death, and significantly, making the solution binding over others. Maharero turns away the people's talk of blood vengeance and focuses on the issue of mistaken identity in a battle. He is said to state that the solution will be that Ovaherero will wear the red and thus avoid any future confusion over their identity in distinction to that of the Nama.

Maharero's proclamation that Mainuwa's death was a mistake and therefore should not call for retribution is powerful, for it appears to have departed from earlier practice. If Vedder is correct, the people who would have sought retribution for Mainuwa would have been people in Mainuwa's matriclan—people potentially in another matriclan from Maharero since such affiliations derive from one's mother's identity. For this reason, and since (as Vedder notes) the chief was not supposed to interfere in such matters, Maharero should have had no say in whether any vengeance was taken for Mainuwa's death. Yet the narratives state that he makes a decisive act against the wishes of the people, and the people abide by his decision.

Maharero is thus unusual in being able to constrain the people; he also is seen to go further to redefine the meaning of the group itself. In redefining the meaning of Mainuwa's death, Maharero redefines the group as one within which vengeance should not be sought. He implies that membership in the matriclan is no longer of singular importance in reckoning responsibility for death—that matriclan identity should be subordinate to a shared identity of a different order. In this moment, he asserts a new kind of authority over a newly defined social group.

Red flag narrative histories, then, tell how Maharero had a new vision of society, how at a time of crisis the wisdom of that vision became clear to others, and what followers should do to demonstrate their commitment to the new moral order. As such, it has some of the classic elements of charismatic prophesy,[28] itself a quintessential example of the imagination of community. When Maharero decrees that Ovaherero should wear the red cloth to distinguish themselves from the Orlams, he asks that they identify *themselves* as members of a restructured, moral community. It is the commitment of troop members to particular social ideals that is being still expressed in the individual's choice to use cloth and color in the flag uniforms.

Oral histories of the other two flags (see Hendrickson 1992) have much in common with that of the Red discussed here, though they also chart the separate identity of each flag and its followers. In Green and White flag histories, the foresight, talent, and intelligence of nineteenth-century chiefs are stressed. The Green flag history tells of the martyr's death of Chief Kahimemua, who directed his people to freedom in Botswana. White flag history explains how Chief Zeraua learned to use firearms and helped free Maharero from subservience to the Orlams.[29] These narratives construct new potentials for the extent of one leader's power in a pastoralist society that makes little provision for the hierarchical or arrangement of positions of power. However, they also define male leadership as responsible to others. They help legitimate new definitions of public authority, in which men turn their individual skills toward making use of new social resources and circumstances for the good of those who depend upon them.

It is important to note that the acts of these visionaries are read into the early colonial past, long before the strictures of formal German colonialism led to the ill-fated Herero revolt, which Europeans and other onlookers see as the defining moment in Herero history. Movement toward social change is said to have originated in several different branches of the Herero-speaking community and has been elaborated into a proliferation of ceremonial events rather than collapsing with the passing of the initial visionaries. The proliferation of bodily markers of commitment to ideals of leadership and community since the nineteenth century suggests that these adjustments in Herero social practice garner considerable support.

Europeans and Their Flags

The importance of bodily symbolism in marking a peculiarly Herero commitment to a new vision of community is underscored by the fact that flags in the European sense were not used by Herero to represent their identity until the early twentieth century. In fact, there is evidence to show that explicit European attempts to inculcate the use of a "national" flag for the purposes of rallying Africans to unified action were essentially ignored by Herero people.

At the time when Maharero is said in the oral histories to have been unifying his people and using a distinctive color to mark them, his European allies were writing in their journals about a flag as representative of the nation, as a rallying point, and as worth fighting for in and of itself. Andersson and Green, as mentioned above, participated in the pivotal battles between newly unified Herero and Orlam forces. Their interest was in defending the town of Otjimbingwe, where Andersson's mining and trading business was located and which had been attacked by the Orlams in 1863 (Goldblatt 1971, 25ff).

These Europeans had been integrated at least temporarily into Herero political alignments of the time. In 1864, when Andersson, Green,[30] and the Ovaherero emerged victorious over the Afrikaner Orlams, Andersson himself was acting as Maharero's military leader (Goldblatt 1971, 33). Having assumed the role of military leader perhaps just before or just after Mainuwa, Andersson was then seriously wounded in the 1864 battle.[31] Maharero assumed the position of overall leader of the united forces just before the battle of Rehoboth, but Andersson himself expected to be offered the role (Lau 1989, 110).

While Andersson was helping to organize the united force against the Orlams, one of his concerns was designing a flag. In his diaries (Lau 1989, 111),

Andersson wrote of developing a flag expressly for the purpose of leading Ovaherero [11 May 1864]:

Baines [see below] suggested a national flag. Thought of the same thing, only did not broach the subject as it seems almost premature . . . Sketch[ed][32] three or four different coloured flags. We must have an eye more to effect than prettiness, as a flag as a rule is rarely exposed to full view, the wind generally causing it more or less to fold, and consequently details are lost. We tried yellow, but [it] neither creates effect nor is it clearly visible at any distance. A red cross on a blue field with a large star appearing just behind the cross looks well and is effective.[33] My wife must make a silken standard if I become the chief of this country. In the meantime we ought to have something for use.

Thomas Baines, an Englishman and painter who traveled in the region in the early 1860s, depicted flags in a painting showing the gathering of African and European allies before the battle of 1864.[34] He renders flags twice—once flying from the front of a wagon where European men sit and again in the hands of a European man in the foreground of the painting. Both flags appear to bear a red cross on a white star on a blue background, as discussed in Andersson's diary, but it is not known whether these flags actually existed or whether they are a product of Baines's artistic vision.

Baines's ideas about the use of a flag are given further testimony in another of his paintings, called "The Otjimbingwe Volunteer Artillery, 1864."[35] It shows Europeans and Africans shooting an unseen enemy while a flag—with the red, white, and blue in one corner and a red field—is held by an African. A European directs the firefight. In this painting, Baines's flag is nearly identical to that of the British. And a card[36] he gave to Andersson is inscribed with the following (Lau 1989, 281–82):

Song of the Otjimbingwe British Volunteer Artillery.
Motto: Defence, and Defiance—1864.
Rule 1: The flag of the Corps shall be the British
flag, and no act contrary to his allegiance to the
British Crown shall be required of any member.

Britannica, the pride of the ocean,
The home of the brave and the free,
The land of the sailor's devotion,
What land can compare, then with thee!
In all countries thy children are scattered,

Yet still to their flag they'll prove true,
Though storm-tossed, or war-worn and tattered,
Three cheers for the Red, White and Blue,
Three cheers for the Red, White and Blue . . .
But we'll rally round the flag of Old England,
And die by the Red, White and Blue.

There is evidence to suggest that some of the nationalist ideology associated
with such flags may have actually been taught to Ovaherero by these men. A few
weeks before the battle at Rehoboth, Andersson writes: "I have reason to believe
Mr. Hahn addressed the assembled chiefs, impressed upon them the necessity
of clinging to me unflinchingly, explaining also the use of the flag, and many
other things" [6 June 1864]. Green described the prominence given the flag (as
it had been envisioned by Andersson) at the start of the 1864 battle (Lau 1989,
242):

> . . . we could observe the enemy's forces in position. We of course drew off
> out of range to examine his different positions, as also to await the arrival
> of our own forces which were left in the rear by our giving chase to the
> horse-men. The wagon soon made its appearance, close after which could
> be seen the Damara [Herero] national flag (the cross and the star), a blue
> ground with a red cross and a white star emerging from the latter, waving
> in front of the black mass of our troops. The oxen were first released from
> the yoke and the wagon stood within rifle range of the enemy with the flag
> transferred and fastened to the front.

Despite these machinations, Ovaherero do not appear to have made their
own European-style flags until well into this century. They were nonetheless
quite capable of using European flags to further their own aims. Pool (1991, 104,
106) cites evidence to show that in 1894, Samuel Maharero and Manasse, another Herero leader of the time, requested German flags to fly over their own
homesteads, presumably to enhance their own reputations as leaders and/or to
intimidate their rivals. Samuel Maharero's request was apparently granted. The
flying of the German flag over central Namibia to symbolize German protection of certain Ovaherero was explicitly mentioned in an 1885 treaty signed by
Maharero and Samuel Maharero, among others (Pool 1991, 63).

Later, it was the British flag that was put to strategic use. In 1923, Frederick
Maharero requested that a British flag be draped across his kinsman Samuel's
coffin to show that the latter had lived and died under that particular banner.[37]
In 1924, Herero petitioners cognizant of the import of cloth banners for Euro-

peans asked to be allowed to "play as soldiers . . . to drill as soldiers in the military . . . we should learn drilling as soldiers as it is very good for us to learn and to know everything under the british flag [sic]."[38]

The earliest archival evidence pertaining to the Herero troops (see Hendrickson 1992; Werner 1990) describes in detail their military drilling, clandestine meetings, use of military titles, and the wearing of military medals and uniforms, but makes no mention of flags per se. When the government first acted in 1928 to ban "any organization which provides for its members wearing uniforms and carrying out drills and parades or military evolutions,"[39] banners were not mentioned by colonial officials.

That Ovaherero continued to brandish European flags when it suited them is apparent in a report filed that same year. In it, a police officer noted that Herero troop members, including "a flag bearer," had been observed drilling at night in Windhoek. He wrote that "in the dark, the flag resembled the German Flag (Three different colours and probably Black, white and red)."[40] It seems likely that this was a salvaged German flag and not a banner constructed for their own purposes by Herero troop members, but we cannot be certain.

A black, white, and red banner is mentioned again in a report from the late 1930s:[41] "Some weeks ago the Hereros held their annual ceremony at the grave of their great chieftain Samuel Maherero [sic] in Okahandja . . . they had been forbidden to march in close formation and to carry the black-white and red flag." The report noted that Ovaherero had come to use these symbolic materials in their own ways and that there had been an official backlash against this:

> As you know, the Hereros had always attended this ceremony in uniform. They wore red socks (red being the tribal colour) coats and jackets in different colours according to their tribal connections . . . as well as German rosettes, black, white and red braid and shining buttons as the old German troops used to wear. The women wore red headcloths and dresses in tribal colours . . . [The Chief Native Commissioner] said that the German uniforms and tokens which they wore by no means made German soldiers of them (which was never intended). He demanded that they should remove the buttons, tokens, rosettes and braid, as the German State did not allow subjects of other states to wear these symbols.

It is not clear when Ovaherero began regularly using European-style banners of their own design, but today the three flag organizations have distinctive banners that are carried by the troops and adorn the ceremony sites. Even these, though, are few in number and handmade without a great degree of standardization. They bear the symbols and acronyms associated with one flag organization, arranged and applied in idiosyncratic ways. They play no special role in the ceremonies, are little discussed, and receive no special reverence. Rather, it is still the massive, dazzling harmony of individuals embodying the flag in their person that practically obliterates the visual presence of banners at these events.

Conclusion

Bodies as flags

Thus, the wearing of colored cloth hatbands as symbols of social affiliation can be traced in oral history and documentary evidence to the second half of the nineteenth century. This practice emerged at a time when the idea of a unified Herero group and of a common enemy were beginning to take shape. In the mid-nineteenth century, new tools, such as guns, raised the possibility for the assertion of different kinds of power, and alliances appeared to make possible new kinds of autonomy. New levels of wealth appeared available in the spoils of raiding and the opportunity for exchange of services and goods with Europeans. New kinds of personal power appeared possessable in the garments of powerful foreigners.

With color, the early Herero interest in clothing as carrying potent personal power was elaborated into a representation of group power. This use of colored cloth and the acceptance of the new idea of community was not immediate. Rather, it developed over decades as relations with others in the region took shape. Later still, as the idea of the unified Herero polity continued to coalesce, the Herero use of colored cloth was codified in the ceremonies of the flag organizations themselves. In these organizations, as in past practice, the collectivity is seen only as the product of mutual individual commitments.

Ovaherero manage the meaning of this past by making this history one of heroic struggles of male leaders successfully adapting to changing times. All three flags celebrate the morality of leaders who use their wits and skills to turn these new resources into advantages for their "children." The flags are voluntary organizations that enact a moral vision of Herero society in which exemplary men and women are ranked and unified in the eyes of the ancestors and fellow, earthly onlookers.

The subtle contest that goes on between old and young, men and women, ranked and unranked participants, troops from different places, and the three flags themselves is muted by more insistent efforts to create a representation of social unity. This same tension is inscribed on the body of each participant. The uniform, which is both the sign of and the ticket to rightful membership in the troops and their ceremonies, records both the individual's achievements within the group and subsumes the individual within the whole, unified body of the celebrants.

The flag organizations, the cloth markers, and the colors *are* the people, unified in their commitments to the whole. Just as one military hero with a colored hatband proclaimed and created his fellowship with other Ovaherero, one uniformed participant distinguishes himself or herself and creates a sense of the unified community at the troop ceremonies. Within a world in which ordinary people can become heroes and heroes are defined by their responsibilities to ordinary people, the morality of the individual *is* the morality of the community and the body of the individual *is* the body of society.

Herero bodily symbolism, and not the depersonalized markers of European allegiance, still expresses this intimate relation of the individual to the collectivity. Bodily expressions of the unified community express both the possibilities for individual agency and the probabilities of belonging to the wider social world. In constructions of colored cloth, an individual remains in contact with, and may produce for him or herself as well as for others, a concrete manifestation of social morality.

These bodily symbols are indices of the individual commitment to shared social values, visions of the past, and images of the future. They express individual intentions to enact a moral ethic that has been critical to group cohesion through a period of growing political centralization. The reasons why Ovaherero were unable to mount an effective allied challenge to German colonial control—a central question in the academic analysis of Herero history— must stem at least in part from the fact that these ideological tensions are only temporarily resolved in social activity like the flag ceremonies.

Bodily symbolism
The differences between the colonial and the Herero idiomatic use of cloth, color, and flags reflect differences in the ways that the relation between the individual and the collectivity were conceived by these social groups. Nonetheless, the common interest in bodily symbolism reflects a common concern with leadership and social cohesion. By examining a history of the use of bodily symbolism, analogies and divergences between culturally specific notions of the relation between the self and society can be investigated.

Exploring these issues is essential for the understanding of colonial histories. The face-to-face relations of early intercultural contact are like those in small-scale societies, where the representation of the bodily self is intimately connected to the imagination of the collectivity, and the symbolic reading of the bodily other is critical to communication about wider social identities.

In the years since 1923, the flag ceremonies have come to be associated with Herero conservatism, both by Ovaherero and by fellow Namibians and tourists alerted by the media to the annual celebrations at Okahandja and Omaruru. Each year, hundreds of spectators line the streets to watch the flag processions go by. Like the Herero long dress, these ceremonies have been come to be seen as "traditional" Herero practice. It seems paradoxical, at first glance, that activities clearly associated with late-nineteenth-century history and not a deeper Herero past should be so taken.

However, it is important to recognize that issues of traditionalism, of ethnic identity, have emerged only since the late-nineteenth-century intercultural contacts and conflicts of the colonial period in Namibia. And since that time, the uniforms and ceremonies associated with the flags have been repeatedly etched upon the landscape and the imagination of a wider Namibian world. It is the visual brilliance and impressive physical presence power of these events that ensures that they are alive in the memory of onlookers and participants alike.

In the construction of body treatments, Herero men and women have been able to express new visions, images, of the individual's relation to the collectivity. These images, specific mental linkages of symbolic form and referent, were characteristic of Herero modes of thought about efficacy, the individual, and the social world. Such images gain currency for individuals when they are materially articulated on the body. They are ideological claims made persuasive by their expression in a bodily metaphor.

However, for others, bodily imagery is impressive because it is concrete, visually powerful, and, above all, remembered. We should seek to understand the pathways between the viewed, experienced, plural, social world and the collective imagination of self and society. In the case discussed here, the idea of the Herero polity has arisen simultaneously with the emergence of new bodily representations of the self and the collectivity. Necessarily, owing to the concreteness of the symbolic media used, the idea of the collectivity, and the idea of Herero traditionalism, have themselves gained authenticity. The repeated construction and use of these material representations over time have lent the weight of time to the ideas. It is by being concretized in material media that shared terms in the imagination of identity can come to be models for, as well as models of, society.

Once when I left Botswana on a long journey to attend one of the Namibian troop celebrations, a woman who had to stay behind wound around my neck a homemade scarf that had been knitted in the colors of the Green flag. Her gesture exemplified the relation of the faithful to the flag, of the individual to the collectivity, for her gift helped me create the flag in my person. In the mundane contexts of domestic life, individuals create the flag in their ideas about it and their instantiation of those ideas, those images, in colored ornaments for the body. In contrast to European ideas about the flag itself as the embodiment of the nation, each Herero flag member is literally in touch with the nation—creates it in their imagination and embodies it in their physical presence. Clothing, color, and ideas about the self and the collectivity are thus linked idiosyncratically in Herero thought and practice. These facts should give us pause in interpreting the apparent transparency of symbols like the new Namibian flag and the political activity that produces them.

Notes

This paper could not have been written without the patient collaboration of George Kazoe Kozonguizi, who shares my interest in the Namibian past. For their comments on this and other drafts of this paper, I extend thanks to George, Ed Wilmsen, Misty Bastian, and the anonymous reviewers for Duke University Press. I am especially grateful to my husband, Dean Jacobson, for his support in the field and at home, and to the many Ovaherero in Namibia and Botswana who were patient teachers and generous friends. Among many others, I thank A. Kaputu, T. Tjirongo, S. Tjivikua, A. Tjirondero, and T. Kamupingene for their help in gathering and interpreting the oral history of the Red flag and K. Ndjarakana for his help with translations.

I am grateful to the governments of Botswana and Namibia for granting me permission to carry out fieldwork in southern Africa between 1987 and 1989. I acknowledge the National Science Foundation, the Wenner-Gren Foundation for Anthropological Research, the Social Science Research Council, and New York University for funding in support of this work.

1   The year 1989 marked the transition to independence, during which the United Nations Transitional Assistance Group (UNTAG) helped prepare the country for its first national elections.

2   The Democratic Turnhalle Alliance was founded in 1977 (see Pütz, von Egidy, and Caplan 1987). It has been a relatively conservative, coalition-based party drawing support from the Herero party NUDO (National Unity Democratic Organization), itself founded in 1964 and associated with the international leadership of the late Clemens Kapuuo.

3   The National Patriotic Front is a new coalition party with Herero leadership associated with SWANU (South West African National Union; founded 1959) and its offshoots.

4   See Hendrickson 1992 for discussion and oral histories pertaining to the wider "flag" organizations that produce the troop ceremonies. Emmet (1986) and Ngavi-

rue (1972, 1990) analyze the troop ceremonies as a form of resistance. Werner (1982, 1989, 1990) discusses the changing role of the ceremonies in the playing out of political relations both inside and outside Herero society. Otto (1979) outlines White flag history.

5   These ceremonies were formerly called "Herero Day" celebrations or the "Truppenspieler," among other terms.

6   Especially, but not exclusively, older people; female membership in the flags outnumbers that of males, but the leaders are predominantly male.

7   While *otjiserandu* and *otjiapa* are derived from standard Otjiherero word roots referring to the colors red and white, *otjingirine* appears to be derived from an English root. *Otjizemba*, "banded thing," is considered the proper name for the White flag. However, this flag is commonly referred to as "the white" or *otjiapa*, a construction parallel to that of the other two terms.

8   The performances in which I participated and upon which this analysis is based were the Red flag in Okahandja, August 1988; the White flag in Omaruru, October 1988; the Green flag in Okahandja, June 1989; the Green flag in Okeseta, August 1989; the Red flag in Okahandja, August 1989.

9   Ritual practitioners must arrive earlier to prepare the way for the participants.

10 It was this crucial difference that many colonial administrators failed to recognize as they kept a suspicious eye on Herero troop activities in the first half of this century (see Hendrickson 1992; Werner 1982, 1990).

11 The Red flag has also been known as "the Red Band," referring to these red pieces of cloth.

12 In archival records, these have been called "Sam Browne" belts (see Hendrickson 1992).

13 Cloth interwoven with gold- or silver-colored thread is especially prized in everyday dresses.

14 This family and their followers should not be confused with the much broader South African Afrikaner cultural group of Dutch descent.

15 Mr. K.T.T., a Red flag member and headman in northwestern Botswana. These and other excerpts are from interviews conducted in 1988–89, in which I solicited information about issues pertaining to clothing and color.

16 Comments of Mr. S.T., a Red flag secretary and member, and former school teacher living outside Okakarara, Namibia.

17 Literally "victory," here used as an abstract, adjectival noun.

18 Comments of Mr. A.K., a Red flag member, government employee, and organizer of many cultural events in Namibia.

19 Photos taken by the Palgrave expedition from the Cape government in South Africa; housed in the National Archives, Windhoek (NAW); copied and reproduced with permission.

20 Posed groupings entitled "Kamaherero and his bodyguard" and "Zeraua and bodyguard" show men's hats with dark-colored hatbands (NAW nos. 2771 and 2773,

respectively). A "Nama school master" (fig. 25) is clearly wearing a white hatband (NAW no. 2829). However, Ovambanderu men are seen in other group photos (NAW nos. 2785, 2772) wearing both dark and light hatbands. A photo dated 1901 (NAW no. 1288) shows Samuel Maharero holding a hat with a dark band, while both the Nama leader Barnabas and the Herero Assa Riarua are holding hats with light bands. A color painting (reprinted by the National Archives, Windhoek) by Thomas Baines depicting a unified force of Ovaherero and Europeans preparing to fight the Afrikaner Orlams in 1864 shows Africans and Europeans wearing a variety of dark and light and even multicolored hatbands.

21   Hahn (1869) wrote that Ovaherero made a distinction between *Ovathorondu* and *Ovatherandu* (black and red) groups amongst themselves, and that the Mbanderu were associated with the red, though not strictly so. Poewe (1985, 128) notes that black was considered Maharero's national color, but her source for this information is unclear. A Herero origin myth (Irle 1906, 76; Vedder [1928] 1966a, 132) links the black with Herero people and red with the Nama. Werner (1990) cites Irle (1906) as the earliest observer who mentions the Herero use of colored cloth; Irle wrote that around the turn of the century Samuel Maharero distributed red hatbands to his followers.

22   Vedder ([1938] 1966b, 332) notes that one group of Nama used a white hatband to signal *un*willingness to fight in one confrontation with the Ovaherero and that Jan Jonker Afrikaner wore a red, not a white, uniform in Windhoek after he assumed leadership of his people in 1863 (339). The use of a white flag for surrender is also mentioned in Mbanderu oral history (Sundermeier n.d., 36, 43). The Nama living in eastern Namibia are said to have been called the Gei-khaua, in part because of the characteristic light brown clothing that their leaders wore (Vedder [1938] 1966b, 172).

23   Excerpted from interviews conducted during 1988–89 in Namibia and Botswana. These texts may constitute a new genre of historical narration, unlike praise songs which have a long history in Herero culture. They were elicited by my requests and given by Ovaherero considered to be experts in the matters of valued historical knowledge.

24   Hendrickson (1992) and Gordon Gibson (personal communication; see also 1952).

25   Mr. K.T.T.

26   Mr. S.T.

27   Mr. A.K.

28   This is even clearer in the Green flag history, in which Chief Kahimemua does not die until the last of the executioners' many bullets are fired by a ranking officer and in which he explicitly prophesies the return of one of his "sons" to Namibia after sending his people to exile in Botswana (Hendrickson 1992).

29   White flag descendants of the leader Zeraua assert that the red cloth was obtained first by Zeraua, who then passed it on to Maharero. Another source (Vedder [1938] 1966b, 339) notes that Zeraua was chosen first to lead the unified Ovaherero because

he was older than Maharero. White flag leaders further assert that Chief Zeraua and his followers adopted white as their own color in 1876, to symbolize peace. Green flag leaders say that their colors of green, black, and white stand for new life, death, and peace, respectively.

30 In organizing this offensive, they were also aided by the missionary Carl Hugo Hahn.

31 The next military leader mentioned in the historical accounts is Riarua, much later in the century. So Mainuwa and perhaps others may have held the position between 1864 and the 1890s, perhaps inactively during the years of peace between 1870 and 1880.

32 Notes by the editor of Andersson's writings are given here in curly brackets.

33 A drawing of a design of the flag is reprinted in Lau 1989 (112).

34 The painting is called "Hugo Hahn addressing the Herero before the battle against the Oorlam/Nama Afrikaners, June 1864." This and the other painting discussed below are included in the reprint set "Namibia in the 1860's as seen and painted by Thomas Baines," published by the National Archives of Namibia, Windhoek, 1988.

35 The Volunteers were an armed group of mercenaries and settlers from the Otjim-bingwe area who were organized by Andersson to defend the town from raids.

36 This card is described by Lau, the editor of Andersson's diaries: "The song is printed on a small card, inscribed at the back: 'C. J. Andersson, with kind remembrance from his friend T. Baines' " (Lau 1989, 281).

37 Report on the burial of Samuel Maharero, Okahandja, by District Commissioner Courtney-Clarke, 1923.

38 By Hans Joel, Luderitzbucht [Luderitz] to The Administrator, Government Buildings, Windhoek, 2 January 1924.

39 From The Secretary for South West Africa in the Office of the Administrator, Windhoek to all Magistrates Confidential, 7 February 1928. All archival documents are from the National Archives, Windhoek, "South West Africa Archives No. 432," vols. 1 and 2. Werner (1990) cites many of the same documents in slightly different ways.

40 From Johannes, statement taken by Constable de Wet, to the Officer-in-Charge, Town & District Police, Windhoek, 6:00 a.m., 22 January 1928.

41 To the Chief Native Commissioner, Windhoek, from the Native Commissioner, Omaruru, 3 April 1939, re: "Herero Troop Movement. (Truppenspielers)."

REFERENCES

Abraham, R. 1958. *A Dictionary of Modern Yoruba.* London: University of London Press.

Afigbo, A. E. 1972. *The Warrant Chiefs: Indirect Rule in Southeastern Nigeria 1891–1929.* New York: Humanities Press.

Allen, J. de Ver. 1974. Swahili Culture Reconsidered: Some Historical Implications of the Material Culture of the Northern Kenya Coast in the Eighteenth and Nineteenth Centuries. *Azania* 9:105–38.

———. 1981. Swahili Culture and the Nature of East Coast Settlement. *International Journal of African Historical Studies* 14:306–34.

———. 1993. *Swahili Origins: Swahili Culture and the Shungwaya Phenomenon.* Athens: Ohio University Press.

Almagor, U. 1985. A Tourist's "Vision Quest" in an African Game Reserve. *Annals of Tourism Research* 12(1):31–48.

Alverson, H. 1978. *Mind in the Heart of Darkness: Value and Self Identity Among the Tswana of Southern Africa.* New Haven: Yale University Press.

Andersson, N., and S. Marks. 1988. Typhus and Social Control: South Africa, 1917–1950. In *Disease, Medicine and Empire: Perspectives on Western Medicine and the Experience of European Expansion,* ed. R. MacLeod and M. Lewis, 257–83. London: Routledge.

Appadurai, A. 1990. Disjuncture and Difference in the Global Cultural Economy. *Public Culture* 2(2):1–25.

———, ed. 1986. *The Social Life of Things: Commodities in Cultural Perspective.* New York: Cambridge University Press.

Appadurai, A., and C. Breckenridge. 1988. Why Public Culture? *Public Culture* 1(1):5–9.

Apter, A. 1991. *Critics and Kings.* Chicago: University of Chicago Press.

Arens, W. 1975. The Waswahili: The Social History of an Ethnic Group. *Africa* 45(4):426–38.

Ash, J., and E. Wilson. 1992. *Chic Thrills: A Fashion Reader.* Berkeley: University of California Press.

Azikiwe, N. 1970. *My Odyssey: An Autobiography.* London: C. Hurst.

Bakengesa, S. K. S. 1974. An Historical Survey of the Coffee Industry in Bukoba District, 1932–1954. M.A. thesis, Department of History, University of Dar es Salaam.

Barber, K. 1991. *I Could Speak Until Tomorrow: Oriki, Women and the Past in a Yoruba Town.* Washington, D.C.: Smithsonian Institution Press.

Barnes, R., and J. Eicher, eds. 1992. *Dress and Gender: Making and Meaning.* Providence, R.I.: Berg.

Barthes, R. [1967] 1983. *The Fashion System.* Trans. M. Ward and R. Howard. London: Hill and Wang.

Bastian, M. L. 1992. The World as Marketplace: Historical, Cosmological and Popular Constructions of the Onitsha Market System. Ph.D. diss., Department of Anthropology, University of Chicago.

Battaglia, D. 1992. The Body in the Gift: Memory and Forgetting in Sabarl Mortuary Exchange. *American Ethnologist* 19:3–18.

Beidelman, T. O. 1968. Some Nuer Notions of Nakedness, Nudity and Sexuality. *Africa* 38(2): 113–131.

———. [1971] 1983. *The Kaguru.* Reprint, Prospect Heights, Ill.: Waveland Press.

———. 1986. *Moral Imagination in Kaguru Modes of Thought.* Bloomington: Indiana University Press.

Bell, Q. 1968. *On Human Finery.* London: Hogarth Press.

Benstock, S., and S. Ferriss, eds. 1994. *On Fashion.* New Brunswick, N.J.: Rutgers University Press.

Berger, J. 1972. *Ways of Seeing.* London: The BBC and Penguin Books.

Bernus, S. 1969. *Particularisme Ethnique en Milieu Urbain: L'Exemple de Niamey.* Paris: Institut d'Ethnologie.

Besmer, F. 1983. *Horses, Musicians, and Gods: The Hausa Cult of Possession—Trance.* South Hadley, Mass.: Bergin and Garvey.

Bhabha, H. K. 1990. The Other Question: Difference, Discrimination and the Discourse of Colonialism. In *Out There: Marginalization and Contemporary Cultures,* ed. Russell Ferguson et al., 71–88. Cambridge, Mass.: MIT Press.

Bickford, K. 1994. The A.B.C.'s of Cloth and Politics in Côte D'Ivoire. *Africa Today* 41(2):5–24.

Blacking, J. 1977. *The Anthropology of the Body.* London: Academic Press.

Bloch, M., and J. Parry. 1982. *Death and the Regeneration of Life.* Cambridge: Cambridge University Press.

Boddy, J. 1989. *Wombs and Alien Spirits: Women, Men, and the Zar Cult in Northern Sudan.* Madison: University of Wisconsin Press.

Boggie, J. 1966. *First Steps in Civilising Rhodesia.* Salisbury, Rhodesia: Kingstons Ltd.

Bourdieu, P. 1977. *Outline of a Theory of Practice.* Translated by R. Nice. Cambridge: Cambridge University Press.

———. 1984. *Distinction: A Social Critique of the Judgement of Taste.* Trans. Richard Nice. Cambridge, Mass.: Harvard University Press.

Bozzoli, B. 1983. Marxism, Feminism and South African Studies. *Journal of Southern African Studies* 9(2):139–177.

Bozzoli, B., with M. Nkotsoe. 1991. *Women of Phokeng: Consciousness, Life Strategy and Migrancy in South Africa 1900–1983.* Johannesburg: Ravan Press.

Brackett, D., and M. Wrong. 1930. Notes on Hygiene Books Used in Africa. *Africa* 3(4): 506–515.

Buchler, J., ed. 1940. *Philosophical Writings of Peirce.* New York: Dover Publications.

Buckley, A. 1985. *Yoruba Medicine.* Oxford: Oxford University Press.

Burke, T. Forthcoming. *Lifebuoy Men, Lux Women: Commodification, Consumption and Cleanliness in Modern Zimbabwe.* Durham, N.C.: Duke University Press.

Burns, C. 1994. Reproductive Labors: The Politics of Women's Health in South Africa, 1900 to 1960. Ph.D. diss., Department of History. Northwestern University.

Butler, J. 1990. *Gender Trouble: Feminism and the Subversion of Identity.* New York: Routledge.

———. 1993. *Bodies That Matter: On the Discursive Limits of "Sex."* New York: Routledge.

Caldwell, J. C., I. O. Orubuloye, and P. Caldwell. 1991. The Destabilization of the Traditional Yoruba Sexual System. *Population and Development Review* 17(2):229–62.

Catechism of Health. 1926. *Rhodesia Native Quarterly* 1:1.

Cesard, E. 1937. Le Muhaya (L'Afrique Orientale). *Anthropos* 32(1–2):15–60.

Chanock, M. 1985. *Law, Custom and Social Order.* Cambridge: Cambridge University Press.

Charles-Roux, E. 1981. *Chanel and Her World.* London: Vendome Press.

Chinodya, S. 1989. *Harvest of Thorns.* Harare, Zimbabwe: Baobab Books.

Chittick, N., and R. Rotberg, eds. 1975. *East Africa and the Orient.* New York: Africana Press.

Cohen, A., and J. L. Comaroff. 1976. The Management of Meaning: On the Phenomenology of Political Transactions. In *Transaction and Meaning: Directions in the Anthropology of Exchange and Symbolic Behavior,* ed. B. Kapferer, 87–108. African Studies Association Vol. 1. Philadelphia: Institute for the Study of Human Issues.

Cohen, E. 1985. The Tourist Guide: The Origins, Structure, and Dynamics of a Role. *Annals of Tourism Research, Special Edition. Tourist Guides: Pathfinders, Mediators and Animators* 12(1):5–29.

Colson, E., and T. Scudder. 1988. *For Prayer and Profit: The Ritual, Economic and Social Importance of Beer in Gwambe District, Zambia.* Stanford, Calif.: Stanford University Press.

Comaroff, J. 1985. *Body of Power, Spirit of Resistance.* Chicago: University of Chicago Press.

———. n.d. The Empire's Old Clothes: Fashioning the Colonial Subject. Unpublished manuscript, University of Chicago.

Comaroff, J., and J. L. Comaroff. 1987. The Madman and the Migrant: Work and Labour in the Historical Consciousness of a South African People. *American Ethnologist* 14(2):191–209.

———. 1989. The Colonization of Consciousness in South Africa. *Economy and Society* 18(3):267–96.

———. 1993. *Modernity and Its Malcontents: Ritual and Power in Postcolonial Africa.* Chicago: University of Chicago Press.

Comaroff, J. L. 1980. Bridewealth and the Control of Ambiguity in a Tswana Chiefdom. In *The Meaning of Marriage Payments,* ed. J. L. Comaroff, 161–95. London: Academic Press.

Comaroff, J. L., and J. Comaroff. 1992. Bodily Reform as Historical Practice. In *Ethnography and the Historical Imagination,* ed. J.L. Comaroff and J. Comaroff, 69–91. Boulder, Colo.: Westview Press.

Cooper, B. 1991. Cloth, Commodity Production and Social Capital: Women in Maradi, Niger 1900–1989. Paper presented at the annual meeting of the African Studies Association, St. Louis, Mo.

Coplan, D. B. 1987. Eloquent Knowledge: Lesotho Migrants' Songs and the Anthropology of Experience. *American Ethnologist* 14(3): 413–31.

———. 1991. Fictions that Save: Migrants' Performance and Basotho National Culture. *Cultural Anthropology* 6(2):164–92.

Cordwell, J. M., and R. A. Schwartz, eds. 1979. *The Fabrics of Culture: The Anthropology of Clothing and Adornment.* The Hague: Mouton.

Culianu, J. 1991. A Corpus for the Body. *Journal of Modern History.* 63(1):61–80.

Cummingham, H. 1980. *Leisure in the Industrial Revolution.* London: Croom Helm.

Curtin, P. D. 1989. *Death by Migration: Europe's Encounter with the Tropical World in the Nineteenth Century.* Cambridge: Cambridge University Press.

Dangarembga, T. 1988. *Nervous Conditions.* London: Women's Press.

Darrah, A. 1980. A Hermeneutic Approach to Hausa Therapeutics: The Allegory of the Living Fire. Ph.D. diss., Department of Anthropology, Northwestern University.

Davis, F. 1992. *Fashion, Culture, and Identity.* Chicago: University of Chicago Press.

de Kadt, E. 1979. *Tourism—Passport for Development?: Perspectives on the Social and Cultural Effects of Tourism in Developing Countries.* Published for the World Bank and UNESCO. New York: Oxford University Press.

de la Mothe, H. D. 1921. *Annual Report on Ekiti Division, Ondo Province,* Ondo Prof 4/1, National Archives, Ibadan.

Delius, P. 1983. *The Land Belongs to Us.* Johannesburg: Ravan Press.

———. 1989. Sebatakgomo: Migrant Organisation, the ANC and the Sekhukhuneland Revolt. *Journal of Southern African Studies* 15(4):581–616.

Denoon, D. 1988. Temperate Medicine and Settler Capitalism: On the Reception of Western Medical Ideas. In *Disease, Medicine and Empire: Perspectives on Western Medicine and the Experience of European Expansion,* ed. R. MacLeod and M. Lewis, 121–38. London: Routledge.

Derrida, J. 1986. *Memories for Paul de Man.* New York: Columbia University Press.

Devisch, R. 1990. The Human Body as a Vehicle for Emotions Among the Yaka of Zaire. In *Personhood and Agency: The Experience of Self and Other in African Cultures,* ed.

M. Jackson and I. Karp, 115–34 Uppsala: Textgruppen i Uppsala. Distributed in the U.S. by Smithsonian Institution Press.

Douglass, M. 1967. Raffia Cloth Distribution in the Lele Economy. In *Tribal and Peasant Economies: Readings in Economic Anthropology*, ed. G. Dalton, 103–22. New York: American Museum of Natural History Press.

———. 1970. *Purity and Danger: An Analysis of Concepts of Pollution and Taboo*. New York: Penguin.

Drechsler, H. [1966] 1980. *Let Us Die Fighting: The Struggle of the Herero and Nama Against German Imperialism (1884–1915)*. Trans. B. Zollner. London: Zed Press.

Drewal, M. T. 1992. *Yoruba Ritual: Performers, Play, Agency*. Bloomington: Indiana University Press.

Eades, J. 1980. *The Yoruba Today*. Cambridge: Cambridge University Press.

Eastman, C. 1971. Who are the Waswahili? *Africa* 41(3):228–36.

Echard, N. 1991a. The Hausa Possession Cult in the Ader Region of Niger: Its Origins and Present-Day Function. In *Women's Medicine: The Zar-Bori in Africa and Beyond*, ed. I. Lewis, A. Al-Safi, and S. Hurreiz, 64–80. Edinburgh: Edinburgh University Press.

———. 1991b. Gender Relationships and Religion: Women in the Hausa Bori of Ader, Niger. In *Hausa Women in the Twentieth Century*, ed. C. Coles and B. Mack, 207–20. Madison: University of Wisconsin Press.

Eco, U. 1986. *Travels in Hyperreality: Essays*. New York: Harcourt, Brace, Jovanovich.

Elias, N. 1978. *The History of Manners*. New York: Pantheon.

Emecheta, B. 1977. *The Slave Girl*. New York: Braziller.

Emmet, T. 1986. Popular resistance in Namibia, 1920–1925. In *Resistance and Ideology in Settler Societies*, ed. T. Lodge, 6–48. Southern Africa Studies Vol. 4, Johannesburg: Ravan Press.

Esterhuyse, J. H. 1968. *South West Africa 1880–1894: The Establishment of German Authority in South West Africa*. Cape Town, South Africa: C. Struik Ltd.

Evans, N. 1976. Tourism and Cross-cultural Communication. *Annals of Tourism Research* 3(4):189–98.

Ewen, S. 1988. *All Consuming Images: The Politics of Style in Contemporary Culture*. New York: Basic Books.

Fadipe, N. A. 1970. *The Sociology of the Yoruba*. Ibadan, Nigeria: University of Ibadan Press.

Faludi, S. 1991. *Backlash: The Undeclared War Against American Women*. New York: Crown.

Feeley-Harnik, G. 1989. Cloth and the Creation of Ancestors in Madagascar. In *Cloth and Human Experience*, ed. A. Weiner and J. Schneider, 73–116. Washington, D.C.: Smithsonian Institution Press.

———. 1991. *A Green Estate: Restoring Independence in Madagascar*. Washington, D.C.: Smithsonian Institution Press.

Feher, M., ed. 1989. *Fragments for a History of the Human Body*. New York: Zone Books.

Ferguson, J. 1992. The Country and the City on the Copperbelt. *Cultural Anthropology* 7(1):80–92.

Flugel, J. C. 1930. *The Psychology of Clothes.* London: Hogarth Press.

Fortes, M. 1973. On the Concept of the Person among the Tallensi. In *La Notion de Personne en Afrique Noire,* ed. G. Dieterlen, 283–319. Paris: Editions de Centre National de la Recherche Scientifique.

Foucault, M. 1979. *Discipline and Punish: The Birth of the Prison.* Trans. A. Sheridan. New York: Vintage Books.

———. 1980. *Knowledge/Power: Selected Interviews and Other Writings 1972–1977.* Brighton, England: Harvester Press.

———. 1980a. *The History of Sexuality Volume 1.* New York: Pantheon.

Freeman-Grenville, G. S. P. 1988. *The Swahili Coast, 2nd to 9th Centuries.* London: Variorum.

Frobenius, L. 1913. The Religion of Possession, Especially among the Houssa Tribes. In *The Voice of Africa: Being an Account of the Travels of the German Inner African Exploration Expedition in the Years 1910–1913,* 560–72. London: Hutchinson.

Fuglesang, M. 1992. No Longer Ghosts: Women's Notions of "Development" and "Modernity" in Lamu Town, Kenya. In *KAM-AP or TAKE-OFF: Local Notions of Development,* ed. G. Dahl and A. Rabo, 123–56. Stockholm: Stockholm Studies in Social Anthropology.

———. 1994. *Veils and Videos: Female Youth Culture on the Kenyan Coast.* Stockholm: Stockholm Studies in Social Anthropology.

Gaines, J. 1990. Introduction: Fabricating the Female Body. In *Fabrications: Costume and the Female Body,* ed. J. Gaines and C. Herzog, 1–27. New York: Routledge.

Gaines, J., and C. Herzog, eds. 1990. *Fabrications: Costume and the Female Body.* New York: Routledge.

Garber, M. 1992. *Vested Interests: Cross-dressing and Cultural Anxiety.* New York: Routledge.

Gelfand, M. 1953. *Tropical Victory: An Account of the Influence of Medicine on Southern Rhodesia, 1890–1923.* Cape Town, South Africa: Juta.

———. 1964. *Mother Patrick and Her Nursing Sisters.* Cape Town, South Africa: Juta.

———. 1971. *Diet and Tradition in African Culture.* London: F. & S. Livingstone.

Gibson, G. 1952. The Social Organization of the Southwestern Bantu. Ph.D. diss., Department of Anthropology, University of Chicago.

Gilman, S. 1985. *Difference and Pathology: Stereotypes of Sexuality, Race and Madness.* Ithaca: Cornell University Press.

Gilmore, D. B. 1980. *The People of the Plain: Class and Community in Lower Andulusia.* New York: Columbia University Press.

Goldblatt, I. 1971. *History of South West Africa.* Cape Town, South Africa: Juta.

Griaule, M. 1965. *Conversation with Ogotemmeli: An Introduction to Dogon Religious Ideas.* New York: Oxford University Press.

Grossberg, L., C. Nelson, and P. Treichler, eds. 1992. *Cultural Studies.* New York: Routledge.

Gugelberger, G. M., ed. 1984. *Nama/Namibia: Diary and Letters of Nama Chief Hendrik Witbooi, 1884–1894.* African Historical Documents Series No. 5, African Studies Center. Boston: Boston University.

Guy, J. 1990. Gender Oppression in Southern Africa's Precapitalist Societies. In *Women and Gender in Southern Africa to 1945,* ed. C. Walker, 33–47. Cape Town, South Africa: David Philip.

Hahn, J. 1869. Die Ovaherero. *Zeitschrift der Gesellschaft für Erdkunde zu Berlin* 4:226–58, 481–511.

Hannerz, U. 1989. Notes on the Global Ecumene. *Public Culture* 1(2):66–75.

———. 1990. Cosmopolitans and Locals in World Culture. *Theory, Culture and Society* 7(2–3):237–51.

———. 1992. *Cultural Complexity: Studies in the Social Organization of Meaning.* New York: Columbia University Press.

Hansen, K. T. 1994. Dealing with Used Clothing: *Salaula* and the Construction of Identity in Zambia's Third Republic. *Public Culture* 6:503–23.

Harries, P. 1989. Exclusion, Classification and Internal Colonialism: The Emergence of Ethnicity among the Tsonga-speakers of South Africa. In *The Creation of Tribalism in Southern Africa,* ed. L. Vail, 82–117. London: James Currey.

Hartwig, G. 1976. *The Art of Survival in East Africa: The Kerebe and Long-Distance Trade, 1800–1895.* New York: Africana.

Harvey, D. 1990. *The Condition of Postmodernity: An Enquiry into the Nature of Cultural Change.* Cambridge, Mass.: Blackwell.

Haug, W. F. 1986. *Critique of Commodity Aesthetic: Appearance, Sexuality, and Advertising in Capitalist Society.* Minneapolis: University of Minnesota Press.

Hay, M. J. 1989. *Western Clothing and African Identity: Changing Consumption Patterns among the Luo. Discussion Papers in the African Humanities, No. 2,* African Studies Center, Boston: Boston University.

Heath, D. 1992. Fashion, Anti-Fashion and Heteroglossia in Urban Senegal. *American Ethnologist* 19(2):19–33.

Hebdige, D. 1979. *Subculture: The Meaning of Style.* London: Methuen.

———. 1988. *Hiding in the Light.* New York: Comedia.

Hendrickson, H. (Anne Alfhild). 1992. Historical Idioms of Identity Representation Among the Ovaherero in Southern Africa. Ph.D. diss., Department of Anthropology, New York University.

———. 1994. A Symbolic History of the "Traditional" Herero Dress in Namibia and Botswana. *African Studies* 53(2):25–54.

Herr, C. 1994. Terrorist Chic: Style and Domination in Contemporary Ireland. In *On Fashion,* ed. S. Benstock and S. Ferriss, 235–66. New Brunswick, N.J.: Rutgers University Press.

Hobsbawm, E., and T. Ranger. 1983. *The Invention of Tradition.* Cambridge: Cambridge University Press.

Hoernle, W. 1937. Social Organisation. In *The Bantu-Speaking Tribes of South Africa,* ed. I. Schapera, 67–94. Cape Town, South Africa: Maskew Miller.

Hofmeyr, I. 1994. *We Spend Our Years as a Tale That Is Told*. Johannesburg: Witwatersrand University Press.

Hollander, A. 1975. *Seeing Through Clothes*. Berkeley: University of California Press.

Hove, C. 1988. *Bones*. Harare: Baobab Books.

Hunt, N. R. 1992. Colonial Fairy Tales and the Knife and Fork Doctrine in the Heart of Africa. In *African Encounters with Domesticity*, ed. K. T. Hansen, 143–71. New Brunswick, N.J.: Rutgers University Press.

Irle, J. 1906. *Die Herero*. Gütersloh, Germany: C. Bertelsmann.

Jackson, M. 1983. Knowledge of the Body. *Man* 18(1):327–45.

———. 1989. *Paths Toward a Clearing: Radical Empiricism and Ethnographic Inquiry*. Bloomington: Indiana University Press.

Jackson, M., and I. Karp, eds. 1990. *Personhood and Agency: The Experience of Self and Other in African Cultures*. Uppsala: Textgruppen i Uppsala. Distributed in the U.S. by Smithsonian Institution Press.

Jacobson-Widding, A. 1990. General Editor's Preface. In *Personhood and Agency: The Experience of Self and Other in African Cultures*, ed. M. Jackson and I. Karp, 9–13. Uppsala: Textgruppen i Uppsala. Distributed in the U.S. by Smithsonian Institution Press.

James, D. 1987. Kinship and Land in an Inter-ethnic Rural Community. M.A. thesis, Department of Anthropology, University of the Witwatersrand.

———. 1994. *Basadi ba baeng*/The Women Are Visiting: Female Migrant Performance from the Northern Transvaal. In *Politics and Performance in Southern Africa*, ed. E. Gunner. Johannesburg: Witwatersrand University Press.

James, W. [1890] 1950. *The Principles of Psychology*, 2 volumes. New York: Dover Publications.

Jameson, F. 1991. *Postmodernism, or, The Cultural Logic of Late Capitalism*. Durham, N.C.: Duke University Press.

Kahari, G. P. 1990. *The Rise of the Shona Novel: A Study in Development, 1890–1984*. Gweru: Mambo Press.

Kahn, A., and L. Holt. 1990. *The A–Z of Women's Sexuality*. New York: Facts on File.

Katjavivi, P. 1988. *A History of Resistance in Namibia*. London: John Currey.

Kienetz, A. 1977. The Key Role of the Orlam Migrations in the Early Europeanization of South-West Africa (Namibia). *International Journal of African Historical Studies* 10(4):553–72.

Kopytoff, I. 1986. The Cultural Biography of Things: Commoditization as Process. In *The Social Life of Things: Commodities in Cultural Perspective*, ed. A. Appadurai, 64–91. New York: Cambridge University Press.

Kroeber, A. 1963. *Style and Civilization*. Berkeley: University of California Press.

Kuper, A. 1982. *Wives for Cattle: Bridewealth and Marriage in Southern Africa*. London: Routledge and Kegan Paul.

Kuper, H. 1973a. Costume and Identity. *Comparative Studies in Society and History* 15(3):348–67.

———. 1973b. Costume and Cosmology: The Animal Symbolism of the *Ncwala*. *Man* 8(4):613–30.

Laqueur, T. 1990. *Making Sex: Body and Gender from the Greeks to Freud*. Cambridge, Mass.: Harvard University Press.

Lass, A. 1988. Romantic Documents and Political Monuments: The Meaning-Fulfillment of History in 19th-Century Czech Nationalism. *American Ethnologist* 15:456–71.

Lau, B., ed. 1989. *Charles John Andersson: Trade and Politics in Central Namibia 1860–1864. Diaries and Correspondence of Charles John Andersson*. Charles John Andersson Papers, Vol. 2. Windhoek, Namibia: Archives Service Division of the Department of National Education.

Leith-Ross, S. 1943. *African Conversation Piece*. London: Hutchinson.

Lloyd, P. C. 1968. Divorce among the Yoruba. *American Anthropologist* 70:67–81.

Mamamane, B. 1982. L'Habillement: Imitation et Complexe. *Sahel Hebdo* 299:11.

Marechera, D. 1978. *The House of Hunger*. London: Heinemann International.

Marshall, R. Forthcoming. "God Is Not a Democrat": Pentecostalism and Democratisation in Nigeria. In *The Churches and Africa's Democratisation*, ed. P. Clifford. London: James Currey.

Masquelier, A. 1992. Encounter with a Road Siren: Machines, Bodies and Commodities in the Imagination of a Mawri Healer. *Visual Anthropology Review* 8(1):56–69.

———. 1993a. Ritual Economies, Historical Mediations: The Poetics and Power of Bori among the Mawri of Niger. Ph.D. diss., Department of Anthropology, University of Chicago.

———. 1993b. Narratives of Power, Images of Wealth: The Ritual Economy of Bori in the Market. In *Modernity and Its Malcontents: Ritual and Power in Postcolonial Africa*, ed. J. Comaroff and J. L. Comaroff, 3–33. Chicago: University of Chicago Press.

———. 1994. Lightning, Death and the Avenging Spirits: Bori Values in a Muslim World. *Journal of Religion in Africa* 24(1):2–51.

———. In press. Consumption, Prostitution and Reproduction: The Poetics of Sweetness in Bori. *American Ethnologist*.

Matory, J. L. 1994. *Sex and the Empire That Is No More: Gender and the Politics of Metaphor in Oyo Yoruba Religion*. Minneapolis: University of Minnesota Press.

Mayer, P., and I. Mayer. 1971. *Townsmen or Tribesmen: Conservatism and the Process of Urbanization in a South African City*. Cape Town, South Africa: Oxford University Press.

Mauss, M. 1973. Techniques of the Body. *Economy and Society* 2:70–88.

———. [1950] 1979. *Sociology and Psychology: Essays*. Trans. B. Brewster. London: Routledge and Kegan Paul.

Mbembe, A. 1992. Provisional Notes on the Postcolony. *Africa* 62:3–37.

McAllister, P. 1980. Work, Homestead and the Shades: The Ritual Interpretation of Labour Migration among the Gcaleka. In *Black Villagers in an Industrial Society: Anthropological Perspectives on Labour Migration in Southern Africa*, ed. P. Mayer, 205–53. Oxford: Oxford University Press.

———. 1991. Using Ritual to Resist Domination in the Transkei. In *Tradition and Transition in Southern Africa: African Studies Fiftieth Anniversary Volume* (ed. A. D. Spiegel and P. McAllister) 50(1–2):129–44.

McCracken, G. 1990. *Culture and Consumption: New Approaches to the Symbolic Character of Consumer Goods and Activities*. Bloomington: Indiana University Press.

McRobbie, A. 1989. Second-Hand Dresses and the Role of the Ragmarket. In *Zoot Suits and Second-Hand Dresses: An Anthology of Fashion and Music*, ed. A. McRobbie, 23–49. Boston: Unwin Hyman.

Merleau-Ponty, M. 1962. *The Phenomenology of Perception*. London: Routledge and Kegan Paul.

Michelman, S. O., and T. Erekosima. 1992. Kalabari Dress in Nigeria. In *Dress and Gender: Making and Meaning*, ed. R. Barnes and J. Eicher, 164–82. Providence, R.I.: Berg.

Middleton, J. 1992. *The World of the Swahili: An African Mercantile Civilization*. New Haven: Yale University Press.

Mkele, N. 1959. Advertising to the Bantu. In *Second Advertising Convention in South Africa*. Durban, South Africa: Society of Advertisers.

Molepo, M. M. 1983. Peasants and/or Proletariat: A Case Study of Migrant Workers at Haggie Rand Limited from Molepo Tribal Village. Honours thesis, Department of Industrial Sociology, University of the Witwatersrand.

———. 1984. The Changing Nature of Labour Migration from the Northern Transvaal with Particular Reference to Molepo Village c. 1900–1940. M.A. thesis, School of Oriental and African Studies, University of London.

Monfouga-Nicolas, J. 1972. *Ambivalence et Culte de Possession: Contribution à l'Etude du Bori Hausa*. Paris: Anthropos.

Monnig, H. O. 1967. *The Pedi*. Pretoria, South Africa: J. L. van Schaik.

Moyo, H. M. D. 1934. Letter to the Editor. *Native Mirror* 2:5.

Mulvey, L. 1975. Visual Pleasure and Narrative Cinema. *Screen* 16:6–18.

Murray, C. 1981. *Families Divided*. Johannesburg: Ravan Press.

Native Economic Commission. 1930–32. Evidence housed in the Church of the Province Library, University of the Witwatersrand.

Ndzou, P. 1935. Letters to the Editors: Digests. *Native Mirror* 2:10.

Ngavirue, Z. 1972. Political Parties and Interest Groups in South West Africa: A Study of a Plural Society. Ph.D. diss., Oxford University.

———. 1990. On Wearing the Victor's Uniforms and Replacing Their Churches—Southwest Africa (Namibia) 1920–50. In *Cargo Cults and Millenarian Movements*, ed. G. W. Trompf, 391–428. New York: Mouton.

Nicolas, G. 1975. *Dynamique Sociale et Appréhension du Monde au Sein d'une Société Hausa*. Paris: Institut d'Ethnologie.

Niehaus, I. 1994. Witch-hunting and Political Legitimacy: Continuity and Change in Green Valley, Lebowa, 1930–91. *Africa* 63(4):498–530.

Nielsen, E. 1990. Handmaidens of the Glamour Culture: Costumers in the Hollywood Studio. In *Fabrications*, ed. J. Gaines and C. Herzog, 160–79. New York: Routledge.

Nurse, D., and T. Spear. 1985. *The Swahili: Reconstructing the History and Language of an African Society, 800–1500*. Philadelphia: University of Pennsylvania Press.

Nyagumbo, M. 1980. *With the People: An Autobiography from the Zimbabwe Struggle*. London: Allison & Busby.

Obiechina, E. 1973. *An African Popular Literature*. Cambridge: Cambridge University Press.

Oguntuyi, A. 1979. *History of Ekiti*. Ibadan, Nigeria: Bisi Books.

Olusanya, P. O. 1967. Cultural Barriers to Family Planning among the Yoruba. *Studies in Family Planning* 37(1):13–16.

Onwuejeogwu, M. A. 1981. *An Igbo Civilization: Nri Kingdom and Hegemony*. London: Ethnographica.

Ortner, S. 1978. The Virgin and the State. *Feminist Studies* 4:19–35.

Osundare, Niyi. 1992. The Nigerian Factor. *Newswatch Magazine*, 12 October, 6.

Otto, A. 1979. Einige Gedanken zur Geschichte und zum Verlauf des Zeraua-Festes der westlichen Herero. *Namibiana* 1(1):39–47.

Pape, J. 1990. Black and White: The "Perils of Sex" in Colonial Zimbabwe. *Journal of Southern African Studies* 16(4):699–720.

Parade [untitled article]. 1991. April, p. 29.

Partington, A. 1992. Popular Fashion and Working-Class Affluence. In *Chic Thrills*, ed. J. Ash and E. Wilson, 145–61. Berkeley: University of California Press.

Peake, R. E. 1984. Tourism and Alternative Worlds: The Social Construction of Reality in Malindi Town, Kenya. Ph.D. diss., School of Oriental and African Studies, University of London.

Peel, J. D. Y. 1978. *Olaju*: A Yoruba Concept of Development. *Journal of Development Studies* 14(2):139–65.

———. 1983. *Ijeshas and Nigerians*. Cambridge: Cambridge University Press.

Pennington, R., and H. Harpending. 1991. How Many Refugees Were There? History and Population Change among the Herero and Mbanderu of Northwestern Botswana. *Botswana Notes and Records* 23:209–20.

Pitje, G. M. 1950. Traditional Systems of Male Education among Pedi and Cognate Tribes. *African Studies* 9(2–4):53–76, 105–24, 194–201.

Poewe, K. 1985. *The Namibian Herero: A History of Their Psychological Disintegration and Survival*. African Studies Vol. 1, Lewiston/Queenston, N.Y.: Edwin Mellen Press.

Pool, G. 1991. *Samuel Maharero*. Windhoek, Namibia: Gamsberg Macmillan.

Pratt, M. L. 1992. *Imperial Eyes: Travel Writing and Transculturation*. London: Routledge and Kegan Paul.

Pütz, J., H. von Egidy, and P. Caplan. 1987. *Political Who's Who of Namibia*. Windhoek, Namibia: Magus.

Rabinbach, A. 1990. *The Human Motor: Energy, Fatigue and the Origins of Modernity*. Los Angeles: University of California Press.

Ranchod-Nilsson, S. 1992. "Educating Eve": The Women's Club Movement and Political Consciousness among Rural African Women in Southern Rhodesia, 1950–1980. In

African Encounters with Domesticity, ed. K. T. Hansen, 195–220. New Brunswick, N.J.: Rutgers University Press.

Reinhardt, L. 1979. Mende Secret Societies and Their Costumed Spirits. In *The Fabrics of Culture: The Anthropology of Clothing and Adornment,* ed. J. Cordwell and R. Schwarz, 231–66. New York: Mouton.

Reining, P. 1967. The Haya: The Agrarian System of a Sedentary People. Ph.D. diss., Department of Anthropology, University of Chicago.

Renne, E. 1986. The Thierry Collection of Hausa Artifacts at the Field Museum. *African Arts* 19(4):54–59.

———. 1991. Water, Spirits and Plain White Cloth: The Ambiguity of Things in Bunu Social Life. *Man* 26:709–22.

———. 1992. Polyphony in the Courts. *Ethnology* 31(3):219–32.

———. 1993. Changes in Adolescent Sexuality and the Perception of Virginity in a Southwestern Nigerian Village. *Health Transition Review* Supplement to Vol. 3:121–33.

Report of the Southern Rhodesian Missionary Conference. 1932. *Native Mirror* 7.

République du Niger. n.d. *Monographie de la Subdivision de Doutchi (entre 1936–1940).* Documents 6.1.6. Niamey: Archives Nationales.

Riesman, P. 1977. *Freedom in Fulani Social Life: An Introspective Ethnography.* Chicago: University of Chicago Press.

———. 1986. The Person and the Life Cycle in African Social Life and Thought. *African Studies Review* 29(2):71–98.

Roach, M. E., and J. B. Eicher, eds. 1965. *Dress, Adornment and the Social Order.* New York: John Wiley and Sons.

Rogers, S. 1975. Female Forms of Power and the Myth of Male Dominance: A Model of Female/Male Interaction in Peasant Society. *American Ethnologist* 2:727–56.

Roseberry, W. 1989. *Anthropologies and Histories: Essays in Culture, History and Political Economy.* New Brunswick, N.J.: Rutgers University Press.

Sahlins, M. 1976. *Culture and Practical Reason.* Chicago: University of Chicago Press.

Salim, A. I. 1973. *The Swahili-speaking Peoples of Kenya's Coast 1895–1965.* Peoples of East Africa Series 4. Nairobi: East African Publishing House.

Schapera, I. 1949. The Ndebele of South Africa. *Natural History* 58:408–14.

———. 1979. Notes on Some Herero Genealogies. *African Studies* 38(10):17–42.

Schmidt, E. 1992. *Peasants, Traders and Wives: Shona Women in the History of Zimbabwe, 1870–1939.* Portsmouth, N.H.: Heinemann Educational Books.

Schmoll, P. 1991. Searching for Health in a World of Dis-ease: Affliction Management among Rural Hausa of the Maradi Valley. Ph.D. diss., Department of Anthropology, University of Chicago.

Schneider, J., and A. Weiner. 1989. Introduction. In *Cloth and Human Experience,* ed. A. Weiner and J. Schneider, 1–29. Washington, D.C.: Smithsonian Institution Press.

Schoss, J. H. 1993. The Wages of Labor: "Good Work" in the Tourist Economy. Paper presented at the 92nd annual meeting of the American Anthropological Association, Washington, D.C.

———. 1995. Beach Tours and Safari Visions: Relations of Production and the Production of Culture in Malindi, Kenya. Ph.D. diss., Department of Anthropology, University of Chicago.

Schultze, L. 1990. On the Muscle. In *Fabrications*, ed. J. Gaines and C. Herzog, 59–78. New York: Routledge.

Setel, P. 1991. "A Good Moral Tone": Victorian Ideals of Health and the Judgment of Persons in Nineteenth-century Travel and Mission Accounts from East Africa. *Working Papers in African Studies No. 150*, African Studies Center. Boston: Boston University.

Shamuyarira, N. M. 1965. *Crisis in Rhodesia*. London: Andre Deutsch.

Sheriff, A. 1987. *Slaves, Spices and Ivory in Zanzibar: Integration of an East African Commercial Empire into the World Economy, 1770–1873*. London: James Currey.

Sibenke, B. 1982. *My Uncle Grey Bhonzo*. Harare, Zimbabwe: Longman Zimbabwe.

Sigauke, M. W. 1939. Do You Shake Hands? *Bantu Mirror*, 2 September, 8.

Silverman, K. 1986. Fragments of a Fashionable Discourse. In *Studies in Entertainment: Critical Approaches to Mass Culture*, ed. T. Modelski, 139–54. Bloomington: Indiana University Press.

Simmel, G. 1904. Fashion. *The International Quarterly* 10:130–55.

Sissa, G. 1990. *Greek Virginity*. Cambridge, Mass.: Harvard University Press.

Smith, V., ed. 1989. *Hosts and Guests: The Anthropology of Tourism*. 2nd ed. Philadelphia: University of Pennsylvania.

Sobantu, J. H. 1933. Letter to the Editor. *Native Mirror* 10:11.

Social Science Research Council. 1954. Summer Seminar on Acculturation—1953. Acculturation: An Exploratory Formulation. *American Anthropologist* 56(6):973–1002.

Spiegel, A. 1990. Cohesive Cosmologies or Pragmatic Practices? *Cahiers d'Etudes Africaines* 117(XXX-I):45–72.

Staunton, I., ed. 1990. *Mothers of the Revolution*. Harare, Zimbabwe: Baobab Books.

Steiner, C. 1984. Another Image of Africa: Toward an Ethnohistory of European Cloth Marketed in West Africa, 1873–1960. *Ethnohistory* 32(2):91–110.

Stepan, N. 1982. *The Idea of Race in Science: Great Britain 1800–1960*. Hamden, Conn.: Archon Books.

Stocking, G. W., Jr. 1987. *Victorian Anthropology*. New York: Free Press.

Stoecker, Helmut, ed. 1986. *German Imperialism in Africa*. Trans. B. Zollner. London: C. Hurst.

Stoller, P. 1986. *The Taste of Ethnographic Things: The Sense in Anthropology*. Philadelphia: University of Pennsylvania Press.

Sundermeier, T. n.d. *The Mbanderu*. Ed. B. Lau, trans. A Heywood. Windhoek, Namibia: Star Binders and Printers.

Sundkler, B. 1974. *Bara Bukoba: Church and Community in Tanzania*. London: C. Hurst.

Swanson, M. 1977. The Sanitation Syndrome: Bubonic Plague and Urban Native Policy in the Cape Colony, 1900–09. *Journal of African History* 18(3): 387–410.

Swantz, M-L. 1985. *Women in Development: A Creative Role Denied?* New York: St. Martin's.

Taylor, L. 1992. Paris Couture, 1940–1944. In *Chic Thrills*, ed. J. Ash and E. Wilson, 127–44. Berkeley: University of California Press.

Thomas, N. 1992. The Inversion of Tradition. *American Ethnologist* 19(2):213–32.

Thomas, T. M. 1872. *Eleven Years in Central South Africa*. London: John Snow.

Thompson, E. P. 1967. Time, Work-Discipline, and Industrial Capitalism. *Past and Present* 38:57–97.

Thompson, R. F. 1966. An Aesthetic of the Cool: West African Dance. *African Forum* 2(2):85–102.

Towner, J. 1985. The Grand Tour: A Key Phase in the History of Tourism. *Annuals of Tourism Research* 12(3):297–334.

Townsend, L. 1974. *Gynaecology for Students*. Melbourne: Macmillan.

Tremearne, A. J. 1914. *The Ban of the Bori: Demons and Demon Dancing in West and North Africa*. London: Heath, Cranton and Ouseley.

True African Ngangas Meet. 1969. *Parade and Foto-Action*, June.

Tucker, R., ed. 1978. *The Marx-Engels Reader*. 2nd ed. New York: W. W. Norton.

Turner, L. 1984. *The Body and Society*. Oxford: Basil Blackwell.

Turner, T. 1980. The Social Skin. In *Not Work Alone*, ed. J. Cherfas and R. Lewin, 112–40. London: Temple Smith.

———. n.d. The Social Skin. Manuscript, University of Chicago.

Tyrrell, B. 1968. *Tribal Peoples of Southern Africa*. Cape Town, South Africa: Books of Africa.

Urry, J. 1990. *The Tourist Gaze: Leisure and Travel in Contemporary Societies*. London: Sage.

Vail, L., and L. White. 1991. *Power and the Praise Poem: Southern African Voices in History*. London: James Currey.

Vaughan, M. 1991. *Curing their Ills: Colonial Power and African Illness*. Stanford, Calif.: Stanford University Press.

Veblen, T. [1899] 1957. *The Theory of the Leisure Class*. Reprint, New York: Mentor.

Vedder, H. [1928] 1966a. The Herero. In *The Native Tribes of South West Africa*, ed. C. H. L. Hahn, H. Vedder, and L. Fourie, 155–211. New York: Frank Cass.

———. [1938] 1966b. *South West Africa in Early Times*. Ed. and trans. C. Hall. New York: Barnes and Noble.

Vlahos, O. 1979. *Body: The Ultimate Symbol*. New York: Lippincott.

Vogel, C. A. M. 1985. Pedi Mural Art. *African Arts* 18(3):78–83.

Wallis, J. P. R., ed. 1945. *The Matabele Journals of Robert Moffat*. 2 vols. No 1: Oppenheimer Series. London: Chatto & Windus.

Wass, B. 1979. Yoruba Dress in Five Generations of a Lagos Family. In *The Fabrics of Culture: The Anthropology of Clothing and Adornment*, ed. J. M. Cordwell and R. A. Schwartz, 331–48. The Hague: Mouton.

Weber, M. 1947. *The Theory of Social and Economic Organization*. Trans. A. M. Henderson and T. Parsons. New York: Free Press.

Weiner, A., 1980. Reproduction: A Replacement for Reciprocity. *American Ethnologist* 7(1):71–85.

———. 1985. Inalienable Wealth. *American Ethnologist* 12:52–65.

———. 1992. *Inalienable Possessions*. Berkeley: University of California Press.

Weiner, A., and J. Schneider. 1986. Cloth and the Organization of Human Experience. *Current Anthropology* 27(2):178–84.

———, eds. 1989. *Cloth and Human Experience*. Washington, D.C.: Smithsonian Institution Press.

Weinstein, D. 1989. The Amnesty International Concert Tour: Transnationalism as Cultural Commodity. *Public Culture* 1(2):60–65.

Weiss, B. 1996. *The Making and Unmaking of the Haya Lived World: Consumption and Commoditization in Everyday Practice*. Durham, N.C.: Duke University Press.

Werner, W. 1982. Truppenspieler in South West Africa. *South West Africa Annual* 1982: 27–30.

———. 1989. The Economic and Social History of the Herero. Doctoral diss., Department of History University of Cape Town.

———. 1990. "Playing Soldiers": The Truppenspieler Movement Among the Herero of Namibia, 1915 to ca. 1945. *Journal of Southern African Studies*, 16(3):476–502.

Williams, R. 1988. *Problems in Materialism and Culture*. London: Verso.

Willis, J. 1993. *Mombasa, the Swahili, and the Making of the Mijikenda*. Oxford: Clarendon Press.

Wilmsen, E. 1989. *Land Filled With Flies: A Political Economy of the Kalahari*. Chicago: University of Chicago Press.

Wilson, E. 1985. *Adorned in Dreams: Fashion and Modernity*. London: Virago.

———. 1990. All the Rage. In *Fabrications*, ed. J. Gaines and C. Herzog, 28–38. New York: Routledge.

———. 1992. Fashion and the Postmodern Body. In *Chic Thrills*, ed. J. Ash and E. Wilson, 3–16. Berkeley: University of California Press.

Wolpe, H. 1972. Capitalism and Cheap Labour Power in South Africa: From Segregation and Apartheid. *Economy and Society* 1(4):425–56.

Wright, L. 1992. In *Chic Thrills*, ed. J. Ash and E. Wilson, 49–57. Berkeley: University of California Press.

Young, I. M. 1994. Women Recovering Our Clothes. In *On Fashion*, ed. S. Benstock and S. Ferriss, 197–210. New Brunswick, N.J.: Rutgers University Press.

Yoshikuni, T. 1989. Black Migrants in a White City: A Social History of African Harare, 1890–1925. Ph.D. diss., Department of History, University of Zimbabwe.

Zimbabwe National Archives (ZNA). Native Affairs Department, Annual Reports. N 9/1/1–2.

———. 1920. Chief Native Commissioner, Correspondence. N 3/9/1–2.

———. 1944. Godlonton Commission on Native Production and Trade. ZBJ 1/2/2.

NOTES ON CONTRIBUTORS

Misty Bastian received her doctoral degree from the University of Chicago and was until recently a Fellow of the Academy Scholars Program at the Center for International Affairs, Harvard University. She is now Assistant Professor of Anthropology at Franklin and Marshall College, Lancaster, Pennsylvania. Her interests include gender, popular culture, religion, and cosmology.

Timothy Burke completed his graduate studies in history at Johns Hopkins and is Assistant Professor of History at Swarthmore College. His book *Lifebuoy Men, Lux Women: Commodification, Consumption and Cleanliness in Modern Zimbabwe* was published in 1996 by Duke University Press. His research interests include consumption and the historiography of southern Africa, as well as the cultural history of Saturday-morning cartoon watching.

Hildi Hendrickson is Assistant Professor of Anthropology at the Brooklyn campus of Long Island University in New York City. She received her Ph.D. in anthropology from New York University. Her research interests include culture change, colonialism, semiotics, ritual, cosmology, and the body, as well as African and Afro-Caribbean dance.

Deborah James teaches anthropology at the University of the Witwatersrand in Johannesburg, South Africa, where she received her doctorate. She is an editor of *African Studies*, and her research interests include the music and popular culture of migration in South Africa.

Adeline Masquelier is Assistant Professor of Anthropology at Tulane University. She has conducted research among the Mawri of Niger and is preparing a book on the bori cult of spirit possession. Her more recent research has focused on the rise of fundamentalists in Niger and the veil of Algerian women in the French colonial imagination. She has published articles on the politics of healing, Islam, religious discourse, and ritual processes in postcolonial Niger.

Elisha Renne received her doctorate in anthropology from New York University and recently taught as a Fulbright Lecturer in the Department of Sociology, Ahmadu Bello

University, Zaria, Nigeria. She is currently affiliated with the Office of Population Research at Princeton University and is teaching at the Woodrow Wilson School of Public and International Affairs. Her research focuses on gender, material culture, and fertility, among other issues. Her book *Cloth That Does Not Die: The Meaning of Cloth in Bunu Social Life* was published in 1995 by the University of Washington Press.

Johanna Schoss recently completed a Ph.D. in anthropology at the University of Chicago with a dissertation entitled "Beach Tours and Safari Visions: Relations of Production and the Production of Culture in Malindi, Kenya." Her research interests include tourism, economic development, the informal economy, and the politics of wildlife conservation. A current project focuses on Kenyan writers and their changing relation to the state and national culture.

Brad Weiss is Assistant Professor of Anthropology at the College of William and Mary in Williamsburg, Virginia, and a graduate of the University of Chicago. His book *The Making and Unmaking of the Haya Lived World: Consumption, Commodities, and Everyday Practice* was published in 1996 by Duke University Press. His research interests include the colonial and neocolonial history of coffee in Tanzania, and the body in space and time.

INDEX

Library of Congress Cataloging-in-Publication Data
Clothing and difference : embodied identities in colonial and post-colonial
Africa / edited by Hildi Hendrickson.
— (Body, commodity, text)
Includes bibliographical references and index.
ISBN 0-8223-1783-4 (cloth : alk. paper). — ISBN 0-8223-1791-5
(paper : alk. paper)
1. Costume—Africa, Sub-Saharan—History—19th century.
2. Costume—Africa, Sub-Saharan—History—20th century.   3. Costume—
Africa, Sub-Saharan—Psychological aspects.   4. Body, Human—Social
aspects—Africa, Sub-Saharan.   5. Identity (Psychology)—Africa, Sub-
Saharan.   I. Hendrickson, Hildi, 1961–   .   II. Series.
GT1580.C56   1996
391'.00967—dc20   95-53957 CIP